GENEALOGICAL GLEANINGS

from

HARFORD COUNTY, MARYLAND

MEDICAL RECORDS

1772-1852

Henry C. Peden Jr.

Colonial Roots
Millsboro, DE
2016

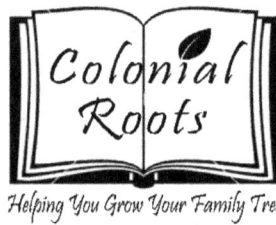

Colonial Roots

Helping You Grow Your Family Tree

ISBN 978-1-68034-353-3

INTRODUCTION

Old medical records, when available, can be useful tools for genealogists, especially in the days before State governments created vital records. The problem is, however, these records are inherently private and are not generally available to the public, although for the 18th and 19th centuries some have been donated to county and state historical societies and university libraries.

Genealogical information has been gleaned for this book from medical records in Harford County, Maryland from 1772 to 1852, primarily from some of the surviving ledgers of Dr. John Archer (1741-1830) and his sons Dr. Robert Harris Archer (1775-1857), Dr. John Archer, Jr. (1777-1830) and Dr. James Archer (1779-1815), and also ledgers of Dr. Alonzo Preston (1796-1801) and Dr. Matthew Johnson Allen (1801-1851). Information has also been gleaned from miscellaneous papers and receipts found in the Archives Department of the Historical Society of Harford County for Dr. Richard N. Allen, Dr. John T. Archer, Dr. Thomas Archer, Dr. Thomas Birckhead, Dr. William M. Dallam, Dr. David Dick, Dr. William L. Horton, Dr. Thaddeus Jewett, Dr. William T. Munnikhuysen, Dr. Jacob A. Preston, Dr. James Reardon, Dr. Richard Sappington, Dr. William Sappington and Dr. James Snow.

Medical treatments and medicines in these records are mostly written in Latin, but there is information in English, fortunately, that is beneficial to researchers, such as names of family members, neighbors, African Americans, locations of residences (mostly Harford County, but some in Baltimore City and Cecil County), occupations, and miscellaneous notes such as "died insolvent" or "debt forgiven" and medical bills that often took years to get paid. In some instances the illness or injury and treatment are written in English and even the full date of birth of a newborn child is given, but not its name. As an aid to researchers I have added additional information in [brackets] from my own research, such as years of birth and death, and I have identified those patients who served either in the Revolutionary War or in the War of 1812.

Dr. John Archer's Ledgers A and B are in the Archives Department of the Historical Society of Harford County, Ledgers D and F are in the Manuscript Division of the Maryland Historical Society, as is the ledger of Dr. John Archer, Jr. Dr. John Archer's Ledger C is in the University Archives and Records Center at the University of Pennsylvania. Dr. Robert H. Archer's Ledger F, his index to Ledger H, his prescription book and a ledger of Dr. James Archer are in the Archives Department of the Historical Society of Harford County. A ledger of Dr. Alonzo Preston and a ledger of Dr. Matthew J. Allen are in the Court Records Department of the Historical Society of Harford County.

Other medical ledgers may exist for these and other early Harford County doctors, but their locations were undetermined at the time of this compilation. Hopefully, my genealogical gleanings from the abovementioned extant medical records will prove helpful for those who are seeking information about their elusive Harford County ancestors.

Henry C. Peden, Jr.
Bel Air, Maryland
October 12, 2016

Genealogical Gleanings
from Harford County, Maryland
Medical Records, 1772-1852

Adair, John, at Cecil Furnace, was treated by Dr. John Archer in 1797 (Ledger I, which is missing, was abstracted by Dr. George W. Archer circa 1890; his notes are in Archives of the Historical Society of Harford County folder "Archer, G. W. Coll. – Ledgers and Day Books")

Adams, Jacob, was visited by Dr. John Archer who treated him in May 1774 and Jun 1774, him and his wife in Jun 1779, his wife in Apr 1782 and him and his wife in Jul 1786 (Ledger B, p. 3; Ledger C, p. 72, noted "debt forgiven by order of testator;" Ledger F, p. 330)

Adams, John, appeared on a list of debts dated 26 Dec 1822 and titled "A List of Allen's Claims" that were due and payable to Dr. Richard N. Allen for services rendered to said Adams [no dates given] (Document filed in Historical Society of Harford County Archives folder "R. N. Allen")

Adams, Walker, was treated by Dr. Robert H. Archer in Nov 1827 (p. 256) [Walker Adams was a War of 1812 veteran.]

Adams, ---- [blank], on H. Stump's place, was visited by Dr. Robert H. Archer who treated his child in Oct 1822 (p. 30; Ledger F, p. 105)

Adkinson, Michael, near William McChanny, was visited by Dr. John Archer who treated him and his wife in 1790 (Ledger F, p. 68) [account continued in Ledger G, which is missing]

Adlam & Hughes, see William Evatt, q.v.

Ady, Miss, was medicated by Dr. Robert H. Archer on 2 Aug 1834 (Rx Book, 1825-1851, p. 112)

Ady, William, see Vincent Richardson and Bazil Buckingham, q.v.

Aiken, William, on B. Silver's place, was visited by Dr. Robert H. Archer who treated him in Jul and Aug 1824 and also treated "Judie" in Jul 1824 (pp. 112, 115, 116, 117; Ledger F, p. 99)

Aisquith, William, see ---- Ascue, q.v.

Aitken, ---- [blank], Frenchman, near P. Thomas, Esq., was treated by Dr. John Archer circa 1798 [no dates or details were given] (Ledger I, which is missing, was abstracted by Dr. George W. Archer circa 1890; his notes are in the Archives of the Historical Society of Harford County folder "Archer, G. W. Coll. – Ledgers and Day Books")

Aitken, Robert, was treated by Dr. Robert H. Archer in Sep 1815 (Ledger F, p. 7)

Albert, John Jacob (Dutch shoemaker), near Mr. Webb's, was visited by Dr. John Archer who inoculated eight of his family in Feb 1776 and treated him in May 1781 (Ledger C, p. 31, noted "debt forgiven by order of testator"); see James Linam, q.v.

Albert, Mr., was treated by Dr. Robert H. Archer in 1823 (p. 90)

Albert, Mrs., see Lloyd Bailey, q.v.

Albert, Philip [1753-1827], was visited by Dr. John Archer who treated him in Jun 1781, his wife in Dec 1782 and him in Jul 1787 (Ledger D, p. 112; Ledger F, p. 347) [account continued in Ledger K, which is missing] [Philip Albert was a Revolutionary War veteran.]

Albert, William [1779-1856], was visited by Dr. James Archer who treated Negro John 16 times in Nov and Dec 1806 for "commotion of the brain" and the treatment was "making an incision into the scalp, blistering, bleedings, various medicines and advice" (p. 1) [William died in Kentucky.]

Aldridge, Sarah, in Bel Air, was visited by Dr. John Archer who treated her and children Gilbert and Betsey in 1794 and 1795 (Ledger I, which is missing, was abstracted by Dr. George W. Archer circa 1890; his notes are in the Archives of the Historical Society of Harford County folder "Archer, G. W. Coll. – Ledgers and Day Books")

Alexander, Charles, see Mrs. Arthur Alexander, q.v.

Alexander, James, on Muddy Creek, was visited by Dr. John Archer who inoculated 7 of his family in 1782 (Ledger D, p. 10) [account continued in Ledger E, which is missing]

Alexander, Mr., near James Clark, Scotsman, in the Barrens [an area in the northwest part of the county near Pennsylvania], was treated by Dr. John Archer in Nov 1786 (Ledger F, p. 134)

Alexander, Mrs. Arthur (widow) was treated by Dr. Robert H. Archer in Sep 1821; also mentioned, and probably treated, her sons Arthur and Charles (Ledger F, p. 4)

Allen, Aaron, was visited by Dr. Parker Forwood who treated his wife in Aug and Sep 1821 in consultation with Dr. Dorsey (Document filed in the Archives of the Historical Society of Harford County folder "R. N. Allen")

Allen, Adeline B., was listed in Dr. Matthew J. Allen's ledger in May 1847 as "one sorrel mare sold me" for $50 and listed other unidentified cash transactions in 1847, 1848 and 1849 (pp. 52, 59)

Allen, Dr., see Robert Gover (miller), Mrs. Creswell, George Bay and Mr. Lingum, q.v.

Allen, Hannah, was treated by Dr. Matthew J. Allen in 1831 and 1834 in Calvert County (p. 26)

Allen, Jane A., was treated by Dr. Matthew J. Allen in 1832-1833 in Calvert County and the account also mentioned Thomas and Samuel Allen, Dr. Dane, L. T. Hodgkins and William Weems; Jane A. Allen had an account in Dr. Matthew J. Allen's medical ledger in Harford County for some non-medical matters between Apr 1844 and Feb 1845 that included "paid John D. Allen, M.D." in May 1844 and "to expenses taking little Addy to relay house" in Jun 1845 (pp. 17, 34)

Allen, John D., see Jane A. Allen and Augustus J. Greme, q.v.

Allen, John G., was mentioned in Dr. Matthew J. Allen's ledger in non-medical matters in 1843, 1844 and 1845 and also mentioned J. Nickle in 1845 (p. 28)

Allen, Moses, "near Jas. Creton," was treated by Dr. John Archer in Dec 1785 (Ledger D, p. 70 noted "debt forgiven as before")

Allen, R. N. and M. J., were treated by Dr. Matthew J. Allen in 1832 in Calvert County and the account also mentioned Dr. Dane, James Spicknall, John French, Charles Graham and William E. Bartlett (pp. 15-16); see Mrs. Stump, q.v.

Allen, Rev., "Yanker," was inoculated by Dr. John Archer in Jan 1795 (Ledger I, which is missing, was abstracted by Dr. George W. Archer circa 1890; his notes are in Archives of the Historical Society of Harford County file "Archer, G. W. Coll. - Ledgers and Day Books") [Dr. George W. Archer also made his own notes: "Who was he? Could it have been Rev. Jno. Allen who had been rector of St. George's since 1792? Then why "Yanker"? The rector was a son of Erin."]

Allen, Richard [1792-1855] (doctor), was treated by Dr. Robert H. Archer eleven times in Sep 1822 (pp. 16, 17, 19; Ledger F, p. 74); see Robert Gover, of Ephraim, and Prush A. Bond, q.v.

Allen, Robert, was treated by Dr. John Archer in Oct 1772 and July 1773 (Ledger B, p. 3)

Allen, Samuel, see Jane A. Allen, q.v.

Allen, Thomas, see Jane A. Allen, q.v.

Allen, William H., was treated by Dr. Matthew J. Allen in 1833 in Calvert County (p. 26)

Allen, William, "at Necks near Griffith's Quarter," was visited by Dr. John Archer who treated him and his wife in July 1789 (Ledger F, p. 331)

Allender, ---- [blank], Mr., at Dismal [swamp at the mouth of Swan Creek], was treated by Dr. Robert H. Archer in Sep 1822 (p. 17; Ledger F, p. 76)

Allender, Mr., at Long Green, was prescribed medicine for his child by Dr. Robert H. Archer on 18 Jun 1830 (Rx Book, 1825-1851, p. 100)

Allender, Nicholas [c1776-1828], was treated by Dr. Robert H. Archer in Sep 1822 (p. 18) [Nicholas Allender was a War of 1812 veteran.]

Allender, Nicholas, was visited by Dr. Matthew J. Allen who treated his daughter in Jul 1845 (p. 51)

Allender, Peggy, see William Allender, q.v.

Allender, William, was visited by Dr. John Archer who treated him in July 1775 and Dec 1778, his wife in Feb 1779, him in Apr 1782 and daughter Peggy in Oct 1788 (Ledger B, p. 8; Ledger C, p. 25, spelled it Allinder; Ledger F, p. 179) [William Allender was a Revolutionary War veteran.]

Allison, James, was visited by Dr. John Archer who treated him in Aug 1772 and at various times between Mar and Nov 1773 and July and Sep 1774, in Mar 1777, Mar 1778, Apr 1781 and Feb 1781, Frank [no relationship was given] in Apr 1783 and him [James] in May 1788 (Ledger B, p. 2; Ledger C, p. 41, Ledger F, p. 203) [James Allison was a Revolutionary War veteran.]

Alloway, Jonathan, was treated by Dr. Robert H. Archer from 24 Feb 1823 to 27 Apr 1823 and "died insolvent" [date of death was not given] (pp. 56, 57; Ledger F, p. 121)

Allston, Mr. (merchant), was treated by Dr. Robert H. Archer in Baltimore before 1822 [no dates or details were given] (Dr. Archer's "Alphabet to Ledger H" is his booklet [filed in the Archives of the Historical Society of

Harford County] that contains his index to Ledger H [which is missing] for his patients in Baltimore before 1822 and Harford County after 1822, according to a notation by Dr. George W. Archer.)

Allum, William (weaver), was treated by Dr. John Archer in May 1778, Apr 1781 and Aug 1783 (Ledger C, p. 106, noted the doctor was paid by Allum "by weaving 26 yards of coarse woolen" in Sep 1783 and the balance of "debt forgiven by order of testator")

Alms House, patients treated by Dr. Matthew J. Allen were Almon and his sister [name not given] and John ---- [blank] in Feb 1848 and a woman ---- [unnamed] in Apr 1848 (p. 72); see Trustees of the Poor, q.v. [Dr. Allen stated he commenced as attending physician here on 7 Feb 1848.]

Altam, Mrs. (widow), was treated by Dr. John Archer at times before 1772 [no dates or details were given] (Ledger B, p. 1)

Ammons, Thomas, at James Rigbie's, was treated by Dr. John Archer in Sep 1782 and Feb 1791 (Ledger D; Ledger F, p. 158) [account continued in Ledger H, which is missing]

Amos, ---- [blank] (blacksmith), was treated by Dr. Robert H. Archer in Baltimore before 1822 [no dates or details were given] (Dr. Archer's "Alphabet to Ledger H" is his booklet [filed in the Archives of the Historical Society of Harford County] that contains his index to Ledger H [which is missing] for his patients in Baltimore before 1822 and Harford County after 1822, according to a notation by Dr. George W. Archer.)

Amos, Aquila, son of Mordecai, was treated by Dr. John Archer in Aug 1786 (Ledger F, p. 33)

Amos, George, appeared on a list of debts dated 26 Dec 1822 and titled "A List of Allen's Claims" that were due and payable to Dr. Richard N. Allen for services rendered [no dates given] by him to Amos (Document filed in Historical Society of Harford County Archives folder "R. N. Allen")

Amos, James, see James Amoss and Aquila Clark, q.v.

Amos, James, Jr., was visited by Dr. John Archer who treated him in Feb 1780, his wife in Feb 1781, an infant in Nov 1781, inoculated Negro Charles in Mar 1782, treated a negro in Mar 1782 and him [James] in Oct 1782 (Ledger D, p. 49) [account continued in Ledger E, which is missing] James Amos, son of James, was treated by Dr. John Archer in Feb 1787 (Ledger F, p. 33); James Amoss, Jr., was treated by Dr. John Archer in Nov 1788 (Ledger F, p. 255) [account continued in Ledger G, which is missing]; James Amos, Jr., of James (sic) was treated by Dr. John Archer circa 1796-1798 [no dates or details were given] (Ledger I, which is missing, was abstracted by Dr. George W. Archer circa 1890; his notes are in Archives of the Historical Society of Harford County folder "Archer, G. W. Coll. – Ledgers and Day Books")

Amos, James, Sr., was visited by Dr. John Archer who treated him in May, Jun, Jul and Oct 1779 and Nov 1782, a negro in May 1791 and reset James' dislocated jaw on 24 May 1791 (Ledger C, p. 71; Ledger D, p. 32) [account continued in Ledger H, which is missing]; James Amoss, Sr. was treated by Dr. John Archer in Mar 1791 (Ledger D)

Amos, James, son of Mordecai, was treated by Dr. John Archer in Aug 1786 (Ledger F, p. 33)

Amos, John Archer [1790-1851], was visited by Dr. Matthew J. Allen who treated him in Dec 1847 and Jan, Mar, Apr and Jun 1848 and his wife in Jun and Sep 1848 (p. 71)

Amos, Joshua, was treated by Dr. Robert H. Archer in Baltimore before 1822 [no dates or details were given] (Dr. Archer's "Alphabet to Ledger H" is his booklet [filed in the Archives of the Historical Society of Harford County] that contains his index to Ledger H [which is missing] for his patients in Baltimore before 1822 and Harford County after 1822, according to a notation by Dr. George W. Archer.)

Amos, Miss, see Negro Aquilla, q.v.

Amos, Mr., was treated by Dr. Robert H. Archer in Baltimore before 1822 [no dates or details were given] (Dr. Archer's "Alphabet to Ledger H" is his booklet [filed in the Archives of the Historical Society of Harford County] that contains his index to Ledger H [which is missing] for his patients in Baltimore before 1822 and Harford County after 1822, according to a notation by Dr. George W. Archer.)

Amos, Mordecai, see Mordecai Amoss, Aquila Amos and James Amos, q.v.

Amos, William, Jr., see William Amoss, q.v.

Amoss, Aquila, was treated by Dr. John Archer in Dec 1785 (Ledger D, p. 70, noted "debt forgiven as before")

Amoss, Elijah, was treated by Dr. John Archer in Mar 1786 (Ledger F, p. 168)

Amoss, James, see Mordecai Amoss and James Amos, q.v.

Amoss, Mordecai [1753-1842], of James, was treated by Dr. John Archer in Jun and Oct 1779, Apr 1780 and Jul 1792 (Ledger C, p. 87, noted "debt forgiven by order of testator;" Ledger F, p. 266) [Mordecai Amoss, of James, was a Revolutionary War veteran.]; see Thomas A. Thompson, q.v.

Amoss, R., see John Flanagan, q.v.

Amoss, Robert (collector), see Matthew McClintock and Thomas Harris, q.v.

Amoss, Robert (esquire), was visited by Dr. John Archer who treated him in Apr 1782 and him and a child in Sep 1788 (Ledger D, p. 38; Ledger F, p. 46); see Samuel Webb, q.v.

Amoss, William [1718-1814], "Quaker preacher," was visited by Dr. John Archer who treated him in Jan 1782, Hanna Rush in Oct 1782 and him, his wife and child in 1793 (Ledger D, p. 117, noted that part of the bill was paid in cash by Hanna Rush in Nov 1782 and it also noted "See F321") [referring to Ledger F, p. 321, where the account listed his name as William Amos, Jr.)

Anderson, Catherine, widow of John, near Cooptown, was visited by Dr. John Archer who treated her in Aug 1774, Mar and May 1780 and Nov 1783, son John in Dec 1783 and her in Jan 1788 and Sep 1789 (Ledger B, p. 104, spelled her name Katherine; Ledger D, p. 50, spelled her name Catherine and noted "debt forgiven as before;" Ledger F, pp. 76, 157)

Anderson, Daniel, was visited by Dr. John Archer who treated him and a child in May 1791 (Ledger F, p. 65) [Daniel Anderson was a Revolutionary War veteran.]

Anderson, Francis, was visited by Dr. Matthew J. Allen who treated a child twice in Mar 1845 and his son twice in Jun 1845 (p. 45)

Anderson, H., Miss, was treated by Dr. Robert H. Archer many times between 16 Oct 1821 and 3 Apr 1822 and he noted in his ledger "by cash recd. of Exr. at twice $22.10" and she was also noted as being deceased, but the date of death was not given; the $40 bill due Dr. Archer was paid by her executor [actually her administrator since she died intestate] on 22 Feb 1823 (pp. 53, 127, listed her name once as Miss H. R. Anderson; Ledger F, pp. 25, 34); see Chamberlaine & Gale, q.v.

Anderson, Hugh, was murdered in 1813: "State vs. Alexander Thompson, filed 26th August 1813, Harford County, to wit. The jurors for the State of Maryland for the Body of Harford County upon their Oath present that Alexander Thompson late of the same County, yeoman, not having the fear of God before his eyes but being moved and seduced by the instigation of the Devil on the ninth day of August in the year of our Lord One thousand eight hundred and thirteen with force and arms at the county aforesaid in and upon one Hugh Anderson in the peace of God and of the said State then and there being feloniously and wilfully *(sic)* and of his malice aforethought did make an assault and that the said Alexander Thompson a certain *(sic)* gun of the value of eight dollars current money then and there charged and loaded with gun powder and divers leaden shot, which gun he the said Alexander Thompson in both his hands, then and there had and held to, against and upon the said Hugh Anderson, then and there feloniously and wilfully *(sic)* and of his malice aforethought did shoot and discharge and that the said Alexander Thompson with the leaden shot aforesaid out of the gun aforesaid then and there by force of the gun powder, shot, discharged, and sent forth as aforesaid him *(sic)* said Hugh Anderson in and upon the left foot of him the said Hugh Anderson near the ancle *(sic)* of him the said Hugh Anderson then and there with the leaden shot aforesaid out of the gun aforesaid by the said Alexander Thompson so as aforesaid shot, discharged and sent forth feloniously, wilfully *(sic)* and of his malice aforethought, did strike, penetrate and wound, giving to the said Hugh Anderson with the leaden shot aforesaid so as aforesaid shot, discharged and sent forth out of the gun aforesaid by the said Alexander Thompson in and upon the left foot of him the said Hugh Anderson near the ancle *(sic)* of him the said Hugh Anderson one mortal wound of the depth of two inches and of the breadth of four inches of which said mortal wound the said Hugh Anderson from the ninth day of August in the year aforesaid until the sixteenth day of August in the year aforesaid did languish and languishing did live on which said sixteenth day of August in the year aforesaid he the said Hugh Anderson did die and so the Jurors aforesaid and upon their Oath aforesaid do say that the said Alexander Thompson him the said Hugh Anderson then and there in manner and form aforesaid, feloniously and wilfully *(sic)* and of his malice aforethought, did kill and murder against the peace, government and dignity of the State." (File 72.28.11 in the Court Records Department of the Historical Society of Harford County)

Anderson, James, was visited by Dr. John Archer who treated him in Feb, Jul and Aug 1781 and him and his wife in Jul 1786 (Ledger D, p. 121, noted "debt forgiven as before;" Ledger F, p. 338)

Anderson, James, near Slate Ridge, was treated by Dr. John Archer in Jun 1787 (Ledger F, p. 334)

Anderson, James, son-in-law of William McComas, in Cooptown, was treated by Dr. John Archer in Jun 1786 (Ledger F, p. 334)

Anderson, James, near Israel Carr's Mill, was treated by Dr. John Archer in 1796 (Ledger I, which is missing, was abstracted by Dr. George W. Archer circa 1890; his notes are in the Archives of the Historical Society of Harford County folder "Archer, G. W. Coll. – Ledgers and Day Books")

Anderson, John [1782-1853] (cooper), was visited by Dr. Robert H. Archer who treated a negro infant in 1825 (p. 153) [John Anderson was a War of 1812 veteran]

Anderson, John, see Catherine Anderson, q.v.

Anderson, John [1792-1854], was visited by Dr. Robert H. Archer who treated a negro child in Sep 1825 ("balance paid by working of Henry") and treated, him [John] in Nov 1827, a child in Apr and Jul 1828, son John in Jul 1828 and him [John Sr.] in Dec 1835 (pp. 253, 270, 284, 287; Ledger F, p. 145) [John Anderson was a War of 1812 veteran]

Anderson, William, was visited by Dr. Matthew J. Allen who treated his wife and child in Apr 1848 (p. 78)

Andrew, John, was mentioned in Dr. Robert H. Archer's ledger in non-medical matters involving masonry work in 1825 and 1827 (Ledger F, p. 151)

Andrews, Dr., see Hugh Jeffrey, q.v.

Annan (Annon, Ammon?), Dr., see John Diemer, James Gallion, James Giles, James Stewart and Reed & Vanbibber, q.v.

Anspauch, ---- [blank], was treated by Dr. Robert H. Archer in Baltimore before 1822 [no dates or details were given] (Dr. Archer's "Alphabet to Ledger H" is his booklet [filed in the Archives of the Historical Society of Harford County] that contains his index to Ledger H [which is missing] for his patients in Baltimore before 1822 and Harford County after 1822, according to a notation by Dr. George W. Archer.)

Antill, John (miller), was visited by Dr. John Archer who treated his child in Nov 1785 and him and his wife in Jul 1787 (Ledger D, p. 124, noted "debt forgiven as before;" Ledger F, p. 342)

Archer, ---- [blank] was treated by Dr. Robert H. Archer in Apr 1846 who simply stated "child sick" ("True Book, 1845, 46, 47" filed in the Archives of the Historical Society of Harford County file "Archer, Dr. Robert H., 1775-1857, Day Book, 1845-47")

Archer, A., Mrs., was prescribed medicine for her son John by Dr. Robert H. Archer on 2 Aug 1834 (Rx Book, 1825-1851, p. 112)

Archer, Betsy, see Paca Smith, q.v.

Archer, Elizabeth, see Samuel Webb, q.v.

Archer, Garretson, see Rachel Archer, q.v.

Archer, John, see A. Archer, John Archer (minor) and George Lochary, q.v.

Archer, John [1741-1810] (doctor), made oath before Ignatius Wheeler, a Justice of the Peace, on 22 Jul 1781 that the information in his ledger was "just and true as they stand stated." [John Archer was a Revolutionary War veteran and a signer of the Bush Declaration on March 22, 1775.]

Archer, John, Jr. [1777-1830] (doctor), was treated by Dr. Robert H. Archer in Apr 1822 and mentioned Thomas Archer's children [names not given] (Ledger F, p. 38) [John Archer, Jr. was a War of 1812 veteran.]; see James Magraw, James Stephenson, George Courtnay, Hugh Smith, Jr., George Gale, George Morrison, Mrs. Stevenson and Mrs. Creswell, q.v.

Archer, John (minor), was mentioned in non-medical matters by Dr. Robert H. Archer in Feb 1822 and Jan 1826 and also mentioned G. Bartol and Mrs. Welch in Apr 1822 and J. Archer, executor of Thomas Archer, dec'd., in 1823-1825 (Ledger F, pp. 8, 39, 156, 157)

Archer, John T., was recorded in Dr. Robert H. Archer's ledger on 13 Feb 1827 as "By cash recd. his proportion of rents for his Father's interest in lands in Mississippi from the time of his death to Feb. 7, 1827" and the amount was $51.18; the same amount and statement as above for Robert H. Archer; on 12 May 1827, it was recorded, "By cash recd. of Exr. of T. A. dec'd. for sales of 3 1/3 shares of stock in your Susqa. Bridge & Bank Co. his portion of twenty shares standing in the name of the decd." and the amount was $41.662/3; the same amount and statement as above for Robert H. Archer except T. A. was T. Archer; on 15 Mar 1828 he recorded "Robert H. Archer, $88.25 "by cash recd. of Exr. his proportion of distributive share of his Father's estate" and the same for John T. Archer; Dr. Archer noted in his medical ledger on 25 Jun 1828 that he had paid $16.00 to "trustees of St. John's College for 2 qtrs. tuition to 30 June" and $60.00 for boarding for 6 months and $40.12 for clothes and shoes for John T. Archer (pp. 214, 226, 267, 284); see Nathaniel W. S. Hays, q.v.

Archer, P. B., Mrs., was treated by Dr. Robert H. Archer after 1822 [no dates or details were given] (Dr. Archer's "Alphabet to Ledger H" is his booklet [filed in the Archives of the Historical Society of Harford County] that contains his index to Ledger H [which is missing] for his patients in Baltimore City before 1822 and in Harford County after 1822, according to a notation by Dr. George W. Archer.)

Archer, Rachel (colored) was treated by Dr. Matthew J. Allen in Apr, May and Sep 1848 (p. 81) [Her name on the account in the ledger was "Garretson Archer or Rachel (colored), Thomas Hays' woman," but a copy of a receipt for $10 was written on a small piece of paper and inserted in the back of the ledger. It spelled her name Rachcel Archer (col'd.) and also Rach. Archer, N.]

Archer, Robert H. (minor), was treated by Dr. Robert H. Archer in Oct 1815 and noted in ledger that Oliver Holmes, dentist [treated Robert in Apr 1823], was paid and a tavern bill was paid to N. Gorsuch in June 1826; he also mentioned non-medical matters involving J. Archer, executor of Thomas Archer, dec'd., in 1823-1825; Dr. Archer also noted in his ledger on 25 Jun 1828 that he paid $27.00 "for sundries in preparation for West Point" for Robert H. Archer and that he had also paid $36.75 for "expences for himself & Thomas who went with him at the particular request of his mother" (pp. 187, 284; Ledger F, p. 15, 39, 158)

Archer, Stevenson [1786-1848], was mentioned in Dr. Robert H. Archer's ledger on 2 Sep 1824 as follows: "The amt. of my distributive share of my father's estate struck this date as per exrs. book, $245.38½." (p. 121; Ledger F, p. 119); S. Archer was prescribed medicine for his wife by Dr. Robert H. Archer on 28 May 1831 (Rx Book, 1825-1851, p. 102) [Stevenson Archer was a War of 1812 veteran.]; see Jarvis Gilbert, q.v.

Archer, Thomas, had an account in Dr. John Archer, Jr.'s ledger that noted payment "for schooling sons John and Robert" on 8 Nov 1819 (p. 39); see Robert H. Archer (minor), John Archer (minor), Mrs. Hurst, Samuel Webb, and St. John's College, q.v.

Archer, Tommy, see James Kelly, q.v.

Armstrong, ---- [blank], Havre de Grace, was treated by Dr. John Archer in 1790 (Ledger F, p. 238)

Armstrong, Isaac, see James Armstrong, q.v.

Armstrong, James, was visited by Dr. John Archer who treated a child in Feb 1773, him in Jun 1775, Nov 1779 and May 1783 (dressing a wound), a daughter and a child [same person?] in Jul 1783 and him in Jul and Sep 1784 (Ledger B, p. 70; Ledger D, p. 37, noted "debt forgiven as before")

Armstrong, James, was prescribed medicine "for Isaac" by Dr. Robert H. Archer on 23 Sep 1802 and medicine for his child on 14 Aug 1803 and was prescribed medicine for him and his child on 1 Jan 1803 (Rx Book, 1802-1804, pp. 5, 29, 53)

Armstrong, Joshua, was treated by Dr. John Archer in Mar 1787 (Ledger F, p. 243)

Armstrong, Mrs., see ---- Saunders, q.v.

Armstrong, Solomon, near the Lower Methodist Meeting, was treated by Dr. John Archer in Dec 1788 (Ledger F, p. 345)

Arnet, Dr., in York County, was consulted by Dr. John Archer in 1792 (Ledger F, p. 25)

Arnold, Ephraim, was treated by Dr. John Archer in Nov 1781 (Ledger D, p. 96, spelled his first name Ephraem and noted "debt forgiven as before")

Arnold, William, at Cumberland Forge, was treated by Dr. John Archer in July 1800 (Ledger F, p. 261) [account continued in Ledger K, which is missing]

Arthur, Joseph, was visited by Dr. Matthew J. Allen who treated him, and a child and infant several times, in Mar 1848 (p. 77)

Arthur, Joshua, see Augustus J. Greme, q.v.

Arthur, Samuel, was treated by Dr. Matthew J. Allen in Sep 1843 (p. 27)

Ashmead, see James Irwine, q.v.

Ashmead, J., see Samuel Corbett, q.v.

Ashmead, Samuel, was treated by Dr. John Archer in Dec 1779 (Ledger C, p. 25, noted "debt forgiven by order of testator") [Samuel Ashmead was a Revolutionary War veteran.]; see Bridget Malady and Hugh Doran, q.v.

Ashmore, John, see William Ashmore, q.v.

Ashmore, William, was visited by Dr. John Archer who treated negroes in Oct 1779, his daughter in Aug 1783 and him and son John in Jan 1790 (Ledger D, p. 31 [account continued in Ledger E, which is missing]; Ledger F, p. 72); see Mrs. McCalla, Joseph Barnett and Simon Nevil, q.v.

Ashton, Joseph, was visited by Dr. Alonzo Preston who treated his wife in 1825 and son Joseph in 1825 and 1827 (p. 50)

Ascue, ---- [blank], son-in-law to Maj. S. Caldwell [his name was actually William Aisquith and he was a son-in-law of Maj. Samuel Calwell], was visited by Dr. John Archer who treated his son William in 1798 (Ledger I, which is missing, was abstracted by Dr. George W. Archer circa 1890; his notes are in the Archives of the Historical Society of Harford County folder "Archer, G. W. Coll. – Ledgers and Day Books")

Atkinson, Isaac, was prescribed medicine on 21 Nov 1804 by Dr. Robert H. Archer (Rx Book, 1802-1804, p. 63); Isaac Atkinson was treated by Dr. Robert H. Archer in Baltimore before 1822 [no dates or details were given] (Dr. Archer's "Alphabet to Ledger H" is his booklet [filed in the Archives of the Historical Society of Harford County] that contains his index to Ledger H [which is missing] for his patients in Baltimore before 1822 and in Harford County after 1822, according to a notation by Dr. George W. Archer.)

Atkinson, Isaac, was visited by Dr. Alonzo Preston who treated his son Israel four times from 23 Jan to 15 Mar 1826 (p. 66)

Ayres, Aquila, see Negro Polydore, q.v.

Babe, John, at Otter Point, was treated by Dr. John Archer in Apr 1782 (Ledger D, p. 127)

Bagley, Orrick, was visited by Dr. Matthew J. Allen who treated his wife in Dec 1843 (p. 29); see Augustus J. Greme, q.v.

Bagley, Samuel, was visited by Dr. Robert H. Archer who treated his wife in Jun 1823 (pp. 78, 79, 81; Ledger F, p. 45)

Bailey, Charles, was treated by Dr. Robert H. Archer from 30 Jul 1822 to 3 Sep 1822 and noted as "died insolvent," but he did not give the date of death (p. 11; Ledger F, p. 60)

Bailey, Daniel, was visited by Dr. John Archer who treated him in Sep 1781, his wife in Dec 1782 and on 26 Mar 1782 "in partu" [in childbirth], him in May 1782, his wife in Sep 1782 and him in Aug 1783 (Ledger D, p. 75, noted "debt forgiven as before") [account continued in Ledger E, which is missing]

Bailey, Francis, see James Bailey, q.v.

Bailey, Gerard, was treated by Dr. John Archer, Jr. in Dec 1817 (p. 24)

Bailey, James, at "York Town [PA], Francis Bailey, Exr.," was treated by Dr. John Archer four times between 26 Feb 1774 and 2 Mar 1774 (Ledger B, p. 85, spelled his name Baily)

Bailey, John [1787-1880], was visited by Dr. Robert H. Archer who treated his son Edward in Oct 1821, him and his wife in July 1822, John Andrew in Oct 1825 and a child in Oct 1843 (p. 8; Ledger F, p. 13, 49) [John Bailey was a War of 1812 veteran.]

Bailey, Josias, was visited by Dr. Robert H. Archer who treated his wife "in partu" [in childbirth] on 29 Nov 1823 and also rendered obstetrical services to her on 1 Dec 1823; treated Negro Tim in Jun, Jul and Aug 1827 and him [Josias] in Aug 1827 and prescribed medicine for a daughter on 22 Jan 1832 (pp. 94, 236, 241, 242; Ledger F, p. 84; Rx Book, 1825-1851, p. 104)

Bailey, Lloyd, was treated by Dr. Robert H. Archer in Oct 1815 and treated by Dr. John Archer, Jr. were his wife in June 1815, sister Sally and boy Frisby in Jan 1816, and mentioned Mrs. Albert in 1815, G. Kidd in 1817 and Mordecai Barnes and James Evans in 1819 (Dr. Robert Archer's Ledger F, p. 18; Dr. John Archer's ledger, p. 12); see James Evans, q.v.

Bailey, Mrs., see Mr. White, q.v.

Bailey, Sally, see Lloyd Bailey, q.v.

Bailey, Samuel, see Platt Whitaker, q.v.

Baker, see Barnaby Bartle, q.v.

Baker, Agness, was treated by Dr. John Archer in Sep 1782 (Ledger D, p. 98, noted "debt forgiven as before" and "now married to Bonar") [Agnes Baker married James Bonar by license dated 1 Apr 1784.]; see Nicholas Baker, q.v.

Baker, Charles, was visited by Dr. John Archer who treated him in Jan and Aug 1782, him, wife and child in Sep 1783 and him in Oct 1783 (Ledger D, p. 115, noted "debt forgiven as before") [Charles Baker was a Revolutionary War veteran.]; see James Perine, q.v.

Baker, Gideon, son of Theophilus, on Winter's Run, was treated by Dr. John Archer in 1787 (Ledger F, p. 272)

Baker, Grafton, was visited by Dr. John Archer who treated him and his wife and a child in 1786 (Ledger F, p. 15)

Baker, Grafton [1781-1851], appeared on a list of debts dated 26 Dec 1822 and titled "A List of Allen's Claims" that were due and payable to Dr. Richard N. Allen for services rendered [no dates] by him to said Baker (Document filed in Historical Society of Harford County Archives folder "R. N. Allen"); Grafton Baker was later visited by Dr. Robert H. Archer who treated him and Grafton Robinson in Jul 1825 (pp. 146-148) [Grafton Baker was a War of 1812 veteran.]

Baker, Henry, was visited by Dr. John Archer, Jr. who treated him and Jerry Baker and his [Henry's] wife in 1816, a child in Nov 1818 and his [Henry's] wife in Jan 1820 (p. 63)

Baker, Jerry, see Henry Baker, q.v.

Baker, John, was visited by Dr. John Archer who treated him in Aug 1781, his wife in Aug 1782 and him in Jun 1783 and Oct 1784 (Ledger D, p. 63) [continued in Ledger G, which is missing]

Baker, Martin, see Constus O'Donnal, q.v.

Baker, Miss, was treated by Dr. Robert H. Archer in Baltimore before 1822 [no dates or details were given] (Dr. Archer's "Alphabet to Ledger H" is his booklet [filed in the Archives of the Historical Society of Harford County] that contains his index to Ledger H [which is missing] for his patients in Baltimore before 1822 and Harford County after 1822, according to a notation by Dr. George W. Archer.)

Baker, Nicholas, was treated by Dr. John Archer in May, June and Sep 1780 (Ledger D, p. 65, did not mention that he had died, but noted "Nicholas Baker was the husband of James Bonar's present wife") [Nicholas Baker was a Revolutionary War veteran.]; see Agnes Baker, q.v.

Baker, Nicholas, "at Boner's Stone House," was visited by Dr. Robert H. Archer who treated his son in Feb and Mar 1827 in consultation with Dr. Dallam (pp. 215, 216, 217); see Jarvis Gilbert, q.v.

Baker, Nicholas, Jr., was visited by Dr. Matthew J. Allen who rendered obstetrical services to his wife on 28 Jan 1845 (p. 43)

Baker, Nicholas, Sr., was treated by Dr. Matthew J. Allen in Feb 1845 (p. 44, noted "paid I believe")

Baker, Theophilus, was treated by Dr. John Archer in Nov and Dec 1781 and Mar and Apr 1782 (Ledger D, p. 94, noted "debt forgiven as before"); see Gideon Baker, q.v.

Baker, Thomas, was treated by Dr. John Archer in Sep 1773 and Feb 1774 (Ledger B, p. 10)

Baker, Widow, see James O'Donal, q.v.

Balderson, Isaiah, was treated by Dr. John Archer in Oct 1782 (Ledger D)

Balderson, Sarah, was treated by Dr. John Archer in Sep and Oct 1780, Aug 1781, May 1782 and Oct 1785 (Ledger D, p. 96)

Baldwin, Marshall, appeared on a list of debts dated 26 Dec 1822 and titled "A List of Allen's Claims" that were due and payable to Dr. Richard N. Allen for services rendered [no dates were given] by him to said Baldwin (Document filed in Historical Society of Harford County Archives folder "R. N. Allen") [Marshall Baldwin was a War of 1812 veteran.]

Balf, Henry, was treated by Dr. John Archer in Apr 1781 (Ledger D, p. 4, "debt forgiven as before")

Ballard, Levin, W., was treated by Dr. Matthew J. Allen in 1823 in Calvert County (p. 8a) [Levin W. Ballard was a War of 1812 veteran.]

Ballard, Mr., see James Stallings, q.v.

Baner, Wm., was prescribed medicine by Dr. Robert H. Archer on 24 Aug 1803 (Rx Book, 1802-1804, p. 54)

Bard, Mr., was prescribed medicine for his wife by Dr. Robert H. Archer on 22 Mar and 3 May 1803 (Rx Book, 1802-1804, pp. 37, 41)

Barker, Joseph, was treated by Dr. Robert H. Archer in Baltimore before 1822 [no dates or details were given] (Dr. Archer's "Alphabet to Ledger H" is his booklet [filed in the Archives of the Historical Society of Harford County] that contains his index to Ledger H [which is missing] for his patients in Baltimore before 1822 and Harford County after 1822, according to a notation by Dr. George W. Archer.)

Barkley, Elizabeth, was treated by Dr. John Archer at various times between Feb 1773 and June 1775 (Ledger B, p. 58, spelled her name Barkly) [but this may actually be Elizabeth Bartly]

Barkley, John, was visited by Dr. John Archer who treated him, his wife and children [unnamed] in 1800 (Ledger F, p. 164); see Betsey Walker, q.v.

Barkley, Mrs., see Hetty Cowenevans, q.v.

Barkley, William, paid Dr. John Archer for treating his brother-in-law's daughter in Cecil County in May 1787 (Ledger F, p. 33, spelled his name Barkly); see James Wilson, q.v.

Barnes, Benjamin, son of James, was treated by Dr. John Archer in Sep 1787 (Ledger F, p. 37) [Benjamin Barnes was a Revolutionary War veteran.]

Barnes, E., see Negro Ned, q.v.

Barnes, Ezekiel, at Widow Wells', was treated by Dr. John Archer in Feb 1786 (Ledger F, p. 122); see Mrs. Barnes, q.v.

Barnes, Gregory Sr. [1765-1846], was visited by Dr. John Archer who treated him in May 1781 and Sep and Oct 1784, his wife in Nov 1784 and him, his wife and daughter Rachel in 1791 (Ledger D, p. 24, transferred to Ledger F, p. 36; both spelled his name Barns); see Richard Barnes, q.v.

Barnes, Gregory, was visited by Dr. Robert H. Archer who treated him and a child in July 1822 and him in Oct 1826 (pp. 10, 206, 207; Ledger F, p. 59); see Mr. Barnes, q.v.

Barnes, Hosea, was visited by Dr. Matthew J. Allen who treated a child (dressed a burn twice) in Aug 1844 (pp. 37 and 74, noted he paid part of the bill in Feb 1848 and the balance in Oct 1848)

Barnes, James, was visited by Dr. John Archer who treated his wife in Dec 1772 and him in Jan 1773 (Ledger B, p. 4, noted as "dead & insolvent," but no date of death was given)

Barnes, James, was treated by Dr. John Archer in Jul 1787 (Ledger F, p. 364, spelled his name Barns) [James Barnes was a Revolutionary War veteran.]; see Benjamin Barnes, q.v.

Barnes, Job, was treated by Dr. John Archer in Nov 1786 (Ledger F, p. 195, spelled his name Barns) [account continued in Ledger G, which is missing]

Barnes, John, see Frances Hollis, q.v.

Barnes, Joseph, was treated by Dr. John Archer in June 1773 (Ledger B, p. 29)

Barnes, Joseph, was visited by Dr. John Archer who treated him and wife in 1793 (Ledger F, p. 20, spelled his name Barns) [account continued in Ledger K, which is missing]

Barnes, Mordecai, see Lloyd Bailey, q.v.

Barnes, Mr., son of Gregory, was treated by Dr. Robert H. Archer in July 1828 (p. 285)

Barnes, Mrs., widow of Ezekiel, was treated by Dr. John Archer in Feb 1786 (Ledger F, p. 243)

Barnes, Rachel, see Gregory Barnes, Sr., q.v.

Barnes, Richard, see Moses Whitlock, q.v.

Barnes, Richard [1762-1830], of Gregory, was treated by Dr. John Archer in 1787 (Ledger F, p. 243)

Barnes, Thomas, was treated by Dr. John Archer in Aug and Oct 1773 (Ledger B, p. 45, spelled his name Barns); see Nicholas Waters and Vincent Goldsmith, q.v.

Barnes, Thomas, appeared on a list of debts dated 26 Dec 1822 and titled "A List of Allen's Claims" that were due and payable to Dr. Richard N. Allen for services rendered [no dates were given] by him to said Barnes (Document filed in Historical Society of Harford County Archives folder "R. N. Allen") [Thomas Barnes was a War of 1812 veteran.]

Barnes, William (ship carpenter), was treated by Dr. John Archer in 1788 (Ledger F, p. 214, spelled his name Barns) [account continued in Ledger G, which is missing]

Barnes, William, see John Williams, q.v.

Barnett, James [1757-1824], near Mr. Webb's, was visited by Dr. John Archer who treated him in Feb 1777 and Dec 1790 and his wife in 1788 and 1789 (Ledger C, p. 9; Ledger F, p. 127, listed him as James Barnet, the Elder); see Patrick Reynolds, David McCoy and James Barnett, Jr., q.v.

Barnett, James, Jr., was treated by Dr. John Archer in Mar 1781 and Sep 1784 (Ledger D, p. 126, noted James Barnett, Sr. was his security)

Barnett, John, near William McComas in Cooptown, was treated by Dr. John Archer in Jun 1786 (Ledger F, p. 339, spelled his name Barnet)

Barnett, Joseph, near William Ashmore, was treated by Dr. John Archer in 1791 (Ledger F, p. 126, spelled his name Barnet)

Barney ---- [blank] (tailor), was treated by Dr. Robert H. Archer in Baltimore before 1822 [no dates or details were given] (Dr. Archer's "Alphabet to Ledger H" is his booklet [filed in the Archives of the Historical Society of Harford County] that contains his index to Ledger H [which is missing] for his patients in Baltimore before 1822 and Harford County after 1822, according to a notation by Dr. George W. Archer.)

Barney, Ann, see John H. Barney, q.v.

Barney, Helen, see John H. Barney, q.v.

Barney, John, was visited by Dr. John Archer who treated him in Aug, Sep and Oct 1778 and Aug 1779, Miss Molly Smith in Oct 1779, a negro in Feb 1780, an infant in May 1781, him [John] in Jul 1781, him and an infant in Aug 1781 and him in Sep 1783 (Ledger C, p. 121, noted "debt forgiven by order of testator")

Barney, John H., was visited by Dr. John Archer who treated him and daughters Helen and Miss Ann at times between 1794 and 1800 [Dr. John Archer noted "Cr. by ferriages" and Dr. George W. Archer later noted "from H." & "to K" after Barney's name] (Ledger I, which is missing, was abstracted by Dr. George W. Archer circa 1890; his notes are in the Archives of the Historical Society of Harford County folder "Archer, G. W. Coll. – Ledgers and Day Books")

Barney, Mr., see Joseph Steele, q.v.

Barrens, Sally, was treated by Dr. John Archer in 1782 (Ledger D, p. 11, "debt forgiven as before")

Barrett, John, near Mr. Clendenin's, was visited by Dr. John Archer who treated his family in 1797 and 1798 (Ledger I, which is missing, was abstracted by Dr. George W. Archer circa 1890; his notes are in the

10

Archives of the Historical Society of Harford County folder "Archer, G. W. Coll. – Ledgers and Day Books") [John Barrett was a Revolutionary War veteran.]

Barrow, James, was treated by Dr. Robert H. Archer after 1822 [no dates or details were given] (Dr. Archer's "Alphabet to Ledger H" is his booklet [filed in the Archives of the Historical Society of Harford County] that contains his index to Ledger H [which is missing] for his patients in Baltimore City before 1822 and in Harford County after 1822, according to a notation by Dr. George W. Archer.)

Barrow, Mrs., at Long Green, was treated by Dr. John Archer in Feb 1788 (Ledger F, p. 159)

Barrow, Widow, see John Lindsey, q.v.

Barry, James, was treated by Dr. Robert H. Archer in Baltimore before 1822 [no dates or details were given] (Dr. Archer's "Alphabet to Ledger H" is his booklet [filed in the Archives of the Historical Society of Harford County] that contains his index to Ledger H [which is missing] for his patients in Baltimore before 1822 and Harford County after 1822, according to a notation by Dr. George W. Archer.)

Barry, John, was prescribed medicine for his wife by Dr. Robert H. Archer on 21 Sep 1802 (Rx Book, 1802-1804, p. 5) and he was treated by Dr. Archer in Baltimore before 1822 [no dates or details were given] (Dr. Archer's "Alphabet to Ledger H" is his booklet [filed in the Archives of the Historical Society of Harford County] that contains his index to Ledger H [which is missing] for his patients in Baltimore before 1822 and Harford County after 1822, according to a notation by Dr. George W. Archer.)

Barry, Lavallin, was prescribed medicine by Dr. Robert H. Archer in Mar 1801 (Rx Book, 1796-1801, pp. 48, 50) [Lavallin or Levallin Barry lived in Baltimore City.]

Bartle, Barnaby, at the Baker's in Havre de Grace, was treated by Dr. John Archer in Jul 1788 (Ledger F, p. 69)

Bartlett, William E., see R. N. and M. J. Allen, q.v.

Bartley, David, was treated by Dr. John Archer in Sep and Oct 1772 (Ledger B, p. 54)

Bartley, Elizabeth, see Elizabeth Barkley, q.v.

Bartley, John, was treated by Dr. John Archer in Aug 1782 (Ledger D, p. 111, spelled his name Bartly and noted "debt forgiven as before")

Bartley, Widow, see James Walker, q.v.

Bartol, G., see John Archer (minor), q.v.

Barton, James, see Polly Smithson, q.v.

Barton, William, was visited by Dr. Matthew J. Allen who rendered obstetrical services to his wife in Apr 1848 [exact date unclear] (p. 78)

Bateman, William (overseer), was visited by Dr. John Archer who treated him and his family in 1798 (Ledger I, which is missing, was abstracted by Dr. George W. Archer circa 1890; his notes are in the Archives of the Historical Society of Harford County folder "Archer, G. W. Coll. – Ledgers and Day Books")

Bates, Mrs., at John McFadon's, was prescribed medicine by Dr. Robert H. Archer on 17 Nov 1804 (Rx Book, 1804, p. 61)

Bathia, Miss, see John Patterson, q.v.

Baxter, John &ca (sic), was treated by Dr. Robert H. Archer in Baltimore before 1822 [no dates or details were given] (Dr. Archer's "Alphabet to Ledger H" is his booklet [filed in the Archives of the Historical Society of Harford County] that contains his index to Ledger H [which is missing] for his patients in Baltimore before 1822 and Harford County after 1822, according to a notation by Dr. George W. Archer.)

Baxter, Mr., near James Quinlan's, was treated by Dr. Robert H. Archer in Nov 1825 (p. 169; Ledger F, p. 149)

Bay, George, "X Roads," was treated by Dr. Robert H. Archer in Sep and Oct 1828 in consultation with Dr. Allen (pp. 297, 298) [George W. Bay was a War of 1812 veteran.]

Bay, Hugh [1758-1818], was treated by Dr. John Archer in Dec 1786 (Ledger F, p. 152) [Hugh Bay was a Revolutionary War veteran.]

Bay, Jen:, see James Holmes, q.v.

Bay, John [1743-1818], was treated by Dr. John Archer in Jul 1775 (Ledger B, p. 47)

Bay, Mr., see Arthur Hague, q.v.

Bay, William [c1715-1773], was treated by Dr. John Archer six times in Sep and Oct 1773 and died testate soon thereafter (Ledger B, p. 90; Baltimore County Will Book 3, p. 262)

Bay, William [1756-1808], of William, was treated by Dr. John Archer in Dec 1777 (Ledger C, p. 86)

Bayard (Byard), Ephraim, was treated by Dr. John Archer in Dec 1780, Jan 1781 and Jun 1788 (Ledger D, p. 111, listed his name as Ephram Byard and noted that Richard Hartgrove was his security; Ledger F, p. 255, spelled his name Ephraem Bayard and indicated he paid his medical bill by rendering services as a wagon maker and wagon repairman) [Ephraim Bayard or Byard was a Revolutionary War veteran.]

Bayard (Byard), James, was visited by Dr. John Archer who treated him and a child in Jan 1790 (Ledger F, p. 319) [James Bayard or Byard was a Revolutionary War veteran.]

Bayless, Benjamin, was visited by Dr. John Archer who treated a child in Sep 1779 and him, his wife and children in Nov 1782 (Ledger D, p. 25, spelled his name Baylis and noted that part of the bill was paid by cash received of N. Baylis and the balance by Hugh Dever's note to Aquila Cain in 1785) [Benjamin Bayless was a Revolutionary War veteran.]

Bayless, Benjamin, Jr., see Samuel Bayless, q.v.

Bayless, Daniel, was treated by Dr. John Archer in Jan 1790 (Ledger F, p. 150) [Daniel Bayless or Baylis was a Revolutionary War veteran.]

Bayless, Elias, see Samuel Bayless, q.v.

Bayless, Jonas, was treated by Dr. John Archer in Aug 1776 and Apr 1781 (Ledger C, p. 54) [Jonas Baylis, sometimes spelled Bayless and Bailess, was a Revolutionary War veteran.]

Bayless, Joseph, was treated by Dr. John Archer in Oct 1780, May 1781 and Jul 1782 (Ledger D, p. 61, spelled his name Baylis and noted that he paid part of the bill on 1 May 1784 and part of it on 28 Nov 1785, but then indicated "debt forgiven as before")

Bayless, Nathaniel [1748-1790], was treated by Dr. John Archer in Jan 1773, Dec 1776 and May 1779 and "Nat. Baylis" was treated in May 1790 (Ledger B, p. 97; Ledger C, p. 65; Ledger F, p. 201) [account continued in Ledger G which is missing] [Nathaniel (Nathan) Baylis, sometimes spelled Bayless and Bailess, was a Revolutionary War veteran.]; see Benjamin Baylis, q.v.

Bayless, Polly, see Samuel Bayless, Sr., q.v.

Bayless, Samuel, was visited by Dr. John Archer who treated him in Jun 1773 and Apr, May and Jul 1775, son Elias and daughter Phebe in Apr 1775, him in Jul 1778, Mar 1780 and Jun 1781, an unnamed negro in Sep 1781 and Oct 1781, his [Samuel's] wife in Oct 1781, a child in Nov 1782 and him and his wife in Nov 1789 (Ledger B, pp. 87, 100 and Ledger C, p. 116, spelled his name Baylis [account continued in Ledger E, which is missing]; Ledger F, p. 323)

Bayless, Samuel, Sr., was visited by Dr. John Archer who treated him and children Samuel, Zephaniah and Polly at various times between 1796 and 1798 (Ledger I, which is missing, was abstracted by Dr. George W. Archer circa 1890 and spelled his name Baylis; his notes are in the Archives of the Historical Society of Harford County folder "Archer, G. W. Coll. – Ledgers and Day Books"); Samuel Baylis was visited by Dr. James Archer who treated him nine times in Mar and Apr 1806 with various medicines, "for bleeding" his daughter Polly in May 1806 and medicating Mrs. Baylis in Jun and Jul 1806 (p. 2)

Bayless, Samuel, of Benjamin Jr., was visited by Dr. John Archer who treated him and his family at various times between 1797 and 1799 (Ledger I, which is missing, was abstracted by Dr. George W. Archer circa 1890 and spelled his name Baylis; his notes are in Archives of the Historical Society of Harford County file "Archer, G. W. Coll. – Ledgers and Day Books")

Bayless, William F. [1814-1873], was visited by Dr. Robert H. Archer who treated his wife on 8 Sep 1847 and he returned on 28 Sep 1847 after she had a difficult birth that he described as follows: "Mrs. Bayless had retained placenta at the fundus uteri with a rotten umbilical cord, copious flooding & syncope. This circumstances was delivered of the placenta & the hemorrhage so copious as to produce [illegible] great & prolonged debility. In this condition precisely according to Dr. Silver's telling to me she expired (sic) [she did not die, so he may have meant she fainted] with her next confinement the placenta undelivered in less than an hour after the birth of the child." Dr. Archer returned on 1 Oct 1847, stayed six days and made the following note: "Four days after delivery while I was with her I was called out of bed to see her that she had fainted – I found her expiring in syncope with copious hemorrhage. Immediately introduced my whole hand into the uterus & emptied it entirely of its contents which was a chamber very full of large coagula. I sat up with her all night, nursed her myself, keeping my hands upon the vulva & abdomen using cold applications & frictions(?), & not wasting (wanting?) these manipulations to to (sic) any one and was the extremity of her care. She was one of those few constitutions which could not with safety with / stood(?) by hemorrhage – Of this I warned Dr. Silver telling him if he had any difficulty [illegible] her after the birth of the child – The labor went on so smoothly & terminated so handsomely that (as he told me) he was put off his guard -- & in half an hour after the birth of the child that she expired / some (sic) uterine hemorrhage the placenta undelivered – All these facts are known to her husband & does he consider me his enemy! – What a crooked

& unreadable world is this!" Dr. Robert H. Archer continued to treat and medicate Mrs. Bayless 18 more times from 1 Oct 1847 to 7 Dec 1847 and many times he remained through the night to care for her. (Document filed in the Archives of the Historical Society of Harford County folder "Archer, Robert H., 1775-1857 – Receipts") [William's full name was William Finney Bayless and Eleanor "Ellen" Brooks (1810-1849), was his first wife. The Maryland Mortality Schedule for the year ending 1 Jun 1850 indicated Ellen Bayless, age 35 *(sic)*, died suddenly in Dec 1849.]

Bayless, Zephaniah, see Samuel Bayless, Sr., q.v.

Beacham, Mrs., see John Herbert, q.v.

Beal, Master, see Reuben H. Davis, q.v.

Bean, William, at T. G. Howard's [Thomas Gassaway Howard], was treated by Dr. John Archer in Nov 1787 (Ledger F, p. 78)

Beatty, Archibald, see Jonathan Fosset, q.v.

Beatty, Dr., was consulted by Dr. John Archer in 1800 (Ledger F, p. 197)

Beatty, Hugh (storekeeper), was treated by Dr. John Archer in Aug 1772 (Ledger B, p. 4); see Andrew Irwine, q.v.

Beatty, James, dec'd., appeared on a list of debts dated 26 Dec 1822 and titled "A List of Allen's Claims" that were due and payable to Dr. Richard N. Allen for services rendered [no dates] by him to the said James (Document filed in Historical Society of Harford County Archives folder "R. N. Allen")

Beatty, Sam, see William Beatty, q.v.

Beatty, William, near Bethel Meeting House, and "son-in-law to Flanagan," was visited by Dr. John Archer who treated him and his son Sam in Aug 1788 (Ledger F, p. 85) [William Beatty was a Revolutionary War veteran.]

Beaver, Charles was visited by Dr. John Archer in Dec 1778 for "ad reduction: tibia" [i. e., reset his broken leg]; treated him in Jan, Feb, Mar and Apr 1779, Dec 1780 and Sep 1783 (Ledger C, p. 75, noted Capt. John Jolly was his security) [Charles Beaver was a Revolutionary War veteran.]

Beck, John, in Bush River Neck, was treated by Dr. John Archer in Apr 1778 (Ledger C, p. 107, noting "debt forgiven by order of testator")

Bell, Becky, see James Bell, q.v.

Bell, Crizzy, see James Bell, q.v.

Bell, David, was treated by Dr. John Archer in May 1786 (Ledger F, p. 271) [account continued in Ledger G, which is missing] [David Bell was a Revolutionary War veteran.]

Bell, James, was visited by Dr. John Archer who treated him, his wife and a child in 1787, him and daughter Crizzy *(sic)* in 1789 and was prescribed medicine for his wife by Dr. Robert H. Archer on 22 Oct 1796 (Ledger F, pp. 18, 71, 188; Rx Book, 1796-1801, p. 10) [account continued in Ledger G, which is missing]; James was visited by Dr. John Archer who treated him and daughters Becky, Molly and Jenny at various times between 1795 and 1797 (Ledger I, which is missing, was abstracted by Dr. George W. Archer circa 1890; his notes are in the Archives of the Historical Society of Harford County file "Archer, G. W. Coll. – Ledgers and Day Books") see Hugh Bennett, q.v.

Bell, Jenny, see James Bell, q.v.

Bell, Molly, see James Bell, q.v.

Belton, Mr., was prescribed medicine by Dr. Robert H. Archer on 21 Nov and 25 Nov 1804 (Rx Book, 1802-1804, pp. 63, 64)

Bemis, Nathaniel S., was treated by Dr. Alonzo Preston in Jan and Feb 1826 (p. 65)

Benjamin, George, was visited by Dr. John Archer, Jr. in June 1815 who treated him and a child and mentioned John Peten and Robert Lowry in 1821 and brother Isaac Benjamin in 1822 (p. 14); see John Cavenaugh, q.v.

Benjamin, Isaac, see George Benjamin, q.v.

Benjamin, Jonathan, was treated by Dr. John Archer in Sep 1778 (Ledger C, p. 123, noted "debt forgiven by order of testator")

Benjamin, William, was treated by Dr. John Archer, Jr. who treated him and a child in 1816 (p. 50)

Bennett, ---- [blank], "in Havre de Grace, now at Hall's Cross Roads," was visited by Dr. John Archer who treated him and his wife in 1787 (Ledger F, p. 72, spelled his last name Bennet)

Bennett, Benjamin, was treated by Dr. John Archer prior to 1772 [no details given] and was charged for 8 years interest on his unpaid bill in 1779 (Ledger B, p. 9, spelled his name Bennet) [Benjamin Bennett was a Revolutionary War veteran.]

Bennett, Hugh (hatter), at James Bell's Crossroads, was treated by Dr. John Archer in 1788 and 1789 (Ledger F, p. 50, spelled his name Bennit, and p. 51, spelled his name Bennet and Bennit)

Bennett, William, at Swan Creek, was treated by Dr. John Archer in 1786 (Ledger F, p. 377)

Berenger, Monsr., was treated by Dr. John Archer at various times between 1797 and 1801 (Ledger I, which is missing, was abstracted by Dr. George W. Archer circa 1890; his notes are in Archives of Historical Society of Harford County folder "Archer, G. W. Coll. – Ledgers and Day Books")

Berry, Richard, at Otter Point, was visited by Dr. John Archer who treated him in May 1782, his wife and child in Jan 1783 and him in Feb 1783 (Ledger D, p. 5, noted "debt forgiven as before") [account continued in Ledger E, which is missing]

Betts, Enoch, was prescribed medicine for his wife by Dr. Robert H. Archer on 17 Dec and 26 Dec 1802 and 28 Jan 1803 (Rx Book, 1802-1804, pp. 27, 31)

Betts, William, near Mr. Wheeler, Jr.'s, was visited by Dr. John Archer on 2 Jan 1778 "to delivering your wife" (Ledger C, p. 98, noted "debt forgiven by order of testator") [William Betts was a Revolutionary War veteran.]

Bevard, George [1796-1869] (cooper), was visited by Dr. Robert H. Archer who treated him seventeen times between 15 Dec 1822 and 28 Apr 1823, his wife in Dec 1822 and Jan and Feb 1823 and "post partu" [i. e., after giving birth] on 17 Mar 1823 and treated again in Apr 1823, a child in Jul 1835 in consultation with Dr. Hopkins and a daughter "moribund" [i. e., near death] on 10 Oct 1847 in consultation with Dr. Ramsay (pp. 43, 47, 52, 58, 65; Ledger F, p. 128)

Bevin, Charles, was visited by Dr. John Archer who treated him and wife in 1795 (Ledger F, p. 83)

Bevin, Edward, was treated by Dr. John Archer in 1788 (Ledger F, p. 323, stated bill was paid by Benjamin Green in 1796)

Biddle, Mrs., had an account with Dr. John Archer [undated, but likely circa 1780] which contained no entries for treatment, yet it noted "debt forgiven as before" (Ledger D, p. 45)

Big Bill, was treated by Dr. Alonzo Preston at various times between 1823 and 1824 (p. 6, noted "R. D. Lee promise to pay" and later noted "paid in full, witness Gorsuch" and initialed by "W.B.B." [i. e., payment was received by Dr. William B. Bond]

Bilings, Widow, see Thomas Hall, q.v.

Billingslea, Josias, was visited by Dr. John Archer who treated him, his wife and son William in 1799 (Ledger F, pp. 49, 56)

Billingslea, Ruth, was treated by Dr. John Archer in Nov 1802 (Ledger F, p. 209)

Billingslea, Sally, see Walter Billingslea, q.v.

Billingslea, Sias, see Cyrus Billingsley, q.v.

Billingslea, Walter [1744-1807], was visited by Dr. John Archer who treated his wife in Dec 1776 and Mar 1778 and him in Apr 1778 (Ledger C, pp. 63, 66, spelled his name Billingsly); he was visited by Dr. John Archer who treated him and his wife in 1805 (Ledger F, p. 39, noted that Mr. McMath was Walter's executor on 22 Dec 1807); he also appeared on a list of debts dated 26 Dec 1822 and titled "A List of Allen's Claims" that were due and payable to Dr. Richard N. Allen for services rendered [no dates were given] by him to said Billingslea (Document filed in Historical Society of Harford County Archives folder "R. N. Allen") [Walter Billingslea was a Revolutionary War veteran.]

Billingslea, Walter [1782-1853] was visited by Dr. Alonzo Preston who treated his daughter Sally in May 1826 and his wife in Oct 1828 (p. 75)

Billingslea, William, see Josias Billingslea, q.v.

Billingsley, Cyrus, was visited by Dr. John Archer who treated him in Oct 1775, him and his wife and daughter in Nov 1775, his wife in Jan 1777, him and his wife in Sep 1777, and inoculated 6 of his family in Apr 1779; treated his wife and son in May 1779 and him in Nov 1782 and Aug 1788 (Ledger C, p. 14, noted that Cyrus "paid 26 dollars in Congress" on 31 Jan 1777) [It is possible that his name was Sias rather than Cyrus.]

Billingsley, Widow, was visited by Dr. John Archer who treated a child in Dec 1776, her [widow] in Jan 1777, a negro child in Jan 1778, a negro infant in Apr 1779, her in Oct 1782 and June 1783, and son Jacob in July 1783 (Ledger C, p. 22)

Birckhead, Matthew, see Capt. John Hall, q.v.

Birckhead, Thomas H., see John Johnson, Capt. John Hall and John McComas Magness, Jr., q.v.

Birckhead, Wm., see Eliza Lewis, q.v.

Bishops, John &ca. *(sic)*, was treated by Dr. Robert H. Archer in Baltimore before 1822 [no dates or details were given] (Dr. Archer's "Alphabet to Ledger H" is his booklet [filed in the Archives of the Historical Society of Harford County] that contains his index to Ledger H [which is missing] for his patients in Baltimore before 1822 and Harford County after 1822, according to a notation by Dr. George W. Archer.)

Black, John N., was visited by Dr. John Archer, Jr. who treated him in Feb 1816, an infant and child Washn. *(sic)* in Jun 1816, and also mentioned John Hassan in Mar 1816 (p. 45) [John N. Black was a War of 1812 veteran]; see Ann Wyatt. Q.v.

Black Bob, see Robert Glover, q.v.

Black Rachel, "at the cross roads," was treated in June 1773 by Dr. John Archer (Ledger B, p. 29)

Blackburn, Brice, was treated by Dr. John Archer in Oct and Nov 1781 and Mar and May 1782 (Ledger D, p. 87, noted bill paid by Robert Blackburn in Dec 1783); see Robert Blackburn, q.v.

Blackburn, John, was visited by Dr. John Archer who treated his son and daughter, a woman and a maid in Sep 1772, a child in Feb 1773, him [John] at various times between Aug 1773 and Feb 1774 and him in Oct 1774 (Ledger B, p. 7, noted "went to the western country," but no date of departure was given); see Robert Blackburn and John Clark, q.v.

Blackburn, John, Jr., was visited by Dr. John Archer who treated his wife in Jun 1778 and Dec 1782, a child in Dec 1778 and him in Mar 1783 (Ledger C, p. 65, noted the medical bill was paid by Robert Blackburn on 3 Dec 1783)

Blackburn, Robert, was visited by Dr. John Archer who treated him before 1772 [no details were given], his wife in Nov 1772 and him at times between Sep 1777 and Sep 1783, and also mentioned Brice, John Blackburn and James McGaw (Ledger B, p. 19; Ledger C, p. 21); see Brice Blackburn and John Blackburn, Jr., q.v.

Blackstone, Elijah, was treated by Dr. John Archer in Oct 1787 (Ledger F, p. 37)

Blake, ---- [blank] (blacksmith), was treated by Dr. Robert H. Archer after 1822 [no dates or details were given] (Dr. Archer's "Alphabet to Ledger H" is his booklet [filed in the Archives of the Historical Society of Harford County] that contains his index to Ledger H [which is missing] for his patients in Baltimore before 1822 and Harford County after 1822, according to a notation by Dr. George W. Archer.)

Blake, Isaac, see Jane Jones and Jinny Jones, q.v.

Blake, Joseph (colonel), was visited by Dr. Matthew J. Allen who treated him and his son Richard in 1823 in Calvert Co. (p. 7b)

Blake, Richard, see Joseph Blake, q.v.

Blaney, John, was visited by Dr. Alonzo Preston who treated his wife at night on 6 Aug 1827 (p. 94)

Blaney, Nat (doctor), was treated by Dr. John Archer in 1786 (Ledger F, p. 73, noted that Dr. Archer was paid "by the profession")

Blaney, Thomas, was treated by Dr. Robert H. Archer in Baltimore before 1822 [no dates or details were given] (Dr. Archer's "Alphabet to Ledger H" is his booklet [filed in the Archives of the Historical Society of Harford County] that contains his index to Ledger H [which is missing] for his patients in Baltimore before 1822 and Harford County after 1822, according to a notation by Dr. George W. Archer.)

Boardsman, Catherine, was visited by Dr. John Archer who treated her in Jul 1781 and inoculated her and her daughter and Cotty *(sic)* Short in Jan 1782 (Ledger D, p. 46, noted that "Catharin" paid for the inoculations, but the balance of "debt forgiven as before"); see William Boardsman, q.v.

Boardsman, William, was visited by Dr. John Archer who treated his wife in Mar, Apr and May 1773, him and wife in May 1774 and June 1775, his wife in Aug 1777 and Aug 1778, Ed Stevenson in Apr 1778, and William in Dec 1778 (Ledger B, p. 11; Ledger C, p. 37, noted Catherine Boardsman paid the bill) [William Boardsman was a Revolutionary War veteran.]

Boarman, Edward, was visited by Dr. Robert H. Archer who treated a negro in Sep 1822 (p. 18; Ledger F, p. 77)

Boarman, Frank, see Robert Boarman, q.v.

Boarman, Mrs., was treated by Dr. Robert H. Archer in July 1825 (p. 142)

Boarman, Robert, son-in-law to Benjamin Wheeler, was visited by Dr. John Archer who treated him and his family at various times between 1797 and 1799 (Ledger I, which is missing, was abstracted by Dr. George W. Archer circa 1890 who noted that Boarman had been misspelled Bowman by Dr. John Archer; Dr. George W. Archer's notes are in the Archives of the Historical Society of Harford County folder "Archer, G. W. Coll. – Ledgers and Day Books"); Robert appeared on a list of debts dated 26 Dec 1822 and titled "A List of Allen's Claims" that were due and payable to Dr. Richard N. Allen for services rendered [no dates given] by him to Boarman (Document in the Archives of the Historical Society of Harford County folder "R. N. Allen")

Boarman, Robert, was visited by Dr. Robert H. Archer in June and July 1825 who treated a negro and Mrs. Boarman with Dr. Forwood, and he was visited by Dr. Matthew J. Allen who treated him in Jan 1844, his wife in Mar 1844, a child and Frank in Apr 1844, a child in Jul 1847, his wife and child in Aug 1847, his wife in Nov 1847 and Mar 1848, his wife and child in Jun 1848 and him in Aug 1848 (Dr. Robert H. Archer's Ledger, p. 138, and his Ledger F, p. 127; Dr. Matthew J. Allen's Ledger, pp. 28, 60) [The following was written on a separate paper dated 24 Nov 1853 that was inserted in the back of Dr. Allen's ledger. The letter, addressed to Major Bond, was signed by I. Day and stated "I have just returned after 3 days ride to look up the Drs. of Dr. Allen and the following is the result." It mentioned several patients, including: "Robert Bowman *(sic)* has agreed to pay $5 per mo. from today."] [Robert Boarman was a War of 1812 veteran.]

Boarman, Sylvester [1746-1811] (reverend), was treated by Dr. John Archer in Aug 1790 and Feb 1791 (Ledger F, pp. 12, 158, misspelled as Bowman) [continued in Ledger H, which is missing]

Bobbet, ---- [blank], was treated by Dr. Robert H. Archer in Baltimore before 1822 [no dates or details were given] (Dr. Archer's "Alphabet to Ledger H" is his booklet [filed in the Archives of the Historical Society of Harford County] that contains his index to Ledger H [which is missing] for his patients in Baltimore before 1822 and Harford County after 1822, according to a notation by Dr. George W. Archer.)

Bodel, Edward (shoemaker), paid by Dr. Robert H. Archer in a non-medical matter in Mar 1827 and treated his wife in Jan and Feb 1828 (pp. 220, 260, 264)

Bodesman, William, see John Moorn, q.v.

Bodkin, Robert, was visited by Dr. John Archer who treated him in Oct 1781 and him and a daughter in Sep 1782 (Ledger D, p. 79, noted "debt forgiven as before") [Robert Bodkin was a Revolutionary War veteran.]

Bodkin, William, was visited by Dr. John Archer who treated him and a child in 1786 (Ledger F, p. 100)

Bolster, William, was treated by Dr. John Archer in 1786 (Ledger F, p. 96)

Bonar, Alex(?), see John Bonar, q.v.

Bonar, Barnet, was visited by Dr. John Archer who treated his daughter in May 1773, him at various times between June 1773 and March 1775, his daughter in Jan 1776 and his son in Dec 1776 (Ledger B, p. 5; Ledger C, pp. 8-9, noted "debt forgiven by order of testator")

Bonar, James, was visited by Dr. John Archer who treated him in Mar 1780, his wife in Sep 1782, and him and a child in 1789 (Ledger D, p. 52, spelled his name Boner and noted "debt forgiven as before" [account continued in Ledger E, which is missing]; Ledger F, p. 14, spelled his name Boner) [continued in Ledger G, which is missing]; see Agness Baker and Nicholas Baker, q.v.

Bonar, John (merchant), was visited by Dr. John Archer who treated him in April and June 1775, inoculated his son William in 1777 and treated him [John] in July 1779 and Mar 1780, him and his wife in Sep 1791 and him and son Alex(?) between 1794 and 1797 (Ledger B, p. 12; Ledger D, pp. 7, 54, spelled his name Boner and noted "debt forgiven as before;" Ledger F, p. 5, spelled his name Boner) [continued in Ledger I, which is missing, but was abstracted by Dr. George W. Archer circa 1890; his notes are in the Archives of the Historical Society of Harford County folder "Archer, G. W. Coll. – Ledgers and Day Books")

Bonar, Matthew, was visited by Dr. John Archer who treated Thomas Kearns in Nov 1773 and him [Matthew] in Oct 1774 and Jun 1775 (Ledger B, p. 10, noted "gone to western country," but gave no date of departure) [Matthew Bonar or Boner was a Revolutionary War veteran.]

Bonar, Robert (tavern keeper), was treated by Dr. John Archer in Dec 1772, June 1773 and Apr 1775 (Ledger B, p. 24)

Bonar, William, was visited by Dr. John Archer who treated him in May and Sep 1774 and his daughter in Sep and Oct 1774 (Ledger B, p. 6) [William Bonar or Boner was a Revolutionary War veteran.]

Bond, Ann, was visited by Dr. Alonzo Preston who treated a black girl named Harriet in Oct 1827, Phebe in Nov and Dec 1827, Rebecca Howard in Mar 1828, Mary Howard in Apr 1828, and her [Ann Bond] in Apr 1828 (p. 100)

Bond, Benjamin (black man), was visited by Dr. Alonzo Preston who treated him at times between 1825 and 1827, his wife in 1825, 1827 and 1827 and Phoebe in 1828 (p. 42, noting "A. W. Bradford witness to promise to pay." Benjamin paid $2 in cash on 14 Dec 1827, paid $5 circa 10 Oct 1828; payment initialed by "W. B. B." [meaning payment was received by Dr. William B. Bond] and Benjamin paid $3 on 5 Aug 1833)

Bond, Benjamin R., see Preston McComas, q.v.

Bond, Betsy, see James Bond, q.v.

Bond, Buckler, was visited by Dr. John Archer who treated his wife in Dec 1776, him in Mar, Aug, Sep and Oct 1780 and Jan, Feb and Jun 1781, his wife in Sep 1781, an infant in Nov 1781 and him in Mar 1782 and Aug 1793 (Ledger C, p. 72; Ledger D, p. 91) [account continued in Ledger E, which is missing]; Ledger F, p. 190, spelled his name Bucklar) [account continued in Ledger I, which is missing] [Buckler Bond was a Revolutionary War veteran.]

Bond, Caroline, see F. A. Bond, q.v.

Bond, Charles, see Thomas T. Bond, q.v.

Bond, Charlotte, see Dennis Bond, q.v.

Bond, Dennis 1760-c1815] (esquire), was visited by Dr. John Archer who treated his daughter Charlotte in 1788, him in 1795, inoculated his children Harriet, Jimmy and Fanny, and treated him and daughters Jane and Harriet at various times between 1795 and 1800 (Ledger F, pp. 5, 28) [account continued in Ledger I, which is missing, but was abstracted by Dr. George W. Archer circa 1890; his notes are in Archives of the Historical Society of Harford County folder "Archer, G. W. Coll. – Ledgers and Day Books")

Bond, E., Dr., see Henry Myers, q.v.

Bond, Elijah, see F. A. Bond, q.v.

Bond, F. A., was visited by Dr. Alonzo Preston who treated him at various times between 1823 and 1828, Jack and three black children in 1824, F. Howard's black children in 1825, F. A. Bond's family, Nancy, Mary, Caroline and Rebecca, in 1826, Master Stansbury, B. Bill and a black boy, Miss Nancy, Jim, Elijah and Caroline and a black girl in 1827, and Miss Caroline in 1828 (p. 46)

Bond, Fanny, see Dennis Bond, q.v.

Bond, Harriet, see Dennis Bond, q.v.

Bond, J., see John Morrice, q.v.

Bond, Jacob, Jr., was visited by Dr. John Archer who treated him in Jun and Sep 1779, Aug 1782 and Jul 1783 and a hired man in Oct 1783 (Ledger C, p. 105; Ledger D, 25, noted "debt forgiven as before")

Bond, Jacob, Sr. [1726-1780], was visited by Dr. John Archer who treated his daughter Sarah four times between 16 Aug 1772 and 6 Jul 1774, and probably him by June 1775, and him in Sep, Oct and Nov 1780 (Ledger B, p. 13; Ledger D, p. 91, noted the £23.10.9 bill was paid in cash by D. Bond on 23 Feb 1796) [Jacob Bond was a Revolutionary War veteran.]

Bond, James, see Mary Moores, q.v.

Bond, James, was visited by Dr. John Archer who treated his sister and a negro in Dec 1781, him in Jan 1782, Miss Betsy in Feb 1782, sister Betsy and a negro in Mar 1782, and sister Betsy in Apr and May 1782 (Ledger D, p. 113) [account continued in Ledger E, which is missing]

Bond, James (captain), at Capt. Sear's in B. Town [Bush Town], was visited by Dr. John Archer who treated him and his wife and daughter Rosan in 1788 (Ledger F, p. 359)

Bond, James (esquire), was treated by Dr. John Archer in July 1794 (Ledger F, p. 213, and continued in Ledger I); James Bond (storekeeper) was treated by Dr. Archer circa 1794-1798 [no dates were given] (Ledger I, which is missing, was abstracted by Dr. George W. Archer circa 1890; his notes are in the Archives of the Historical Society of Harford County folder "Archer, G. W. Coll. – Ledgers and Day Books")

Bond, James, son of William, was visited by Dr. John Archer who treated him and a child in 1788 (Ledger F, p. 333)

Bond, Jane, was treated by Dr. Alonzo Preston in Aug 1825 (p. 49, noted bill was paid in Jul 1827); see Dennis Bond, q.v.

Bond, Jim, see F. A. Bond, q.v.

Bond, Jimmy, see Dennis Bond, q.v.

Bond, John, see John Stevenson, q.v.

Bond, John, son of John, was treated by Dr. John Archer in May 1780 (Ledger D, p. 68) [account continued in Ledger H, which is missing]

Bond, John, son of Samuel, was treated by Dr. Robert H. Archer in Baltimore before 1822 [no dates or details were given] (Dr. Archer's "Alphabet to Ledger H" is his booklet [filed in the Archives of the Historical Society of Harford County] that contains his index to Ledger H [which is missing] for his patients in Baltimore before 1822 and Harford County after 1822, according to a notation by Dr. George W. Archer.)

Bond, John, of Samuel, was treated by Dr. John Archer in 1795 (Ledger I, which is missing, was abstracted by Dr. George W. Archer circa 1890; his notes are in the Archives of the Historical Society of Harford County file "Archer, G. W. Coll. – Ledgers and Day Books")

Bond, Josh. B., was treated by Dr. Alonzo Preston on 9 Nov and 10 Nov 1827 and he paid the bill in full on 3 Mar 1831 (p. 49)

Bond, Mary, see F. A. Bond, q.v.

Bond, Nancy, Miss, was treated by Dr. John Archer in Jun 1781, Dec 1782 and Feb 1783 (Ledger D, p. 35) [account continued in Ledger E, which is missing]; see F. A. Bond, q.v.

Bond, Nathan, see Thomas T. Bond, q.v.

Bond, Nathaniel, was treated by Dr. John Archer in Jun 1782 (Ledger D, p. 89, noted "By transfer to Ledger E, fol. 10, to Capt. Hall's acct.") [Ledger E is one of the missing ledgers.]

Bond, Phoebe, see Benjamin Bond, q.v.

Bond, Priscilla, Miss, was treated by Dr. John Archer in Apr 1781 (Ledger D, p. 26, noted "debt forgiven as before")

Bond, Prush A. (Negro), was mentioned in a letter from Dr. Richard N. Allen to James Moores, Esq., Bel Air, MD, dated 24 May 1834, in which the doctor informed Mr. Moores that "Prush A. Bond, col^d man, owes me $5, the amount of a year's attendance, by agreement, for which I rendered him the value of at least $30 in service. You will oblige by obtaining his assumption, and if possible, getting the amt. from him. He paid me $5 for services in a former year." (Document filed in Historical Society of Harford County Archives folder "R. N. Allen"); Prush A. Bond was later visited by Dr. Matthew J. Allen who treated his grandson in Aug and Sep 1847, his wife in May and Aug 1847 and him in Jun and Oct 1847 (p. 63) [The following statement was written on a separate page dated 24 Nov 1853 that was inserted in the back of Dr. Allen's ledger. The letter, addressed to Major Bond, was signed by I. Day and stated "I have just returned after 3 days ride to look up the Drs. of Dr. Allen and the following is the result." It mentioned several patients, including this one: "Negro Prush Bond says he does not owe one cent, that he has petitioned twice since the debt has been contracted."]

Bond, Ralph, was treated by Dr. John Archer in July 1788 (Ledger F, p. 28) [account continued in Ledger G, which is missing]

Bond, Rebecca, see F. A. Bond, q.v.

Bond, Richard, was treated by Dr. Robert H. Archer in Baltimore before 1822 [no dates or details were given] (Dr. Archer's "Alphabet to Ledger H" is his booklet [filed in the Archives of the Historical Society of Harford County] that contains his index to Ledger H [which is missing] for his patients in Baltimore City before 1822 and in Harford County after 1822, according to a notation by Dr. George W. Archer.)

Bond, Rosan, see James Bond, q.v.

Bond, Rose (Negro), at Magraw's, was treated by Dr. Matthew J. Allen in Jun 1848 (p. 86)

Bond, Samuel, was visited by Dr. John Archer who treated a child in Dec 1781 and Jan 1782 and him in Oct 1782 (Ledger D, p. 108, noted "debt forgiven as before")

Bond, Samuel, was treated by Dr. John Archer in July 1799 (Ledger F, p. 268) [account continued in Ledger K, which is missing]

Bond, Samuel, was treated by Dr. Robert H. Archer after 1822 [no dates or details were given] (Dr. Archer's "Alphabet to Ledger H" is his booklet [filed in the Archives of the Historical Society of Harford County] that contains his index to Ledger H [which is missing] for his patients in Baltimore City before 1822 and in Harford County after 1822, according to a notation by Dr. George W. Archer.)

Bond, Samuel, was treated at various times from 1821 to 1825 [no dates or details were given] by Dr. Alonzo Preston and also treated him in Jan 1826 (p. 61, indicated the bill was for $6.00 and the doctor noted in his ledger that Bond "says he has paid this acct.")

Bond, Samuel, see John Bond, q.v.

Bond, Sarah, see Jacob Bond, q.v.

Bond, Thomas, Sr., was treated by Dr. John Archer in May 1788 (Ledger F, p. 85) [continued in Ledger I, which is missing]

Bond, Thomas S., see Wm. W. Hall and Bennet Vansickle, q.v.

Bond, Thomas T. [1792-1875], was visited by Dr. Alonzo Preston who treated his children [no names given] in Feb 1827 and Nathan and Charles Bond in 1828 (p. 84) [His full name was Thomas Talbott Bond and he was a War of 1812 veteran.]

Bond, William, see James Bond, q.v.

Bond, William (esquire), was treated by Dr. John Archer in Apr 1787 (Ledger F, p. 263)

Bond, William, was treated by Dr. Robert H. Archer in Baltimore before 1822 [no dates or details were given] (Dr. Archer's "Alphabet to Ledger H" is his booklet [filed in the Archives of the Historical Society of Harford County] that contains his index to Ledger H [which is missing] for his patients in Baltimore before 1822 and in Harford County after 1822, according to a notation by Dr. George W. Archer.)

Bond, William, of Joshua, was visited by Dr. John Archer who treated his sisters in Feb and June 1773 in consultation with Dr. Haslet, his mother in July 1773, a negro in Feb 1775, and him in Oct 1781, Dec 1783 and Mar and Jul 1784 (Ledger B, p. 33; Ledger D, p. 85, noted the "debt forgiven as before")

Bond, William, of Samuel, was treated by Dr. John Archer in May 1793 (Ledger F, p. 338)

Bond, William B. (doctor), was treated by Dr. Alonzo Preston in 1823 and by Dr. Matthew J. Allen who rendered obstetrical services to his wife on the night of 9 Nov 1844 and treated her again in Mar 1845; treated him and a negro woman in Apr 1847 and him thirteen times between 18 May and 8 Jun 1848; Dr. Bond was listed as William B. Bond, Esq., in 1852 (Dr. Preston's Ledger, p. 3; Dr. Allen's Ledger, pp. 41, 70, and p. 82 noted that part of the bill was paid "my (sic) order to James Herron" and p. 96 noted Bond paid part of the bill on 25 May 1852); see Abraham Spicer, Thomas A. Hays, Howard Whitaker, Margaret Love, Samuel Brown, John Henderson, Abraham Jarrett, Parker Moores, Sophia Norris, Humphrey Wilson, Big Bill, Henry Dorsey, Bernard Mitchell, Benjamin Bond and Mrs. Stump, q.v.

Bond, Z. O., see John Forwood, of Jacob, q.v.

Boner, see Carvel Hall, Mr. Gilbert, Nicholas Baker and James Coale and also see Bonar, q.v.

Boots, Mr. ---- [first name blank, but possibly Samuel] (merchant), in Havre de Grace, was treated by Dr. John Archer in 1797 (Ledger I, which is missing, was abstracted by Dr. George W. Archer circa 1890; his notes are in the Archives of the Historical Society of Harford County folder "Archer, G. W. Coll. – Ledgers and Day Books")

Bosley, William, was treated by Dr. Robert H. Archer in Baltimore before 1822 [no dates or details were given] (Dr. Archer's "Alphabet to Ledger H" is his booklet [filed in the Archives of the Historical Society of Harford County] that contains his index to Ledger H [which is missing] for his patients in Baltimore before 1822 and Harford County after 1822, according to a notation by Dr. George W. Archer.)

Booth, Mr. ("P. Actor"), was visited by Dr. Alonzo Preston who treated him in Mar 1825, a black child in Nov 1826 and a child of "Mr. Booth, play actor" in Jan 1828 (p. 31, noting "1830, June 21st paid" and initialed by "Wm. B. B." (p. 260) [payment received by Dr. William B. Bond]

Bosley, William, was visited by Dr. John Archer who treated him in Sep 1781, his wife in Mar 1782, him and his daughter in Jul 1783 and him in Aug, Oct and Nov 1783 (Ledger D, p. 76, noted "debt forgiven as before")

Bottee, Peter, was treated by Dr. Robert H. Archer in Baltimore before 1822 [no dates or details were given] (Dr. Archer's "Alphabet to Ledger H" is his booklet [filed in the Archives of the Historical Society of Harford County] that contains his index to Ledger H [which is missing] for his patients in Baltimore before 1822 and Harford County after 1822, according to a notation by Dr. George W. Archer.)

Botts, Betsy, see Sarah Botts, q.v.

Botts, Eliza, see Sarah Botts, q.v.

Botts, George, was treated by Dr. John Archer in Nov 1772, Nov 1774, Mar and May 1781 and Jan 1784 (Ledger B, p. 19; Ledger D, p. 128, noted the bill was paid in full in cash on 19 Feb 1784) [George Botts was a Revolutionary War veteran.]

Botts, John [c1755-c1805], was treated by Dr. John Archer in 1790 (Ledger F, p. 284) [account continued in Ledger I, which is missing] [John Botts was a Revolutionary War veteran.]

Botts, Sarah, was visited by Dr. John Archer who treated her and daughters Betsy and Eliza in 1791 (Ledger F, pp. 224, 364) [continued in Ledger H, which is missing]; see Betsey Saunders, q.v.

Bouldin, Ann, Mrs., at Ring Factory [on Winters Run, west of Bel Air], was visited by Dr. Matthew J. Allen who treated her son in Nov 1847 and Jun 1848 and children [unnamed] in Sep 1848 and her [Ann} in Oct 1848 (pp. 68, 87)

Bouls, Thomas, was visited by Dr. John Archer who treated him and his wife and child in 1786 (Ledger F, p. 84)

Boushangue, John (shoemaker), was treated by Dr. John Archer in Feb 1775, in 1776 and Jan 1778 and mentioned his wife's account amount (6 sh.) that was transferred from another ledger; he was visited by Dr. John Archer who treated him in May and Jun 1782 and Jan 1788 and him and his wife in 1789 (Ledger B, p.

66; Ledger C, p. 1; Ledger D, p. 120, spelled his name Boshang [account continued in Ledger E, which is missing]; Ledger F, p. 138, spelled his name Bushang) [account continued in Ledger G, which is missing]

Bowen, Captain, was treated by Dr. Robert H. Archer in Baltimore before 1822 [no dates or details were given] (Dr. Archer's "Alphabet to Ledger H" is his booklet [filed in the Archives of the Historical Society of Harford County] that contains his index to Ledger H [which is missing] for his patients in Baltimore before 1822 and Harford County after 1822, according to a notation by Dr. George W. Archer.)

Bowen, Charlotte, was treated by Dr. Matthew J. Allen in Feb 1845 (p. 44)

Bowen, William, at Mudtown [now called Aldino], was visited by Dr. Robert H. Archer who treated his wife several times in Mar and Apr 1826, "in partu" [in childbirth] on 13 May 1826, and treated her again in June 1826, and a negro in Aug 1828; William was noted as "died a drunkard insolvent" [date of death not given] (pp. 176, 180, 181, 182, 186, 189, 291; Ledger F, p. 140)

Bower, Elisha, was treated by Dr. Robert H. Archer in Jun 1826 (p. 190)

Bowers, George, was prescribed medicine for his child by Dr. Robert H. Archer on 5 Aug 1802 (Rx Book, 1802-1804, p. 8)

Bowles, Thomas, was treated by Dr. John Archer in Nov 1781 and Apr and May 1782 (Ledger D, p. 104, spelled his name Bowls and noted a charge by Archer "to 5 bushels of wheat from Veech" and a partial payment "by 3 bushels of wheat received of you for ___ [blank] Veech") [account continued in Ledger E, which is missing]; see John Porter, q.v.

Bowman, see John Smith, of Jabish, q.v.

Bowman, Henry [1762-1836] (chair maker), was visited by Dr. John Archer who treated him in Sep 1795 and him and his family at various times between 1795 and 1798 (Ledger F, p. 252) [account continued in Ledger I, which is missing, but was abstracted by Dr. George W. Archer circa 1890; his notes are in the Archives of the Historical Society of Harford County file "Archer, G. W. Coll. – Ledgers and Day Books")

Bowsen, Benjamin (Negro), at Cumberland Forge, was visited by Dr. John Archer who treated him and his family circa 1794 [no dates were given] (Ledger I, which is missing, was abstracted by Dr. George W. Archer circa 1890; his notes are in the Archives of the Historical Society of Harford County folder "Archer, G. W. Coll. – Ledgers and Day Books") [Dr. George W. Archer added his own note in which he asked the question "Was Bowsen's Hill named for him?"]

Boy Frisby, see Lloyd Bailey, q.v.

Boyce, Benjamin, was treated by Dr. John Archer in Mar 1798 (Ledger F, p. 238)

Boyce, R., see Benedict Hall, q.v.

Boyce, William, was treated by Dr. John Archer in Jan 1781 (Ledger D, p. 117, noted "debt forgiven as before")

Boyd, Alexander, was visited by Dr. John Archer, Jr. who treated him in Oct 1815 and his wife in Apr 1817 (p. 30); see Thomas Huggins & Co., q.v.

Boyd, H., see John McCullough, q.v.

Boyd, James, see Thomas Huggins & Co., q.v.

Boyd, John, was treated by Dr. John Archer in Aug 1786 (Ledger F, p. 22)

Bradford, A. W., see Benjamin Bond, q.v.

Bradford, Charles, see Samuel Bradford, q.v.

Bradford, Dr., see William Slade, q.v.

Bradford, F. S., see Henry G. Watters, q.v.

Bradford, G., see Mrs. Crawford, q.v.

Bradford, James, north side of Deer Creek, was visited by Dr. John Archer who treated him and his family at various times in 1797 and 1798 (Ledger I, which is missing, was abstracted by Dr. George W. Archer circa 1890; his notes are in the Archives of the Historical Society of Harford County folder "Archer, G. W. Coll. – Ledgers and Day Books")

Bradford, Mr., see ---- Ross, q.v.

Bradford, S., see Henry G. Watters, q.v.

Bradford, Samuel [1774-1849], was visited by Dr. Alonzo Preston who treated him before 1826 [no details were given], his wife several times in 1826, and him and son Charles in 1827 (p. 64) [Samuel Bradford was a War of 1812 veteran.]; see William Bradford and Aquila Preston, q.v.

Bradford, William [1739-1794] (captain), was treated by Dr. John Archer in 1788 (Ledger F, p. 239, indicated his executor on 4 Feb 1802 was [son] Samuel Bradford) [William Bradford was a Revolutionary War veteran and a signer of the Bush Declaration on March 22, 1775.]

Bradford, William, Jr., was visited by Dr. John Archer who treated him and his wife in Nov 1781, him in Dec 1781 and Jan 1782, wife in Mar 1782, child in Aug 1782 and infant in Mar 1783 (Ledger D, p. 99, noted "debt forgiven as before") [continued in Ledger E, which is missing]

Bradford, William, was treated by Dr. Robert H. Archer in Baltimore before 1822 [no dates or details were given] (Dr. Archer's "Alphabet to Ledger H" is his booklet [filed in the Archives of the Historical Society of Harford County] that contains his index to Ledger H [which is missing] for his patients in Baltimore before 1822 and Harford County after 1822, according to a notation by Dr. George W. Archer.)

Bradley, Edward, was treated by Dr. John Archer in Oct 1790 (Ledger F, p. 195)

Bradley, Thomas M., at Ring Factory [on Winters Run, west of Bel Air], was treated by Dr. Matthew J. Allen in Aug 1848 (p. 91, listed him as Thos. M. Bradly)

Bramble, Thomas, was visited by Dr. Matthew J. Allen who treated his wife eight times in May and Jun 1848 (p. 83, noted that part of the bill was paid on 13 Nov 1852)

Brannon, Caleb, was treated by Dr. John Archer in Sep 1780 (Ledger D, p. 94, noted "debt forgiven as before")

Brannon, John, was visited by Dr. Robert H. Archer who treated his daughter Sally six times in May and June 1828 and she was also prescribed medicine on 6 Aug 1829 (pp. 276, 278, 279, 281, 283; Rx Book, 1825-1851, p. 95)

Brannon, Mr., son-in-law to Richard Coale, was visited by Dr. Robert H. Archer who treated his wife in Oct 1822 and a "child at Richard Coale's" in Mar 1824 (pp. 29, 99; Ledger F, p. 100, listed him as ----- [blank] Brannon, Jr.)

Brannon, Patrick, was visited by Dr. John Archer who treated him in Mar and May 1773 and Oct 1774, a child in Aug 1776 and him in Mar 1786 (Ledger B, p. 35, and Ledger C, p. 53, both spelled his name Brannen; Ledger F, p. 155, spelled his name Brannin)

Brannon, Sally, see John Brannon, q.v.

Brannon, William, was treated by Dr. John Archer in Oct 1796 (Ledger F, p. 210)

Brazier, Robert, was visited by Dr. John Archer who treated an infant in Feb 1775 (Ledger B, p. 66)

Breedenbaugh, John, was prescribed medicine for his wife by Dr. Robert H. Archer on 26 Aug 1803 and medicine for him on 17 Sep 1803 (Rx Book, 1802-1804, pp. 54, 56)

Brevard, Charles, was treated by Dr. John Archer in Aug 1782 and May 1788 (Ledger D, p. 96, spelled his name Bravard and noted "debt forgiven as before;" Ledger F, p. 74)

Brevard, James, was treated by Dr. John Archer in 1802 (Ledger F, p. 109) [account continued in Ledger L, which is missing]

Brian, Thomas (miller), was treated by Dr. John Archer between 1795 and 1801 (Ledger I, which is missing, was abstracted by Dr. George W. Archer circa 1890; his notes are in the Archives of the Historical Society of Harford County folder "Archer, G. W. Coll. – Ledgers and Day Books")

Briarly, Hugh, see Hugh Bryarly, q.v.

Brice, Thomas, was visited by Dr. John Archer who treated his maid in Aug and Sep 1774 (Ledger B, p. 43) [Thomas Brice was a signer of the Bush Declaration on 22 Mar 1775.]

Brice, Widow, was visited by Dr. John Archer who treated her in Dec 1775 and inoculated three of her family, and treated her in May 1779 (Ledger C, p. 16)

Brice, William, was visited by Dr. John Archer who treated him and wife in 1774 (Ledger B, p. 59)

Bridge, James, was visited by Dr. John Archer who treated an infant in Dec 1775 (Ledger B, p. 88)

Brison, Master, see Reuben H. Davis, q.v.

Bristor, Dr., see James McGaw, q.v.

Brook, James, see William Brook, q.v.

Brook, William, was visited by Dr. Robert H. Archer who treated him in Jul 1822, a daughter in Aug 1823, son James five times in Oct 1826, a negro seven times in Jul 1827 and a negro in Jul 1828 (pp. 202-204, 238-240, 286; Ledger F, p. 55) [William Brook was a War of 1812 veteran.]

Brooke, C., see William Stokes, q.v.

Brooks, Eleanor (Ellen), see William F. Bayless, q.v.

Brooks, Isaac, was prescribed medicine by Dr. Robert H. Archer on 13 Mar 1801 and medicine for his child on 13 Jul 1803 (Rx Book, 1796-1801, p. 46; Rx Book, 1802-1804, p. 50)

Brooks, Kitty, Miss, was treated by Dr. John Archer in Jan 1791 and Nov 1792 (Ledger F, p. 170, and p. 189 spelled her name Ketty) [account continued in Ledger H, which is missing]

Brooks, Mrs., widow of Richard, was treated by Dr. John Archer in 1796 (Ledger I, which is missing, was abstracted by Dr. George W. Archer circa 1890; his notes are in the Archives of the Historical Society of Harford County folder "Archer, G. W. Coll. – Ledgers and Day Books")

Brooks, Richard, was prescribed medicine by Dr. Robert H. Archer on 8 May 1796 (Rx Book, 1796-1801, p. 4); see Mrs. Brooks, q.v.

Brooks, Richard O., "from ye west," brother-in-law to Joseph Wheeler, was treated by Dr. John Archer in 1795 and 1796 (Ledger I, which is missing, was abstracted by Dr. George W. Archer circa 1890; his notes are in the Archives of the Historical Society of Harford County file "Archer, G. W. Coll. – Ledgers and Day Books")

Brooks, William, was visited by Dr. Robert H. Archer who treated an "African at Bailey's" in Jul 1822 and an unnamed negro in Jul 1828 (pp. 8, 286)

Brooks, William, was visited by Dr. Robert H. Archer who treated his wife many times in Jul and Aug 1823 (pp. 85-87)

Broughton, Dr., see James Magraw and George Gale, q.v.

Brown, see William Webb, q.v.

Brown, ---- [blank] (drayman), was treated by Dr. Robert H. Archer in Baltimore before 1822 [no dates or details were given] (Dr. Archer's "Alphabet to Ledger H" is his booklet [filed in the Archives of the Historical Society of Harford County] that contains his index to Ledger H [which is missing] for his patients in Baltimore before 1822 and Harford County after 1822, according to a notation by Dr. George W. Archer.)

Brown, Augustus, at B. Town [Bush Town], was treated by Dr. John Archer in Jun 1786 and May 1787 (Ledger F, pp. 273, 292)

Brown, Elisha, was mentioned by Dr. Robert H. Archer in a non-medical matter as "paid him in full in Port Deposit" [on the Susquehanna River in Cecil County] in May 1827 (p. 228)

Brown, Eliza, see Freeborn Brown, q.v.

Brown, Franklin, see Simon Brown, q.v.

Brown, Freeborn, was visited by Dr. John Archer who treated him in June 1775 and Sep and Oct 1780, a child in Feb 1781, him in Apr and Aug 1781, a child in May 1782, him in Sep 1781, inoculated 5 of his family in 1782, treated him, his wife and infant in Apr 1786 and him, his wife and daughter Eliza in Apr 1788 (Ledger B, p. 55; Ledger D, p. 97 [account continued in Ledger E, which is missing]; Ledger F, pp. 120, 138) [account continued in Ledger G, which is missing] [Freeborn Brown was a Revolutionary War veteran.]; see Catherine Smith, Mrs. Brown, Negro Dick, Garrett Brown and Abram Steel, q.v.

Brown, Freeborn, was visited by Dr. Robert H. Archer who treated him in July 1822, a negro girl in Nov 1822, other unnamed "Africanos" in Dec 1822 and Jan 1823, negroes Sam, Sal and Jacob in Jan 1823, an unnamed negro in May 1825, daughter Mary Brown in Sep 1825 and him in Oct 1825; Freeborn was prescribed medicine for a negro on 6 May 1825 and for himself on 18 Sep 1825; Mrs. Brown, widow, was treated in April 1827; Dr. Archer recorded on 8 Apr 1828 that "Freeborn Brown, decd., $62.69 by cash in full of that a/c recd. of Miss Mary Brown" (Ledger, pp. 8, 35, 36, 44-49, 131, 156, 163, 270; Rx Book, 1825-1851, pp. 77, 84; Ledger F, p. 53); see Mrs. Brown, q.v.

Brown, Garrett, was treated by Dr. John Archer in Nov 1781, Aug 1784 (visit and dressing) and April 1786 (Ledger D, p. 94, noted "charge to Freb: Brown;" Ledger F, p. 181)

Brown, George, son-in-law to Simon Denny, was visited by Dr. John Archer who treated his wife and child in 1789 and treated him in 1804 (Ledger F, p. 124)

Brown, J., see Martin Rigdon, q.v.

Brown, James, was treated by Dr. John Archer in April 1788 (Ledger F, p. 240)

Brown, John, at Bynum Run, was visited by Dr. John Archer who treated him in Aug 1778 and Feb 1779 and his children [no names were given] in Apr 1780 (Ledger C, p. 118, noted "debt forgiven by order of testator")

Brown, John, at Jos. Dallam's place, was treated by Dr. John Archer in Nov 1786 (Ledger F, p. 312)

Brown, John, was prescribed medicine by Dr. Robert H. Archer on 30 Jan 1801 (Rx Book, 1796-1801, p. 29)

Brown, John, was visited by Dr. Alonzo Preston who treated him in 1825 and his wife several times from April to June 1825; part of the bill was received and paid in cash "through the hands of N. S. Hays" on 18 Jun 1825 (p. 34)

Brown, John (Negro), was treated by Dr. John Archer, Jr. in Feb 1817 (p. 71; Ledger F, p. 71)

Brown, John (Negro), was treated by Dr. Robert H. Archer in Baltimore before 1822 [no dates or details were given] (Dr. Archer's "Alphabet to Ledger H" is his booklet [filed in the Archives of the Historical Society of

Harford County] that contains his index to Ledger H [which is missing] for his patients in Baltimore before 1822 and Harford County after 1822, according to a notation by Dr. George W. Archer.)

Brown, John (potter), was treated by Dr. Robert H. Archer in Baltimore before 1822 [no dates or details were given] (Dr. Archer's "Alphabet to Ledger H" is his booklet [filed in the Archives of the Historical Society of Harford County] that contains his index to Ledger H [which is missing] for his patients in Baltimore before 1822 and Harford County after 1822, according to a notation by Dr. George W. Archer.)

Brown, John (saddler), in Brown's Neck, was visited by Dr. John Archer who treated his family on 22 Jun 1775, a daughter and a negro wench on 28 Jun 1775 and a daughter and son in 1780 (Ledger B, p. 5, noted $12.00 paid "to boarding of son as per agreement" in 1780)

Brown, Joseph, was prescribed medicine by Dr. Robert H. Archer for his child circa Dec 1804 [exact date was not given] (Rx Book, 1802-1804, p. 67)

Brown, Joshua [1751-1819], on Gunpowder Neck, was visited by Dr. John Archer who treated an infant in Jan 1782 (Ledger D, p. 114, noted "debt forgiven as before")

Brown, Joshua, son of John, was treated by Dr. John Archer in Jan 1774 (Ledger B, p. 1)

Brown, Mahala (colored), was treated by Dr. Matthew J. Allen in Sep and Oct 1847 (p. 66)

Brown, Mary, Miss, was treated by Dr. Robert H. Archer in June and July 1826 and in Aug and Sep 1828 and was prescribed medicine for herself and a negro by Dr. Archer on 3 Jul 1829 and medicine for herself on 2 Aug 1834 (pp. 188, 192, 193, 294, 297; Rx Book, 1825-1851, pp. 95, 112); see Freeborn Brown and Samuel Brown, q.v.

Brown, Mortimer, was treated by Dr. Matthew J. Allen in May 1844 (p. 35, noted he paid part of the bill in Jul 1853 and part of it by cash in Sep 1853)

Brown, Mr., was prescribed medicine by Dr. Robert H. Archer circa Dec 1804 [exact date not given] (Rx Book, 1802-1804, p. 68)

Brown, Mrs. (widow), mother of Freeborn Brown, was treated by Dr. John Archer four times in June 1774 and he also treated a negro wench at that time (Ledger B, p. 55)

Brown, Mrs., widow of Freeborn, was visited by Dr. Robert H. Archer who treated her and Negro Poll and Negro Wash in 1826 (pp. 178, 186, 199, 200)

Brown, Mrs., widow of Samuel, was treated by Dr. John Archer in Feb and Mar 1780 (Ledger D, p. 46, noted "debt forgiven as before")

Brown, Parker, see Simon Brown, q.v.

Brown, Patty, at John Gibbs, was treated by Dr. John Archer in Jun 1782 (Ledger D, p. 82, noted "debt forgiven as before")

Brown, Peregrine, was treated by Dr. Matthew J. Allen in 1823 in Calvert County (p. 4a)

Brown, Samuel [1769-1835], was visited by Dr. Alonzo Preston who treated him, his wife and family and a black girl in 1826 and him [Samuel] in 1828; W. B. Bond noted the bill was paid on 6 Apr 1831; Samuel was prescribed medicine for his daughter Mary by Dr. Robert H. Archer on 20 May and 13 June 1832, for a negro on 10 Dec 1832, and for a child on 15 Oct 1833 and 16 Apr 1834 (Dr. Preston, p. 67; Dr. Archer's Rx Book, 1825-1851, pp. 105, 106, 108, 109, 110)

Brown, Simon [1777-1860s], appeared on a list of debts dated 26 Dec 1822 and titled "A List of Allen's Claims" that were due and payable to Dr. Richard N. Allen for services rendered [no dates were given] by him to said Simon (Document filed in Historical Society of Harford County Archives folder "R. N. Allen"); Simon Brown, son-in-law of Reuben Jones, was visited by Dr. Robert H. Archer who treated his son in Apr 1823, him and his daughter in June and July 1824, son Franklin in Apr and Sep 1826 and son Parker in Oct 1826 (pp. 62, 63, 110, 112, 199, 205; Ledger F, p. 155) [Simon Brown was a War of 1812 veteran.]

Brown, Thomas, at Mr. Phillips', was treated by Dr. John Archer in 1780 (Ledger D, p. 69, noted "debt forgiven as before")

Brown, Thomas, was prescribed medicine by Dr. Robert H. Archer on 21 Aug 1802 (Rx Book, 1802-1804, p. 15)

Brown, William (joiner), was treated by Dr. John Archer in Nov 1774 (Ledger B, p. 1)

Brown, William, at Binams Run [Bynum Run], was treated by Dr. John Archer in Jul 1781 and Apr 1783 (Ledger D, p. 7, noted "debt forgiven as before")

Brown, William, was visited by Dr. Robert H. Archer who treated his son William in Apr 1825, him at times from Dec 1825 to Sep 1826, Negro Nat twelve times in Aug 1828, him [William] in Sep 1828, Negro Essex in Sep and Oct 1828, a child in Oct 1828 and his wife in Nov 1828 (pp. 128, 171-173, 288-291, 295, 297-300; Ledger F, p. 108) [William Brown was a War of 1812 veteran.]

Brown, William, was visited by Dr. Matthew J. Allen who treated his wife in Feb 1845 (p. 44, noted part of bill paid in 1852 "by cash per Mortimer") [William Brown was a War of 1812 veteran.]

Browning, Milcah, see Mrs. Browning, q.v.

Browning, Mrs., widow of Thomas, near Bush [Bush Town or Harford Town], was visited by Dr. John Archer who treated her, daughter Milcah and son Thomas in June 1787 (Ledger F, p. 313)

Browning, Peregrine, "B. Town" [Bush Town or Harford Town], was visited by Dr. John Archer who treated him and his wife in 1787 (Ledger F, p. 305)

Browning, Thomas, was treated by Dr. John Archer in May and Sep 1780 and Jan and Aug 1781 (Ledger D, p. 67, noted "debt forgiven as before") [Thomas Browning was a Revolutionary War veteran.]; see Mrs. Browning, q.v.

Brownley, Arthur, was visited by Dr. John Archer who treated his wife in May 1782 (Ledger D, p. 111, noted "debt forgiven as before")

Brownley, Dr., see Timothy Cain and George Chauncey, q.v.

Brownley, Jacky, see Joseph Brownley, q.v.

Brownley, Joseph, was visited by Dr. John Archer who treated him and a "domestic" in Jan 1773, him [Joseph] in Feb 1774, Ned in Jul 1777, him [Joseph] in Sep 1777, child in Apr 1778, wife in June and July 1778, him in Nov 1778, May, Jul 1779 and Aug 1779, and Mar and Nov 1780, and his wife on 20 Apr 1781 "obstetricand" [in childbirth]; treated Thomas Richard in Aug 1781 and a negro in Oct 1781; inoculated daughter Nancy in Oct 1781; treated him [Joseph] in May 1782, daughter Nancy in Jun 1782, an infant in Aug 1782, him and Nelly [no relationship given] in Sep 1782, Thomas Richard in Oct 1782, daughter Sally in 1788, him [Joseph] in Oct 1789 and him and children Sally, Joseph, Jacky, Thomas, Nancy and Nelly at times between 1794 and 1798 [no dates were given] (Ledger B, p. 8, and Ledger C, p. 47, spelled his name Brownlee; Ledger D, p. 5 [continued in Ledger E, which is missing]; Ledger F, p. 291) [continued in Ledger G, which is missing]; Ledger I, which is missing, was abstracted by Dr. George W. Archer circa 1890; his notes are in the Archives of the Historical Society of Harford County folder "Archer, G. W. Coll. – Ledgers and Day Books")

Brownley, Nancy, see Joseph Brownley, q.v.

Brownley, Nelly, see Joseph Brownley, q.v.

Brownley, S., Miss, was prescribed medicine by Dr. Robert H. Archer on 5 May 1799 (Rx Book, 1796-1801, p. 14); Miss Sally Brownley was treated by Dr. Archer in Baltimore before 1822 [no dates or details were given] (Dr. Archer's "Alphabet to Ledger H" is his booklet [filed in the Archives of the Historical Society of Harford County] that contains his index to Ledger H [which is missing] for his patients in Baltimore City before 1822 and in Harford County after 1822, according to a notation by Dr. George W. Archer.)

Brownley, Sally, see Joseph Brownley and Miss S. Brownley, q.v.

Brownley, Thomas, see Joseph Brownley, q.v.

Bryarly, ---- [blank], of Hugh, son-in-law to Patrick Scott, was treated by Dr. John Archer in 1795 (Ledger I, which is missing, was abstracted by Dr. George W. Archer circa 1890 and spelled his name Bryerly; his notes are in the Archives of the Historical Society of Harford County folder "Archer, G. W. Coll. – Ledgers and Day Books")

Bryarly, ---- [blank], was treated by Dr. John Archer in Dec 1776 and Jan 1777 (Ledger C, p. 81, spelled his name Bryerly)

Bryarly, Carol, see Priscilla Bryarly, q.v.

Bryarly, Charles, see Priscilla Bryarly, q.v.

Bryarly, David, see Robert Bryarly, q.v.

Bryarly, Dr., see Hugh Dever, q.v.

Bryarly, Harriet, see Priscilla Bryarly, q.v.

Bryarly, Hugh, was visited by Dr. John Archer who treated him and his family between 1795 and 1801 and noted "Cr. by cash of Robert Bryarly, 1803" (Ledger I, which is missing, was abstracted by Dr. George W. Archer circa 1890 and spelled Hugh's name Briarly; Dr. George W. Archer's notes are in the Archives of the Historical Society of Harford County folder "Archer, G. W. Coll. – Ledgers and Day Books"); see ---- Bryarly, q.v.

Bryarly, James, see Robert Bryarly, q.v.

Bryarly, John (saddler), was treated by Dr. John Archer at various times between 1797 and 1800 (Ledger I, which is missing, was abstracted by Dr. George W. Archer circa 1890; his notes are in the Archives of the Historical Society of Harford County folder "Archer, G. W. Coll. – Ledgers and Day Books")

Bryarly, Priscilla, was visited by Dr. Alonzo Preston who treated her at times in 1824 and 1825 and her husband and Carol, Charles, Harriet and a black child in 1825 (pp. 11-13, noted medical bills amounting to $52.43 were paid on 4 May 1825 by W. D. Lee, administrator of P. Bryarly)

Bryarly, Robert, was visited by Dr. John Archer who treated him in Feb 1795 and inoculated his children Wakeman, David, Thomas, James and Sally (Ledger F, p. 80 spelled his name Bryerly, but spelled the children's names Bryarly) [account continued in Ledger G, which is missing]; see Hugh Bryarly, Negro Cass, Negro Dinah and Negro Hagar, q.v.

Bryarly, Sally, see Robert Bryarly, q.v.

Bryarly, Thomas, see Robert Bryarly, q.v.

Bryarly, Wakeman, see Robert Bryarly, q.v.

Bryden, James, "(Baltimore) [innkeeper] (A.C.)" *(sic)*, was visited by Dr. John Archer who treated his son James in 1798 (Ledger I, which is missing, was abstracted by Dr. George W. Archer circa 1890; his notes are in the Archives of the Historical Society of Harford County folder "Archer, G. W. Coll. – Ledgers and Day Books")

Buchanan, Walter, was treated by Dr. John Archer in Sep 1786 (Ledger F, p. 53)

Buck, John, was prescribed medicine for a boy by Dr. Robert H. Archer on 16 Aug 1802 (Rx Book, 1802-1804, p. 13); John Buck was treated by Dr. Archer in Baltimore before 1822 [no dates or details were given] (Dr. Archer's "Alphabet to Ledger H" is his booklet [filed in the Archives of the Historical Society of Harford County] that contains his index to Ledger H [which is missing] for his patients in Baltimore City before 1822 and in Harford County after 1822, according to a notation by Dr. George W. Archer.)

Buck, William, was prescribed medicine for his wife by Dr. Robert H. Archer on 14 Jun 1803 (Rx Book, 1802-1804, p. 44) William Buck was treated by Dr. Archer in Baltimore before 1822 [no dates or details were given] (Dr. Archer's "Alphabet to Ledger H" is his booklet [filed in the Archives of the Historical Society of Harford County] that contains his index to Ledger H [which is missing] for his patients in Baltimore City before 1822 and in Harford County after 1822, according to a notation by Dr. George W. Archer.)

Buckingham, see James Patten, q.v.

Buckingham, Bazil, son-in-law of William Edy [name also spelled Ady in other county records], was treated by Dr. John Archer in 1797 (Ledger I, which is missing, was abstracted by Dr. George W. Archer circa 1890; his notes are in the Archives of the Historical Society of Harford County folder "Archer, G. W. Coll. – Ledgers and Day Books")

Buckingham, Viney, Miss, was treated by Dr. John Archer in Apr 1788 (Ledger F, p. 196, and p. 240 noted that her account had been transferred to James Moores, tailor's account)

Buckley, Daniel, was murdered in 1787: "Harford County to wit: The Jurors of the State of Maryland for the body of Harford County aforesaid upon their oath present that Stephen Jones, late of the County aforesaid, yeoman, not having the fear of God before his eyes but being moved and seduced by the instigation of the Devil on the twenty third day of April in the year of our Lord Seventeen hundred and Eighty Seven with force and arms at Harford County aforesaid in and upon one Daniel Buckley in the peace of God and our said State then and there being feloniously, wilfully *(sic)* and of his malice aforethought did make an assault and that he the said Stephen Jones with his fists and with his feet by kicking and striking in and upon the head, back, sides, brest *(sic)* and belly of him the said Daniel Buckley then and there feloniously, wilfully *(sic)* and of his malice aforethought did strike, thrust and kick, giving to the aforesaid Daniel Buckley then and there with his fists and feet aforesaid in and upon the head, neck, sides, breast and belly of him the said Daniel Buckley divers mortal wounds and bruises each wound and bruise being of the length of four inches and of the breadth of three inches which said mortal wounds and bruises the said Daniel Buckley instantly died and so the Jurors aforesaid upon their oath foresaid do say that the said Stephen Jones the said Daniel Buckley in a manner and form aforesaid feloniously, wilfully *(sic)* and of his malice aforethought did kill and murder against the peace, government and dignity of the State of Maryland." (File 11.05.1 in the Court Records Department of the Historical Society of Harford County)

Buckley, Philip, was treated by Dr. John Archer in Sep 1788 (Ledger F, p. 238)

Buckmaster, James, was treated by Dr. Matthew J. Allen in 1832 in Calvert Co. and also mentioned James A. D. Dalrumple (p. 22)

Buckulow, Mrs., was visited by Dr. John Archer who treated a child in Aug 1780 (Ledger D, p. 90) [account continued in Ledger E, which is missing]

Bull, Abram, see William Bull, q.v.

Bull, Bennett, see Jacob Bull, Sr., q.v.

Bull, Edmund, was treated by Dr. Robert H. Archer after 1822 [no dates or details were given] (Dr. Archer's "Alphabet to Ledger H" is his booklet [filed in the Archives of the Historical Society of Harford County] that contains his index to Ledger H [which is missing] for his patients in Baltimore before 1822 and Harford County after 1822, according to a notation by Dr. George W. Archer.); see William Bull, Jacob Bull and John Bull, q.v.

Bull, Edward, was treated by Dr. John Archer in Sep 1774 (Ledger B, p. 45); see Jacob Bull and John Bull, q.v.

Bull, Edward [1753-1808], of Jacob, was treated by Dr. John Archer in May 1786 (Ledger F, p. 292) [Edward Bull, of Jacob, was a Revolutionary War veteran.]

Bull, Frances (widow), was visited by Dr. John Archer who treated her and a child in 1786 and her in 1789 (Ledger F, p. 7, and p. 193 indicated Henry Waters, Jr. was her executor in June 1795); see John Bull, q.v.

Bull, Hannah, Miss, "of John," was treated by Dr. John Archer from 1794 to 1797 (Ledger I, which is missing, was abstracted by Dr. George W. Archer circa 1890; his notes are in the Archives of the Historical Society of Harford County folder "Archer, G. W. Coll. – Ledgers and Day Books")

Bull, Henry, see William Bull, q.v.

Bull, J., see ---- Wix, q.v.

Bull, Jacob, see Edward Bull and William Bull, q.v.

Bull, Jacob [1757-1803], son of Edmund and brother to John, was visited by Dr. John Archer who treated his wife in Dec 1781 and him in Oct 1802 (Ledger D, p. 116, noted that he paid the bill in full in cash in Dec 1784) (Ledger F, p. 237) [account continued in Ledger L, which is missing]

Bull, Jacob, Sr., was visited by Dr. John Archer who treated a child in May 1779 and inoculated Bennett and James in 1782 (Ledger C, p. 72)

Bull, James, see William Bull and Jacob Bull, Sr., q.v.

Bull, John, see Samuel Bull, q.v.

Bull, John, at Scott's Old Fields [now Bel Air], was visited by Dr. John Archer who treated him, his wife and a child in 1789 (Ledger F, p. 380) [account continued in Ledger H, which is missing]; see William Bull and Hannah Bull, q.v.

Bull, John, was visited by Dr. John Archer who treated his wife in Sep 1774 and Sep and Oct 1779, Samuel Ruff in Feb 1780, a child in Mar 1780 and him 14 times between Feb and Aug 1782 (Ledger B, p. 62; Ledger D, p. 12, noted Frances Bull, executrix, paid part of the bill on 4 Dec 1783 and Henry Waters, Jr., exec. of Mrs. Frances Bull, dec'd., paid the balance in June 1795)

Bull, John, of Edmund, was treated by Dr. John Archer at various times between 1796 and 1798 (Ledger I, which is missing, was abstracted by Dr. George W. Archer circa 1890; his notes are in the Archives of the Historical Society of Harford County folder "Archer, G. W. Coll. – Ledgers and Day Books"); see Jacob Bull, q.v.

Bull, John, of Edward, was visited by Dr. John Archer who treated him and inoculated his daughter in Nov 1781 (Ledger D, p. 96, noted "debt forgiven as before")

Bull, John (fan maker), son of John, was treated by Dr. John Archer at various times between 1794 and 1806 and noted in his ledger "Cr. by a fan, $30" (Ledger I, which is missing, was abstracted by Dr. George W. Archer circa 1890; his notes are in the Archives of the Historical Society of Harford County file "Archer, G. W. Coll. – Ledgers and Day Books")

Bull, John (innkeeper), was visited by Dr. John Archer who treated him and his daughter Nancy at various times between 1797 and 1799 (Ledger I, which is missing, was abstracted by Dr. George W. Archer circa 1890; his notes are in the Archives of the Historical Society of Harford County folder "Archer, G. W. Coll. – Ledgers and Day Books")

Bull, Nancy, see John Bull and William Bull, q.v.

Bull, Phebe, see William Bull, q.v.

Bull, Rachel, was treated by Dr. John Archer (tooth extraction) on 25 Dec 1781 (Ledger D, p. 108, noted "debt forgiven as before") [account continued in Ledger E, which is missing]

Bull, Richard, was treated by Dr. John Archer in May, Jun and Aug 1780, Nov 1783 and Nov 1789 (Ledger D, p. 69, noted "debt forgiven as before;" Ledger F, p. 193, indicated that his executor in 1795 was Henry Waters, Jr.)

Bull, Richard (blacksmith), in Abingdon, was visited by Dr. John Archer who treated him and infant in 1787 (Ledger F, p. 36)

Bull, Sally, was visited by Dr. Alonzo Preston who treated her child in May 1826 (p. 75)

Bull, Samuel, of John, was treated by Dr. John Archer between 1795 and 1799 (Ledger I, which is missing, was abstracted by Dr. George W. Archer circa 1890; his notes are in Archives of the Historical Society of Harford County file "Archer, G. W. Coll. - Ledgers and Day Books")

Bull, Susannah, was visited by Dr. John Archer who treated her in May 1779, a negro in May 1780, her in Oct 1780 and Mar 1781, a daughter in May 1781, her [Susannah] in Dec 1781, inoculated 9 of her family in Dec 1782, and treated a negro in Apr 1783 (Ledger C, p. 127) [account continued in Ledger E, which is missing]

Bull, Walter, son of William, was visited by Dr. John Archer who treated him, his wife and child in 1794 (Ledger F, p. 164) [account continued in Ledger I, which is missing, but was abstracted by Dr. George W. Archer circa 1890 who noted Walter was treated from 1794 to 1802 by Dr. John Archer; Dr. George W. Archer's notes are in the Archives of the Historical Society of Harford County folder "Archer, G. W. Coll. - Ledgers and Day Books"]

Bull, Widow, see George Rawlins, q.v.

Bull, William, see Walter Bull, q.v.

Bull, William, near Smith's Mill, was visited by Dr. John Archer who treated him and son Edmund in Mar 1787 and Apr 1790 and Mrs. Bull in July 1802 (Ledger F, pp. 21, 67)

Bull, William, was visited by Dr. James Archer who treated him and his sister Nancy several times in Oct 1806 and treated a negro child in Nov 1806 (pp. 3, 4)

Bull, William, was visited by Dr. Alonzo Preston who treated him in 1823, a black child in 1824, his wife and sons Henry and James in 1826, sons James, John and Jacob in 1827, son William in Nov 1827 (amputated a finger and visited him 7 times), and daughter Phebe in 1828; William was also treated by Dr. Robert H. Archer in Oct 1828 (Dr. Preston, pp. 1, 92; Dr. Archer, p. 299)

Bull, William, was prescribed medicine by Dr. Robert H. Archer on 2 Jun 1842 (Rx Book, 1825-1851, p. 118)

Bull, William, of Abram, was treated by Dr. John Archer in Sep 1785 and Dec 1792 (Ledger D, p. 97, noted "debt forgiven as before;" Ledger F, p. 21)

Bull, William, of Jacob, was treated by Dr. John Archer in Jun 1788 (Ledger F, p. 216)

Bull, William, of John, was treated by Dr. Robert H. Archer after 1822 [no dates or details were given] (Dr. Archer's "Alphabet to Ledger H" is his booklet [filed in the Archives of the Historical Society of Harford County] that contains his index to Ledger H [which is missing] for his patients in Baltimore City before 1822 and in Harford County after 1822, according to a notation by Dr. George W. Archer.)

Bunting, Billy Drew (widow), was treated by Dr. John Archer in Jul 1789 (Ledger F, p. 167)

Burgess, Joseph, was treated by Dr. John Archer in Apr, Jul, Aug and Sep 1774 (Ledger B, p. 43)

Burk, James, see William G. Burk, q.v.

Burk, Peter, was treated by Dr. John Archer in Aug 1781 (Ledger D, p. 37, noted the bill was settled)

Burk, William, see William G. Burk, q.v.

Burk, William G., was visited by Dr. Matthew J. Allen who treated his wife and a child [daughter?] in Dec 1847, son in Jan 1848, James [son?] in Oct 1848 and son William in Jun 1848 (p. 71 spelled his name Burke, and p. 86 spelled it Burk); see James Lytle and John McCullough, q.v.

Burkins, Charles, see John Forwood, q.v.

Burkins, Edward, see Isaac Burkins, q.v.

Burkins, Isaac [c1777-1834], was visited by Dr. Alonzo Preston who treated his son Edward twice in Feb 1825 (p. 27, misspelled his name Berkins) [Isaac Burkins was a War of 1812 veteran.]

Burkins, Jacob, was visited by Dr. John Archer, Jr. who treated him, his wife and child in Sep 1817 and his wife in Sep 1819 (p. 75, spelled his name Berkins)

Burkins, Mr., at John Forwood's, was treated by Dr. John Archer in Sep 1781 (Ledger D, p. 71, misspelled his name as Berkin and noted "debt forgiven as before")

Burling, Richard, "Bal. Town" [Baltimore], "for son at Mrs. Giles," was treated by Dr. John Archer in Jul 1787 (Ledger F, p. 340)

Bunting, William, was visited by Dr. John Archer who treated a negro in Dec 1781, Mrs. Bunting in Sep 1782, him and his son in Dec 1782 and him in Aug 1783 and Apr 1784 (Ledger D, p. 103, noted "debt forgiven as before")

Burnett, Isaiah, was visited by Dr. Alonzo Preston who treated a child on 22 Aug and 31 Aug 1826 (p. 82, noting the bill was $5.15 and "19ᵗʰ Jul 1831 paid $5.18¾" including interest)

Burney, Mrs. (widow), was treated by Dr. John Archer in Sep and Oct 1779 and Jan and Mar 1784 (Ledger D, p. 16, noted "debt forgiven as before")

Burnside, Sh.(?), in Havre de Grace, was treated by Dr. John Archer, Jr. in Apr 1815 and mentioned Burnside & Hogg in Oct 1815 (pp. 5, 16)

Burrill, Thomas & Co., was mentioned in Dr. Robert H. Archer's ledger in Sep 1815 (p. 8)

Burrough, John, see Callendar Patterson, q.v.

Burrows, Betsey, see John Burrows, q.v.

Burrows, Capt., in Wilson & Stump's employ, was treated by Dr. John Archer in July 1788 (Ledger F, p. 59)

Burrows, John, was visited by Dr. John Archer, Jr. who treated him in Mar 1817, a child in Aug 1820 and his wife in Sep 1820; John Burrows (blacksmith) was visited by Dr. Robert H. Archer who treated him, son John and daughter Betsey in Mar 1823 (Dr. John Archer, Jr., p. 76; Dr. Robert H. Archer, Ledger F, p. 37)

Burrows, Mrs., was listed in Dr. John Archer, Jr.'s ledger and her account "since her husband's death" mentioned son William in July 1816 and daughter Polly in Mar 1817 (p. 58)

Burrows, Polly, see Mrs. Burrows, q.v.

Burrows, William, see Mrs. Burrows, q.v.

Burton, William, was visited by Dr. Matthew J. Allen who treated and rendered obstetrical services to his wife on 1 Apr 1848 (p. 78)

Bussey, Benedict, see Edward Bussey, q.v.

Bussey, Bennett [1745-1827] (esquire), was visited by Dr. John Archer who treated him and his son Clement in 1797 (Ledger F, p. 291, listed them as Bennet Bussy and Clemmont Bussy) [account continued in Ledger I, which is missing] [Bennett Bussey was a Revolutionary War veteran.]; see Negro Gamboe, q.v.

Bussey, Betsy, Miss, was treated by Dr. Matthew J. Allen in Jul 1848 (p. 90)

Bussey, Edward, was treated by Dr. John Archer in Apr 1787 (Ledger F, p. 265) [Edward Bussey was a Revolutionary War veteran.]

Bussey, Edward, was treated by Dr. Robert H. Archer in Baltimore before 1822 [no dates or details were given] (Dr. Archer's "Alphabet to Ledger H" is his booklet [filed in the Archives of the Historical Society of Harford County] that contains his index to Ledger H [which is missing] for his patients in Baltimore before 1822 and Harford County after 1822, according to a notation by Dr. George W. Archer.); Edward Bussey was visited by Dr. Alonzo Preston in Harford County and he treated his son Benedict on 15 Sep 1825 and 18 Aug 1827 (p. 56)

Bussey, Edward, was visited by Dr. Matthew J. Allen who treated his son in Jan 1844 and him [Edward] in Jan and Feb 1844 (p. 30)

Bussey, Elizabeth, appeared on a list of debts dated 26 Dec 1822 and titled "A List of Allen's Claims" that were due and payable to Dr. Richard N. Allen for services rendered [no dates were given] by him to said Bussey (Document filed in Historical Society of Harford County Archives folder "R. N. Allen"); Elizabeth was also visited by Dr. Alonzo Preston who treated a negro man named Samuel in Dec 1825 (p. 61)

Bussey, Harriet, see Julia Bussey, q.v.

Bussey, Jesse (esquire), was treated by Dr. John Archer in Sep 1791 (Ledger F, p. 370, indicated the bill was paid by Bennett Jarrett in 1809) [Jesse Bussey was a Revolutionary War veteran.]

Bussey, Julia, Mrs., was visited by Dr. Matthew J. Allen who treated her son in Jan 1844, daughter Mary twenty-eight times between 5 Jul and 21 Aug 1847 and daughter Harriet once in Mar 1848 (p. 30, listed her as Mrs. Edward Bussey, but then Edward was lined out, and the account was continued to pp. 58 and 62 which listed her as Mrs. Julia Bussey)

Bussey, Julian, Miss, was treated by Dr. Robert H. Archer after 1822 [no dates or details were given] (Dr. Archer's "Alphabet to Ledger H" is his booklet [filed in the Archives of the Historical Society of Harford County] that contains his index to Ledger H [which is missing] for his patients in Baltimore City before 1822 and in Harford County after 1822, according to a notation by Dr. George W. Archer.)

Bussey, Mary, see Julia Bussey, q.v.

Bussey, Robert, was treated by Dr. Matthew J. Allen "for fistula in ano" in Sep 1847 (p. 67)

Bussey, Ruth (widow), near C. Town [Cooptown], was treated by Dr. John Archer in Oct 1793 (Ledger F, p. 331) [account continued in Ledger I, which is missing]

Butler, Lewis, was visited by Dr. Robert H. Archer who treated a child in Mar 1826, his wife twice in Jun 1828 and him [Lewis] in Jul 1828 (pp. 276, 282, 283, 285)

Butler, Mr., was treated by Dr. John Archer in Aug 1781 (Ledger D, p. 55, noted the "debt forgiven as before")

Butler, Mr., was visited by Dr. Robert H. Archer who treated a child in Mar 1828 (p. 266)

Butler, Thomas, on Belle Farm, "son-in-law to McAtee," was treated by Dr. John Archer in 1795 (Ledger I, which is missing, was abstracted by Dr. George W. Archer circa 1890; his notes are in the Archives of the Historical Society of Harford County file "Archer, G. W. Coll. – Ledgers and Day Books")

Butler, Thomas, appeared on a list of debts dated 26 Dec 1822 and titled "A List of Allen's Claims" that were due and payable to Dr. Richard N. Allen for services rendered [no dates were given] by him to said Butler (Document filed in Historical Society of Harford County Archives folder "R. N. Allen"); Thomas was treated by Dr. Robert H. Archer in Oct 1823 in consultation with Dr. Street (p. 86; Ledger F, p. 58)

Byard, Ephram, see Ephraim Bayard, q.v.

Byard, James, see James Bayard, q.v.

Byford, Moses, was treated by Dr. John Archer in Sep 1779 and Apr and May 1780 (Ledger D, p. 20, noted "debt forgiven as before")

Cagle, John &ca (sic), was treated by Dr. Robert H. Archer in Baltimore before 1822 [no dates or details were given] (Dr. Archer's "Alphabet to Ledger H" is his booklet [filed in the Archives of the Historical Society of Harford County] that contains his index to Ledger H [which is missing] for his patients in Baltimore before 1822 and Harford County after 1822, according to a notation by Dr. George W. Archer.)

Cain, Aquila, was treated by Dr. John Archer in 1786 (Ledger F, p. 367); see Benjamin Bayless, q.v.

Cain, Betsy, see James Cain, q.v.

Cain, Dennis, was visited by Dr. John Archer who treated him, his wife and an infant in 1788 (Ledger F, p. 329, spelled his name Caine and noted account was paid by Philip Quinlan on 18 Oct 1793)

Cain, Dennis, Mrs. (widow), was visited by Dr. John Archer who treated her in Jul 1780 and son Timothy in Jul 1781 (Ledger C, p. 57; Ledger D, p. 79, noted "debt forgiven as before")

Cain, Edward [1753-1832], was treated by Dr. Robert H. Archer in May 1827 and was visited by Dr. Alonzo Preston who treated a child in May 1828; he was prescribed medicine by Dr. Archer on 28 Mar 1832 (Dr. Archer, p. 223, wrote "(Revolutionary)" after his name; Dr. Alonzo Preston's ledger, p. 102, marked the account as "Denied;" Dr. Robert H. Archer's Rx Book, 1825-1851, p. 105) [Edward Cain, sometimes spelled Kain, was a Revolutionary War veteran.]

Cain, Elizabeth, was visited by Dr. Alonzo Preston who treated him and a black girl in 1825 (p. 47); see Matthew Cain, q.v.

Cain, James, was visited by Dr. John Archer who treated him in Jan 1777, his wife in Jan 1778, him in Jul 1778 and Jul 1779, an infant in Sep 1779, him and a child in Jul 1780, him in Nov and Dec 1780 and May 1782, him and a child in Aug 1783, him, his wife and son William in 1786, him and an infant in Nov 1789 and him and children Matthew, Betsey and Molly between 1795 and 1797 (Ledger C, p. 70, spelled his name Caine; Ledger D, p. 75, noted that part of the bill was paid by Edward Flanagan on 29 Nov 1783 [account continued in Ledger E, which is missing]; Ledger F, p. 105) [account continued in Ledger G, which is missing] (Ledger I, which is missing, was abstracted by Dr. George W. Archer circa 1890 [who stated James died 18 Apr 1797] and noted the debt was "forgiven" by the doctor; Dr. George W. Archer's notes are in the Archives of the Historical Society of Harford County folder "Archer, G. W. Coll. – Ledgers and Day Books") [James Cain was a Revolutionary War veteran.]

Cain, Jane, Mrs., widow of John, was treated by Dr. Robert H. Archer in Mar 1824 and Oct 1825 in consultation with Dr. Bristor and Dr. Preston; mentioned "hiring her girl Maria" in Aug 1824 and "hiring her woman Minta" in Sep 1825; Jane was treated by Dr. Alonzo Preston from 5 Oct 1825 to 7 Dec 1825 and also treated several times by Dr. Robert Archer on 16 Oct 1825); Jane was visited many times by Dr. Preston, ran up $36.10 in medical bills and he noted in his ledger that she "refuses to pay." (Dr. Preston, p. 58; Dr. Archer, pp. 99, 163-166, and Ledger F, p. 127)

Cain, John, was treated by Dr. Robert H. Archer in Baltimore before 1822 [no dates or details were given] (Dr. Archer's "Alphabet to Ledger H" is his booklet [filed in the Archives of the Historical Society of Harford County] that contains his index to Ledger H [which is missing] for his patients in Baltimore before 1822 and Harford County after 1822, according to a notation by Dr. George W. Archer.)

Cain, John (deceased), appeared on a list of debts dated 26 Dec 1822 and titled "A List of Allen's Claims" that were due and payable to Dr. Richard N. Allen for services rendered [no dates given] by him (Document filed in Historical Society of Harford County Archives folder "R. N. Allen")

Cain, John, see John Caine, q.v.

Cain, M., see George Lochary, q.v.

Cain, Matthew [1781-1859], was visited by Dr. Robert H. Archer who treated Negro Dan in Nov 1822 and visited by Dr. Alonzo Preston who treated daughter Elizabeth in Sep 1826 (Dr. Archer, p. 25, Ledger F, p. 117; Dr. Preston, p. 84, noted the medical bill was $2.00 and then marked the account as "Denied") [Matthew Cain was a War of 1812 veteran.]; see James Cain, q.v.

Cain, Molly, see James Cain, q.v.

Cain, Rebecca, see Timothy Cain, q.v.

Cain, Timothy, was visited by Dr. John Archer who treated him in Jun 1776, daughter Rebecca in Jul 1776, him in Oct 1778 and him and his wife in Jun 1786 (Ledger C, p. 57, noted "debt forgiven by order of testator;" Ledger F, p. 6, indicated he was "dead and poor," but gave no death date)

Cain, Timothy, at Hall's X Roads, was treated by Dr. Robert H. Archer in Sep 1822 in consultation with Dr. Brownley (p. 18, and Ledger F, p. 78); see Mrs. Cain, q.v.

Cain, William, see James Cain, q.v.

Caine, John, near Hickory, was treated by Dr. John Archer circa 1796-1798 [no dates or details were given] (Ledger I, which is missing, was abstracted by Dr. George W. Archer circa 1890; his notes are in the Archives of the Historical Society of Harford County folder "Archer, G. W. Coll. – Ledgers and Day Books"); see John Cain and John Jackson, q.v.

Calaghan, John, was prescribed medicine for his wife by Dr. Robert H. Archer on 22 Sep 1802 (Rx Book, 1802-1804, p. 5)

Caldwell, John, was visited by Dr. John Archer who treated him in Jul 1779 and inoculated him and 5 of his family in 1782 (Ledger D, p. 2, noted he paid £3.16.7 in cash on 4 Jan 1783, but also noted "debt forgiven as before")

Caldwell, John [1779-1865], was treated by Dr. Alonzo Preston in Aug 1825 and his medical bill was paid "by tayloring" on 5 Dec 1825 (p. 52) [John Caldwell was a War of 1812 veteran.]

Caldwell, Mary Ann, see Mary Hassan, q.v.

Caldwell, Mr. (cabinet maker), was visited by Dr. Robert H. Archer who treated a child in July 1824 and his wife and child in Aug 1829 (p. 112; Ledger F, p. 100)

Caldwell, Thomas, was treated by Dr. John Archer in Jan 1788 (Ledger F, p. 312)

Caldwell, Thomas, in Baltimore, was visited by Dr. John Archer who treated his family in 1796 and 1797 (Ledger I, which is missing, was abstracted by Dr. George W. Archer circa 1890; his notes are in Archives of the Historical Society of Harford County folder "Archer, G. W. Coll. – Ledgers and Day Books"); see Thomas Calwell, q.v.

Caldwell, William, in Bel Air, was treated by Dr. John Archer in 1796 and 1797 (Ledger I, which is missing, was abstracted by Dr. George W. Archer circa 1890; his notes are in the Archives of the Historical Society of Harford County folder "Archer, G. W. Coll. – Ledgers and Day Books")

Callahan, Edmund (schoolmaster), was treated in Jan 1777 by Dr. John Archer (Ledger C, p. 24)

Callendar, William, was treated by Dr. John Archer, Jr. in Nov 1815 and the ledger also mentioned "wood delivered to school Chesapeake Academy" in Jan 1822 (p. 35)

Callender, Robert, was treated by Dr. John Archer in Oct 1775 (Ledger B, p. 13)

Calwell, A., see Luther A. Norris, q.v.

Calwell, Mary Ann, Miss, was treated by Dr. Robert H. Archer in Aug and Nov 1824 and was prescribed medicine on 28 May 1825 and 22 Dec 1825; she was treated in June 1825 and Oct 1825 and in Nov 1827 and paid her $6 bill in full on 6 Mar 1828; she was treated again on 4 Apr 1828 and prescribed medicine on 8 Sep 1828 (pp. 134, 165, 254, 266, 270, 294; Rx Book, 1825-1851, pp 79, 92, but p. 85 and Ledger F, p. 61, both misspelled her name Caldwell while Ledger F, p. 38 listed her as Miss Maryann Calwell); see Mary Hassan, q.v.

Calwell, Mr., was prescribed medicine by Dr. Robert H. Archer on 28 Jan 1803 (Rx Book, 1802-1804, p. 30)

Calwell, Mr., was prescribed medicine for his child by Dr. Robert H. Archer on 10 Aug 1829 (Rx Book, 1825-1851, p. 95)

Calwell, Samuel [c1739-1800], "for James Tagart," was visited by Dr. John Archer who treated Samuel Caldwell *(sic)* and James Tagart in May 1774, Jacob Tagart in July 1774 and William Tagart in Dec 1774 (Ledger B, p. 22, misspelled his name Caldwell); Maj. Samuel Caldwell [actually Calwell], was visited by Dr. John Archer who treated his family in 1796 (Ledger I, which is missing, was abstracted by Dr. George W. Archer circa 1890; his notes are in Archives of the Historical Society of Harford County folder "Archer, G. W. Coll. – Ledgers and Day Books") [Samuel Calwell was a Revolutionary War veteran and a signer of the Bush Declaration on March 22, 1775.]; see James Tagart, q.v.

Calwell, Samuel, was treated by Dr. Robert H. Archer in Baltimore before 1822 [no dates or details were given] (Dr. Archer's "Alphabet to Ledger H" is his booklet [filed in the Archives of the Historical Society of Harford County] that contains his index to Ledger H [which is missing] for his patients in Baltimore before 1822 and Harford County after 1822, according to a notation by Dr. George W. Archer.)

Calwell, Thomas [1765-1828], was prescribed medicine for Jo.(?) by Dr. Robert H. Archer on 7 Jul 1803 (Rx Book, 1802-1804, p. 48); Thomas Calwell [merchant] was treated by Dr. Archer in Baltimore before 1822 [no dates or details were given] (Dr. Archer's "Alphabet to Ledger H" is his booklet [filed in the Archives of the Historical Society of Harford County] that contains his index to Ledger H [which is missing] for his patients in Baltimore before 1822 and Harford County after 1822, according to a notation by Dr. George W. Archer.) [Thomas Calwell, of Baltimore Town, was a Revolutionary War veteran.]

Campbell, Collin, was treated by Dr. John Archer in Aug 1772 (Ledger B, p. 65)

Campbell, Jacob, see John Campbell, q.v.

Campbell, John, near Peach Bottom [on the Susquehanna River], was visited by Dr. John Archer who treated him, his wife and sons William, Thomas and Jacob in 1790 (Ledger F, p. 279) [account continued in Ledger G, which is missing]

Campbell, Thomas, see John Campbell, q.v.

Campbell, William, see John Campbell and James Moores, q.v.

Canan, ---- [blank], was visited by Dr. Alonzo Preston who treated his wife and child in 1826 and a child in 1827 (p. 71)

Cannon, Moses, near Philip Gover's place, was visited by Dr. John Archer who treated a child in 1786 and him in Apr 1787 (Ledger F, pp. 105, 311) [account continued in Ledger K, which is missing]

Cantlin (Cantling), Robert, was visited by Dr. Matthew J. Allen who treated his wife in May, Jun and Jul 1840, but this account was not listed in his ledger. Allen appeared before Sylvester Macatee, a Justice of the Peace, on 7 Dec 1842 and swore an oath that the account was just and true and he had not received payment for his services. The following statement was written on a separate piece of paper, dated 24 Nov 1853, and inserted in the back of Dr. Allen's ledger. The letter, addressed to Major Bond, was signed by I. Day and stated "I have just returned after 3 days ride to look up the Drs. of Dr. Allen and the following is the result." The letter included several patients and among them noted that "Robt. Cantling is gone to N.J."]

Captain Quint, see Mr. Monk, q.v.

Carlin, James (cordwainer), living at Lester Carlin's, was treated by Dr. John Archer in 1797 (Ledger I, which is missing, was abstracted by Dr. George W. Archer circa 1890; his notes are in the Archives of the Historical Society of Harford County folder "Archer, G. W. Coll. – Ledgers and Day Books")

Carlin, Lester, see James Carlin, q.v.

Carlin, William (tailor), was treated by Dr. John Archer in Aug 1775 (Ledger B, p. 104, listed him as William Carlan, taylor)

Carlisle, John, was treated by Dr. Thomas Archer at times before Dec 1804 as noted in a complaint filed by the doctor who stated, in part, he "performed and bestowed in and about the visiting of prescribing and furnishing physic to and for the said John Carlisle in his lifetime labouring and languishing under divers diseases, maladies and disorders." He also noted that John Carlisle died testate on 1 Oct 1805. (Court Record File 39.24.4C at Historical Society of Harford County)

Carlton, William, on Spesutia Island, was treated by Dr. John Archer in Sep 1790 (Ledger F, p. 235)

Carmichael, Alexander, son of Thomas, was treated by Dr. John Archer in July 1786 (Ledger F, p. 239, misspelled his name Charmichael)

Carmichael, Hugh, was treated by Dr. John Archer in Sep 1781 (Ledger D, p. 72, noted "debt forgiven as before")

Carmichael, John, was treated by Dr. John Archer in July 1786 (Ledger F, p. 366, spelled his name Charmichael)

Carmichael, Thomas, was treated by Dr. John Archer in Oct and Dec 1779 (Ledger D, p. 28, spelled his name Carmichel) [account continued in Ledger E, which is missing]; see Alexander Carmichael, q.v.

Carmine, Elizabeth, see Susan Carmine, q.v.

Carmine, Joseph(?), see Susan Carmine, q.v.

Carmine, Susan, at Ring Factory [on Winters Run, west of Bel Air], was visited by Dr. Matthew J. Allen who treated her children Soph. *(sic)* and Elizabeth in Aug 1848 (p. 91)

Carnicle, George, see George McCarnicle, q.v.

Carr, Ann, Mrs., was treated by Dr. Matthew J. Allen in 1832 in Calvert County (p. 25)

Carr, Israel, see James Anderson, q.v.

Carr, Robert, see Robert Kerr, q.v.

Carr, William (miller), at Forwood's Mill, was treated by Dr. John Archer in 1788 (Ledger F, p. 279)

Carroll, James, Jr., was visited by Dr. John Archer who treated him, his wife and his son in 1787 and treated him [James] in 1796 (Ledger F, p. 107, spelled his name Carrol) [account continued in Ledger K, which is missing]

Carroll, John, was treated by Dr. John Archer in Jul 1782 (Ledger D, p. 42, spelled his name Carrel and noted "debt forgiven as before")

Carroll, John, near the Stone House, was treated by Dr. John Archer in Sep 1788 (Ledger F, p. 288, listed his name as "Jno. Carrol")

Carroll, Peter, see Aquila Clark and Elizabeth Hitchcock, q.v.

Carson, James, was visited by Dr. John Archer who treated him in Oct 1781, his sister in Feb 1782 and him in Mar 1787 (Ledger D, p. 80, noted "debt forgiven as before;" Ledger F, p. 252)

Carson, John, was treated by Dr. Robert H. Archer in Baltimore before 1822 [no dates or details were given] (Dr. Archer's "Alphabet to Ledger H" is his booklet [filed in the Archives of the Historical Society of Harford County] that contains his index to Ledger H [which is missing] for his patients in Baltimore City before 1822 and in Harford County after 1822, according to a notation by Dr. George W. Archer.)

Carsons, James, was treated by Dr. Matthew J. Allen in Apr and May 1848 (p. 80)

Carter, Samuel, was visited by Dr. John Archer who treated him and a child in 1790 (Ledger F, p. 66)

Carter, Samuel, at Stafford Mills, was treated by Dr. John Archer in Sep 1793 (Ledger F, p. 216)

Carter, Samuel, at Stump's Mill, was visited by Dr. John Archer who treated his wife and child in Sep and Oct 1783 (Ledger D, p. 18) [account continued in Ledger E, which is missing]

Caruthers, Robert (miller), at William Wilson's, was treated by Dr. John Archer in Nov 1789 (Ledger F, p. 228)

Carver, Henry [1761-1818] (blacksmith), in Havre de Grace, was visited by Dr. John Archer who treated him and child in Aug 1791 (Ledger F, p. 332) [continued in Ledger H, which is missing]

Cashmore, Cornelius, was treated by Dr. John Archer in Mar 1786 (Ledger F, p. 199)

Caskey, William, Mrs., see William Montgomery, q.v.

Caswell, William, see Robert Craswell, q.v.

Catterton, James, was treated by Dr. Matthew J. Allen in 1823 in Calvert County (p. 9b)

Catterton, Jeremiah, was visited by Dr. Matthew J. Allen who treated him and daughter Nancy in 1823 in Calvert Co. (p. 11a)

Catterton, Nancy, see Jeremiah Catterton, q.v.

Caulston, Patty, was prescribed medicine by Dr. Robert H. Archer on 14 Aug 1802 (Rx Book, 1802-1804, p. 12)

Causten, John, was treated by Dr. Robert H. Archer in Baltimore before 1822 [no dates or details were given] (Dr. Archer's "Alphabet to Ledger H" is his booklet [filed in the Archives of the Historical Society of Harford County] that contains his index to Ledger H [which is missing] for his patients in Baltimore before 1822 and Harford County after 1822, according to a notation by Dr. George W. Archer.)

Cavenaugh, John, was visited by Dr. John Archer, Jr. who treated him and a child in Jan 1816, "daughter White" in Jun 1816, son John in Feb 1817, a grandchild in Nov 1817 and Negro Stephen in Feb 1819; mentioned Negro Ned hired in 1817 and George Benjamin in 1819 (p. 43); see Budd White, q.v.

Cecil Furnace account, mentioned Samuel Coale in Nov 1815, Negro Dan in 1818, John Conway in Feb 1819, Negro Nat in 1819 and William G. Walmsley in Dec 1819 (p. 37)

Ceeders, Joseph (tailor), was treated by Dr. John Archer in Oct 1786 (Ledger F, p. 88)

Chalk, Elizabeth, was treated by Dr. John Archer in Oct and Nov 1781 (Ledger D, p. 82, noted "debt forgiven as before")

Chalk, Tudor, see Widow Lisby, q.v.

Chamberlaine, Anna, see Henry Chamberlaine, q.v.

Chamberlaine, George, see Henry Chamberlaine, q.v.

32

Chamberlaine, Henrietta, see Henry Chamberlaine, q.v.

Chamberlaine, Henry, was visited by Dr. Robert H. Archer who treated him in Sep 1815, his wife in Sep 1815 and Jul 1827, son Henry in Aug 1816, Aug 1818 and Aug 1821, Negro Phil in Nov 1816, an infant in Sep 1817, a child in Dec 1817 and Aug 1818, daughter Anna in Jun 1819 and Aug 1821, son George in Aug 1821, Susan Moore in Aug 1821, daughter Henrietta in Aug 1821 and Aug 1822, his wife in Aug 1821 and Feb 1823, son George in Jul 1825, and his [Henry's] wife in Jun 1827 (pp. 13, 54, 144, 232; Ledger F, p. 114, listed as H. Chamberlaine); see Chamberlain & Gale and Thomas Hugins, q.v.

Chamberlaine, John, near Griffith Gittings' Mill, was visited by Dr. John Archer who treated him and his wife in 1792 (Ledger F, p. 28, spelled his name Chamberlain)

Chamberlaine & Gale, had an account with Dr. Robert H. Archer that mentioned George Gale in Oct 1816 and Miss H. Anderson and Henry Chamberlaine in Nov 1816 (p. 46; Ledger F, p. 20)

Chamberlane ---- [blank], was treated by Dr. Robert H. Archer in Baltimore before 1822 [no dates or details were given] (Dr. Archer's "Alphabet to Ledger H" is his booklet [filed in the Archives of the Historical Society of Harford County] that contains his index to Ledger H [which is missing] for his patients in Baltimore before 1822 and Harford County after 1822, according to a notation by Dr. George W. Archer.)

Chambers, Jim (Negro), was treated by Dr. Robert H. Archer after 1822 [no dates or details given] (Dr. Archer's "Alphabet to Ledger H" is his booklet [filed in the Archives of the Historical Society of Harford County] that contains his index to Ledger H [which is missing] for his patients in Baltimore before 1822 and Harford County after 1822, according to a notation by Dr. George W. Archer.)

Chancey, George, was visited by Dr. John Archer who treated him in 1789 and also treated a child named Lytle (Ledger F, p. 77) [account continued in Ledger G, which is missing]

Chancy, Thomas, near Roger Matthews, was treated by Dr. John Archer in 1786 (Ledger F, p. 102)

Chandlee, James, was treated by Dr. John Archer in Feb 1788 (Ledger F, p. 280)

Chandlee, William, was treated by Dr. Robert H. Archer in Mar 1816 (Ledger F, p. 13)

Chandler, William, had a non-medical account in Dr. John Archer, Jr.'s ledger that mentioned "cash paid to your father" on 26 Jun 1819 (p. 11)

Chapman, Mary, was treated by Dr. John Archer in Apr 1788 (Ledger F, p. 160, indicated that her account was charged to Harford County) [account continued in Ledger G, which is missing]

Chapel, John, was treated by Dr. Robert H. Archer in Baltimore before 1822 [no dates or details were given] (Dr. Archer's "Alphabet to Ledger H" is his booklet [filed in the Archives of the Historical Society of Harford County] that contains his index to Ledger H [which is missing] for his patients in Baltimore before 1822 and Harford County after 1822, according to a notation by Dr. George W. Archer.)

Chappell, William, miller at Cox's, was treated by Dr. John Archer in 1794 (Ledger I, which is missing, was abstracted by Dr. George W. Archer circa 1890; his notes are in the Archives of the Historical Society of Harford County folder "Archer, G. W. Coll. – Ledgers and Day Books")

Chapple, William, was treated by Dr. John Archer in April 1782 (Ledger D, p. 39, and noted "debt forgiven as before")

Chapple, William, was visited by Dr. James Archer who treated him for cholera in July 1806 (p. 5)

Chase, Sam (Negro), was prescribed medicine by Dr. Robert H. Archer on 14 Sep 1803 (Rx Book, 1802-1804, p. 55)

Chauncey, George, was visited by Dr. Richard Sappington who treated "Lady" on 5 Dec 1812, "Lady from Paca's Farm" on 17 Dec 1812 and "Lady" in Jan and Feb 1813, son Maxwell in Apr 1813, "ad visitand ten miles post mort son" [son had died] on 1 May 1813, an infant in Jan 1814, him [George] in Mar 1815 in consultation with Dr. Brownley, and son William in Aug 1815; on the reverse of the document: "Acct., Major George Chauncey" (Document filed in Historical Society of Harford County Archives folder "Sappington, Dr. Richard – Accounts, 1783-1830," spelled his name Chauncy and Chauncey) [George Chauncey was a War of 1812 veteran.]

Chauncey, Maxwell, see George Chauncey, q.v.

Chauncey, William, see George Chauncey, q.v.

Cherevoy, John P., was treated by Dr. John Archer, Jr. in Dec 1817 (p. 11)

Cherry, Charlotte, Mrs., was visited by Dr. Matthew J. Allen who treated a negro girl Emma several times in Nov 1847 and her [Charlotte] several times in Mar 1848 (pp. 68, 76, noted that part of the bill was paid in cash on 23 Aug 1853)

Chesapeake Academy, see Charles Rutter, q.v.

Chew, Capt., see Thomas Huggins & Co., q.v.

Chew, Cassandra, Miss, was treated by Dr. Robert H. Archer in Oct and Nov 1823 and July and Oct 1825 and July and Aug 1826; she was listed as Miss C. Chew on 6 Sep 1826 when medicine was prescribed by Dr. Archer (pp. 87, 89, 92-95, 139, 140, 162, 193, 195, 198, 201; Ledger F, p. 76, 155; Rx Book, p. 86); see Mrs. Chew, q.v.

Chew, Edward, was visited by Dr. Robert H. Archer who treated "niece Chew" in Sep and Oct 1826 and his sister Margaret in Oct 1826 (pp. 201, 203)

Chew, Carson, John, was treated by Dr. Robert H. Archer in Baltimore before 1822 [no dates or details were given] (Dr. Archer's "Alphabet to Ledger H" is his booklet [filed in the Archives of the Historical Society of Harford County] that contains his index to Ledger H [which is missing] for his patients in Baltimore before 1822 and Harford County after 1822, according to a notation by Dr. George W. Archer.)

 Edward M., was visited by Dr. Robert H. Archer who treated a negro in May and June 1827 (p. 230)

Chew, Elizabeth, see Nathaniel Chew, q.v.

Chew, Henrietta, see Nathaniel Chew, q.v.

Chew, John A., account in the ledger of Dr. Robert H. Archer mentioned George Bartol on 26 Dec 1821 (Ledger F, p. 28)

Chew, Margaret, Miss, was treated by Dr. Robert H. Archer in Oct and Nov 1826 (pp. 208, 209); see Edward Chew, q.v.

Chew, Miss, see Richard Johns, q.v.

Chew, Mrs., was visited by Dr. Robert H. Archer who treated a negro in Jun 1823 and daughter Cassandra in Aug, Sep and Oct 1823, once in consultation with Dr. Worthington; Mrs. Chew died before 20 Dec 1825 at which time Dr. Archer was paid $16 in cash by her executor S. Worthington (pp. 93, 94, 95, 173; Ledger F, p. 48)

Chew, Nathaniel, account in the ledger of Dr. Robert H. Archer mentioned in 1822 son Washington, daughters Elizabeth and Henrietta, and negroes Charles, Lyd and D. (Ledger F, p. 31)

Chew, Richard, was treated by Dr. John Archer in Apr 1780 and also listed "Ferrying: 20 Dollars" as part of the account due (Ledger D, p. 60, noted "debt forgiven as before") [Richard Chew was a Revolutionary War veteran.]

Chew, Suckey, was treated by Dr. John Archer in May and July 1778 (Ledger C, p. 78, account was titled "Suckey Chew … [spacing] … Jos. Miller" and noted "debt forgiven by order of testator")

Chew, Thomas, see William Morgan, q.v.

Chew, Thomas S. [1757-1821], was visited by Dr. John Archer who treated him and his son William at various times in 1797 and 1798 (Ledger I, which is missing, was abstracted by Dr. George W. Archer circa 1890; his notes are in Archives of the Historical Society of Harford County folder "Archer, G. W. Coll. – Ledgers and Day Books") [His full name was Thomas Sheredine Chew.]

Chew, Washington, see Nathaniel Chew, q.v.

Chew, William, see Thomas S. Chew, q.v.

Cheyney, E., Miss, was prescribed medicine by Dr. Robert H. Archer on 15 Oct 1833 (Rx Book, 1825-1851, p. 108)

Childs, James, see Hannah Childs, q.v.

Childs, Hannah, Mrs., at Ring Factory [on Winters Run, west of Bel Air], was visited by Dr. Matthew J. Allen who treated her son James in Dec 1847 (tooth extraction) and treated her and son in Aug 1847 and her son in Sep 1847 (p. 92)

Childs, Martha, Miss, at Ring Factory [on Winters Run, west of Bel Air], was treated by Dr. Matthew J. Allen in Nov and Dec 1847 and Oct 1848 (pp. 68, 94)

Chillson, David, at G. P. Neck [Gunpowder Neck], was visited by Dr. John Archer who treated him and a child in 1787 (Ledger F, p. 305)

Chinoweth, Arthur, was treated by Dr. Robert H. Archer in Baltimore before 1822 [no dates or details were given] (Dr. Archer's "Alphabet to Ledger H" is his booklet [filed in the Archives of the Historical Society of Harford County] that contains his index to Ledger H [which is missing] for his patients in Baltimore before 1822 and Harford County after 1822, according to a notation by Dr. George W. Archer.)

Chipman, Daniel (stone cutter), near Dublin, son-in-law to Mrs. McCann, was visited by Dr. Robert H. Archer who treated him, his wife and a child in June and July 1823; paid $3 to Dr. Archer on 13 Jul 1825 who noted it was a "counterfeit note & returned" and noted on 5 Aug 1825 that $3 "to counterfeit bank note returned recd. on 13th ultimate by W. Hopkins" (pp. 81, 82, 83, 84, 142, 149; Ledger F, p. 52, 58, noted "dead and insolvent," but no date of death was given)

Christey, Charles, Dutchman near Stafford, was treated by Dr. John Archer in Dec 1782 (Ledger D, p. 53, noted "debt forgiven as before")

Christie, Charles, was visited by Dr. John Archer who treated him and his wife in 1791 (Ledger F, p. 317); see Gabriel Christie, q.v.

Christie, Gabriel [c1756-1808] (esquire), was visited by Dr. John Archer who treated him in Oct 1780, an infant in Oct 1892, him and his son Charles in 1790 and him [Gabriel] in 1797 (Ledger D, p. 100, noted "debt forgiven as before" [account continued in Ledger E, which is missing]; Ledger F, pp. 311, 314) [Gabriel Christie, of Havre de Grace, was a Revolutionary War veteran.]

Christie, Sam (Negro), was treated by Dr. Robert H. Archer after 1822 [no dates or details were given] (Dr. Archer's "Alphabet to Ledger H" is his booklet [filed in the Archives of the Historical Society of Harford County] that contains his index to Ledger H [which is missing] for his patients in Baltimore before 1822 and Harford County after 1822, according to a notation by Dr. George W. Archer.)

Churchman, Enoch [1762-1842], was prescribed medicine for his wife by Dr. Robert H. Archer on 13 Aug 1802 and medicine for Tony (Negro?) on 9 Apr 1803 (Rx Book, 1802-1804, pp. 12, 39); Enoch was treated by Dr. Robert H. Archer in Baltimore before 1822 [no dates or details were given] (Dr. Archer's "Alphabet to Ledger H" is his booklet [filed in the Archives of the Historical Society of Harford County] that contains his index to Ledger H [which is missing] for his patients in Baltimore City before 1822 and Harford County after 1822, according to a notation by Dr. George W. Archer); see James McGlaughlin, q.v.

Churchman, William, was treated by Dr. John Archer in 1797 (Ledger I, which is missing, was abstracted by Dr. George W. Archer circa 1890 who made his own note that he "probably died in September of this year."] Dr. George W. Archer's notes are in the Archives of the Historical Society of Harford County folder "Archer, G. W. Coll. – Ledgers and Day Books")

Clark, ----, brother of Robert, was visited by Dr. John Archer who treated him in Sep 1777, a child in Oct 1777 and Jan 1782, and him in Apr 1783 and June 1788 (Ledger C, p. 19)

Clark, Aquila, near James Amos, was visited by Dr. John Archer who treated him in Aug 1779 and Peter "Carol:" [Carroll] in Sep 1779 (Ledger D, p. 4, noted "debt forgiven as before") [Aquila Clark was a Revolutionary War veteran.]

Clark, Caesar (Negro), on Smithson's place, was visited by Dr. Robert H. Archer who treated a child in Aug 1824 and son John in Jun and Jul 1825 and Aug 1826; account was paid in full in Aug 1826; Caesar was prescribed medicine for a child by Dr. Archer on 29 May 1825 and medicine for himself on 7 June and 7 July 1825 [but was not identified as a negro in Dr. Archer's prescription book] (pp. 138, 142, 197; Ledger F, p. 106; Rx Book, 1825-1851, pp. 80, 81) "Cesar Clark" also appeared on a list of debts dated 26 Dec 1822 and titled "A List of Allen's Claims" that were due and payable to Dr. Richard N. Allen for services rendered [no dates were given] by him to said Clark (Document filed in Historical Society of Harford County Archives folder "R. N. Allen")

Clark, Charity, see David Clark, q.v.

Clark, David (surveyor), was visited by Dr. John Archer who treated him in Feb and Sep 1781 and Apr and May 1782, inoculated 4 of his family in 1782, and treated his wife in May 1784 and him in Sep 1784 (Ledger D, p. 121) [account continued in Ledger E, which is missing]; treated him, his wife and daughter in 1792 (Ledger F, p. 92) [continued in Ledger H, which is missing] and him and children Charity, Thomas, Joseph and Patty between 1794 and 1796 (Ledger I, which is missing, was abstracted by Dr. George W. Archer circa 1890; his notes are in the Archives of the Historical Society of Harford County folder "Archer, G. W. Coll. – Ledgers and Day Books")

Clark, Francis, see William Garret, q.v.

Clark, James, was visited by Dr. John Archer who treated his wife in Mar 1773 (Ledger B, p. 89)

Clark, James (Scotsman), see Mr. Alexander, q.v.

Clark, John, see Caesar Clark and William McMath, q.v.

Clark, John, at John Blackburn's, was treated by Dr. John Archer on 21 Sep 1774 (Ledger B, p. 102)

Clark, John (Negro), was treated by Dr. Robert H. Archer in May 1822 (Ledger F, p. 45); see Caesar Clark and Thomas Jenkins, q.v.

Clark, John (schoolmaster), at Otter Point, was visited by Dr. John Archer who treated him in Jan 1774, Sep 1780, Oct 1780 and Sep 1780, "James at Otter Point" in Sep 1780, him [John] in Oct 1780 and Sep 1781, his wife in Dec 1782 and him and a child in Aug 1784 (Ledger B, p. 1; Ledger C, p. 116, noted "1782, paid by your account for school keeping;" Ledger D, p. 95 [account continued in Ledger E, which is missing]

Clark, John, "son-in-law to wid. Andrew Deaver," was treated by Dr. John Archer between 1794 and 1798 (Ledger I, which is missing, was abstracted by Dr. George W. Archer circa 1890; his notes are in the Archives of the Historical Society of Harford County folder "Archer, G. W. Coll. – Ledgers and Day Books")

Clark, Joseph, see David Clark, q.v.

Clark, Lawrence, was visited by Dr. John Archer who treated him in Nov 1772, him, his wife and sister-in-law in Jan 1774, him in Sep and Nov 1780, his son in Jun 1785 and him [Lawrence] in Apr 1786 (Ledger B, p. 1; Ledger D, p. 96, noted "debt forgiven as before;" Ledger F, p. 216)

Clark, Michael, at Widow McGaw's, was treated by Dr. John Archer in Jan 1776 and in Jan 1777 (Ledger C, p. 22, noted "debt forgiven by order of testator")

Clark, Patty, see David Clark, q.v.

Clark, Ralph, was visited by Dr. Robert H. Archer who treated his wife "in partu" [in childbirth] on 4 Aug 1822 (p. 12; Ledger F, p. 45) [Ralph Clark was a War of 1812 veteran.]

Clark, Rev. Mr., was treated by Dr. John Archer in Aug 1780 and Jul 1782 (Ledger D, p. 62, noted "debt forgiven as before")

Clark, Robert, on Deer Creek, was treated by Dr. John Archer in Nov 1778, Mar and Apr 1779 and Aug 1780 (Ledger C, p. 124, noted "debt forgiven by order of testator"); [Robert Clark was a Revolutionary War veteran.]; see ---- Clark, q.v.

Clark, Thomas, was visited by Dr. Robert H. Archer who treated his wife in Aug 1822 and him in Apr and May 1824 (pp. 12, 105, 106; Ledger F, p. 66) [Thomas Clark was a War of 1812 veteran.]; see David Clark, q.v.

Clark, William, was visited by Dr. John Archer who treated him in Aug 1782 and son William in Mar 1783 (Ledger D, p. 28)

Clark, William, was treated by Dr. John Archer in Aug 1794 (Ledger F, p. 172) [account continued in Ledger I, which is missing] [William Clark was a Revolutionary War veteran.]

Clarke, Jane, see John Clarke, q.v.

Clarke, John, was visited by Dr. Matthew J. Allen who treated daughter Jane in Aug and Sep 1848 (p. 92) [Account was initially written in the name of "Jane Clarke, Harriet Green's daughter." The doctor then lined out Jane's name, but did not line out the words "Harriet Green's daughter" and he then changed the account to "John Clarke" and treatment was rendered to "daughter Jane."]

Clarkson, ---- [blank], was visited by Dr. Alonzo Preston who treated a child in 1827 (p. 89)

Clendenin, Adam, see James Clendenin, q.v.

Clendenin, David, was treated by Dr. John Archer at various times between 1796 and 1801 (Ledger I, which is missing, was abstracted by Dr. George W. Archer circa 1890 who noted "no wife or child mentioned;" his notes are in the Archives of the Historical Society of Harford County folder "Archer, G. W. Coll. – Ledgers and Day Books"); see James Clendenin, q.v.

Clendenin, Ellen, Miss, was treated by Dr. Robert H. Archer after 1822 [no dates or details were given] (Dr. Archer's "Alphabet to Ledger H" is his booklet [filed in the Archives of the Historical Society of Harford County] that contains his index to Ledger H [which is missing] for his patients in Baltimore before 1822 and Harford County after 1822, according to a notation by Dr. George W. Archer.)

Clendenin, James [1737-1795], was visited by Dr. John Archer who treated him in Apr and Jul 1781, Mar 1782, an infant in Sep 1782, George Ferril or Fervil(?) and James' daughter in Jun 1783 and him [James], a child in Dec 1790, him in 1795 and his sons David and Adam at various times between 1795 and 1802 (Ledger D, p. 39, spelled his name Clendennon [account continued in Ledger E, which is missing]; Ledger F, p. 64 [account continued in Ledger H, which is missing]; Ledger I, which is missing, was abstracted by Dr. George W. Archer circa 1890 and noted "Cr. by tickets in the Bethel Lottery £4.10;" his notes are in the Archives of the Historical Society of Harford County file "Archer, G. W. Coll. – Ledgers and Day Books") [Dr. George Archer's own note stated "He was Mrs. H. G. Watters' grandfather." James Clendenin was a Revolutionary War veteran.]; see Elizabeth Gilcrease, Robert Glascow and Richard Cooley, q.v.

Clendenin, Nelly, Miss, was treated by Dr. John Archer in 1796 (Ledger I, which is missing, was abstracted by Dr. George W. Archer circa 1890; his notes are in the Archives of the Historical Society of Harford County file "Archer, G. W. Coll. – Ledgers and Day Books")

Clerk, John, was treated by Dr. John Archer in May 1786 (Ledger F, p. 59); John Clerk, Rock Run miller, was visited by Dr. John Archer who treated him and his family in 1797 (Ledger I, which is missing, was abstracted by Dr. George W. Archer circa 1890; his notes are in the Archives of the Historical Society of Harford County file "Archer, G. W. Coll. – Ledgers and Day Books")

Clifford, Mr., see Jacob Giles, Jr., q.v.

Clindennan, see James Watson, q.v.

Clinging, Jane, daughter to Widow Gilmore, was treated by Dr. John Archer in Apr 1788 (Ledger F, p. 282)

Clingman, John, was treated by Dr. Robert H. Archer in 1815 (Ledger F, p. 6)

Cloman, Eliza, see John Cloman, q.v.

Cloman, James, see John Cloman, q.v.

Cloman, John (shoemaker), was visited by Dr. Robert H. Archer who treated his wife during the night of 24 Nov 1822 and rendered obstetrical services; treated his wife in Nov 1823, daughter Eliza in Aug 1825, him [John] in Sep 1825, son James in Mar 1826 and him [John] in Aug 1827 (pp. 38, 94, 147, 156, 242, 243; Ledger F, p. 123); see Thomas Huggins and A. P. Moores, q.v.

Close, George, was treated by Dr. John Archer in Feb 1780 (Ledger D, p. 87, noted "debt forgiven as before")

Close, Peter, was treated by Dr. John Archer in July 1773 (Ledger B, p. 91)

Coale, also see Cole, q.v.

Coale, Benjamin, near Hall's X Roads, was visited by Dr. Robert H. Archer who treated his wife "in partu" [in childbirth] on 3 Nov 1827 (p. 256)

Coale, Betsey, see James Coale and Jonathan Coale, q.v.

Coale, Daniel (Negro), near Finney's, was visited by Dr. Robert H. Archer who treated his wife in Aug 1823, Aug 1824, Feb 1825 and Aug 1828 (pp. 90, 115, 125, 295; Ledger F, p. 82)

Coale, Dr., see Isaac Coale, Samuel Cox and Jesse Hartley, q.v.

Coale, Edward, see Jonathan Coale, q.v.

Coale, Ellis, see Skipwith Coale, q.v.

Coale, Ephraim (blacksmith), was visited by Dr. John Archer who treated him and a child in 1790 (Ledger F, p. 378)

Coale, Frederick, see Jonathan Coale, q.v.

Coale, Isaac, was visited by Dr. Robert H. Archer who treated him and his wife on 23 Oct and 24 Oct 1822, in consultation with Dr. Coale and Dr. Worthington, and she was noted as "Mrs. Coale, widow of Isaac" on 26 Oct 1822 (pp. 31-32; Ledger F, p. 111)

Coale, James, who lived below Boner's Stone House, was treated by Dr. John Archer in Oct 1787 (Ledger F, p. 31)

Coale, James, was visited by Dr. Robert H. Archer who treated his sister Betsey in Apr 1827 in consultation with Dr. Worthington (p. 222)

Coale, Jonathan, was visited by Dr. John Archer who treated him in 1794 and 1795 and inoculated children Frederick, Thomas, Betsey and Edward in 1795 (Ledger I, which is missing, was abstracted by Dr. George W. Archer circa 1890; his notes are in the Archives of the Historical Society of Harford County folder "Archer, G. W. Coll. – Ledgers and Day Books")

Coale, Joseph, see Samuel Coale, q.v.

Coale, Louisa, see William Coale, q.v.

Coale, Philip, was treated by Dr. John Archer in Apr 1788 and Apr 1791 (Ledger F, pp. 157, 195, 207) [account continued in Ledger H, which is missing]; see Philip Cole, q.v.

Coale, Richard, was treated by Dr. John Archer in 1797 and 1798 (Ledger I, which is missing, was abstracted by Dr. George W. Archer circa 1890; his notes are in the Archives of the Historical Society of Harford County file "Archer, G. W. Coll. – Ledgers and Day Books"); see Mr. Brannon, q.v.

Coale, Samuel, was visited by Dr. John Archer who treated him and son Joseph at various times between 1796 and 1799 (Ledger I, which is missing, was abstracted by Dr. George W. Archer circa 1890; his notes are in the Archives of the Historical Society of Harford County folder "Archer, G. W. Coll. – Ledgers and Day Books")

Coale, Samuel, was visited by Dr. John Archer, Jr. who treated him and a child in May 1817 (p. 78); see Cecil Furnace, q.v.

Coale, Sarah, see William Coale, Sr., q.v.

Coale, Skipwith, was visited by Dr. John Archer who treated him and his wife in 1793 and him and his son Gilbert at various times between 1796 and 1799 (Ledger F, p. 4) [continued in Ledger H, which is missing] (Ledger I, which is missing, was abstracted by Dr. George W. Archer circa 1890 and spelled his name Coal; his notes are in the Archives of the Historical Society of Harford County folder "Archer, G. W. Coll. – Ledgers and Day Books"); see Negro Sam, q.v.

Coale, Skipwith, had an account in the ledger of Dr. Robert H. Archer that mentioned James Jackson and Ellis Coale in Sep 1821 (Ledger F, p. 6); see Joseph Moore, q.v.

Coale, Susan, see William Coale, q.v.

Coale, Thomas, see Jonathan Coale, q.v.

Coale, William, see Samuel Rodgers and Alexander Finley, q.v.

Coale, William, was visited by Dr. John Archer, Jr. who treated his daughter in May 1817, his wife in Dec 1817, him and a child in Feb 1819, William Hughes in May 1820, a child named Atleo or Atlas(?) in Aug 1820 and daughter Louisa in Sep 1821 (p. 51)

Coale, William, at Deer Creek, was visited by Dr. John Archer who treated his wife and "Johannem Mitchel" in Dec 1776, him in Jan 1777 and Apr 1781, his mother in May 1781, his wife in Jun 1781, him in May 1781 and him and daughter Susan in Jul 1791 (Ledger C, p. 71; Ledger D, p. 25 [account continued in Ledger E, which is missing]; Ledger F, p. 161) [account continued in Ledger H, which is missing]

Coale, William, in Belle Aire [Bel Air], was treated by Dr. John Archer in 1787 (Ledger F, p. 215)

Coale, William, was visited by Dr. Robert H. Archer who treated a child in Oct 1825 and his wife in Mar 1828 (pp. 161, 268)

Coale, William of William, was visited by Dr. John Archer who treated his children in Jul 1777 and him in Jul 1779 and 1782 [date not given] (Ledger C, p. 36)

Coale, William, of William, was visited by Dr. Robert H. Archer who treated him in Oct 1825 and his wife and child in Mar 1828 (Ledger F, p. 43)

Coale, William, Jr., was visited by Dr. Alonzo Preston who treated him in 1825, wife and Acy (Asy?) and Jane several times from 1825 to 1827, and a child in 1827 (p. 17)

Coale, William, Sr., was visited by Dr. John Archer who treated two children in Dec 1776, him and son Billy [also shown as Guliel: which is a Latin abbreviation for William] in Jan 1777, him in Apr 1781 and daughter Sarah in Feb 1782 (Ledger C, p. 78)

Cole, also see Coale, q.v.

Cole, Joseph, was visited by Dr. Matthew J. Allen who treated his son in Jan and Feb 1844 and him, his son and children [names not given] in Jun 1845 (pp. 29, 49); see Augustus J. Greme, q.v.

Cole, Mr., at Israel Morris', was treated by Dr. John Archer in Apr 1786 (Ledger F, p. 212)

Cole, Skipwith, of William, was treated by Dr. John Archer in Mar and Aug 1782 and Mar 1783 (Ledger D, p. 122, noted "debt forgiven as before")

Cole, Philip, of William, was visited by Dr. John Archer who treated him in Oct 1779 and Apr and Aug 1781, his wife in Nov 1781, a child in Mar 1782 and him in Dec 1783 and Dec 1784 (Ledger D, p. 32, noted account taken to Ledger F); see Philip Coale and Negro Jim, q.v.

Cole, William, see Philip Cole and Skipwith Cole, q.v.

Colegate, Robert, Englishman, was visited by Dr. John Archer who treated him and children "M." and "L." at various times between 1795 and 1799 (Ledger I, which is missing, was abstracted by Dr. George W. Archer circa 1890; his notes are in the Archives of the Historical Society of Harford County file "Archer, G. W. Coll. – Ledgers and Day Books")

Coleman, Becky, see John Coleman, q.v.

Coleman, Charles, was treated by Dr. John Archer in Feb 1786 (Ledger F, p. 119)

Coleman, James (blacksmith), was visited by Dr. John Archer who treated his wife in Sep 1781 (Ledger D, p. 75, noted "debt forgiven as before")

Coleman, John [1758-1816] (reverend), was visited by Dr. John Archer who treated him and daughter Becky in 1795 (Ledger F, p. 201; Ledger I, which is missing, was abstracted by Dr. George W. Archer circa 1890; his notes are in the Archives of the Historical Society of Harford County file "Archer, G. W. Coll. – Ledgers and Day Books") [John "Parson" Coleman was a Revolutionary War veteran.]

Coleman, Mary (colored), was treated by Dr. Matthew J. Allen in Feb 1845 (p. 45)

Coleman, Susanna, was treated by Dr. John Archer in Mar 1782 (Ledger D, p. 85, noted "debt forgiven as before")

Collins, Henry (ship carpenter), was visited by Dr. John Archer who treated him and a child in 1786 (Ledger F, p. 41)

Collins, Joseph, was treated by Dr. John Archer before 1772 [no dates were given] and in May, Aug and Sep 1773 (Ledger B, p. 16)

Collock, Robert, was treated by Dr. John Archer in 1786 (Ledger F, p. 171)

Combess, Uty, was treated by Dr. John Archer in 1790 (Ledger F, p. 103) [account continued in Ledger G, which is missing] [Utey Combess was a Revolutionary War veteran.]

Compton, Mr., was prescribed medicine "for Boy" by Dr. Robert H. Archer on 19 Oct 1804 (Rx Book, 1802-1804, p. 59)

Conelton, Mathew, see James Tourk, q.v.

Conklin, Mathew, see Hannah Forwood, q.v.

Conley, Jean, was visited by Dr. John Archer who treated a child in Aug 1780 (Ledger D, p. 88, and "debt forgiven as before")

Conn, Mrs., was treated by Dr. Robert H. Archer in Baltimore before 1822 [no dates or details given] (Dr. Archer's "Alphabet to Ledger H" is his booklet [filed in the Archives of the Historical Society of Harford County] that contains his index to Ledger H [which is missing] for his patients in Baltimore City before 1822 and in Harford County after 1822, according to a notation by Dr. George W. Archer.)

Conn, Robert (pedagogue), near Winters Run, was treated by Dr. John Archer in Mar 1786 and several times in 1798 and was prescribed medicine by Dr. Archer on 13 Sep 1804 (Ledger F, p. 262, entered his name as Mr. Conn, but written in another handwriting in the account was the name Robert Conn; Dr. John Archer's Rx Book, 1802-1804, p. 58, also listed him as Robert Conn; Ledger I, which is missing, was abstracted by Dr. George W. Archer circa 1890; his notes are in the Archives of the Historical Society of Harford County folder "Archer, G. W. Coll. – Ledgers and Day Books"); see Arnold Rush, q.v.

Connaway, Nicholas, was treated by Dr. John Archer in Sep 1780 and Oct 1783 (Ledger D, p. 99, noted "debt forgiven as before")

Connell, Dennis, was prescribed medicine by Dr. Robert H. Archer on 27 Jan 1801 and 30 Jan 1801 (Rx Book, 1796-1801, p. 29)

Connoly, Bartholomew (pedagogue), at "W. Hall," was treated by Dr. John Archer in 1795 (Ledger I, which is missing, was abstracted by Dr. George W. Archer circa 1890; spelled his name Barth^w. Connally; Dr. George Archer's notes are in the Archives of the Historical Society of Harford County folder "Archer, G. W. Coll. – Ledgers and Day Books")

Connoly, Daniel (shoemaker), was treated by Dr. Matthew J. Allen in Nov 1843 (p. 27)

Connoly, Francis, was treated by Dr. John Archer before 1772, but no dates or details were given (Ledger B, p. 17)

Connoly, Ignatius, was visited by Dr. Matthew J. Allen who treated him and also a child in Mar 1848 (p. 77)

Connoly, Margaret, at James Fisher's, was treated by Dr. John Archer in Sep 1782 (Ledger D, p. 23, noted "debt forgiven as before")

Connor, Edward (shoemaker), was treated by Dr. John Archer before 1772 [no dates or details given] and also treated a "man" in Oct 1772 and Jan 1773 (Ledger B, p. 21, spelled his name Connar)

Connor, Michael, was treated by Dr. John Archer in Jun 1781 (Ledger D, p. 49, spelled his name Conner and noted "debt forgiven as before")

Conway, John, see Cecil Furnace, q.v.

Conway, Lawrence, was visited by Dr. John Archer who treated his wife in May 1781 and extracted his tooth in May 1781 and her tooth in 1784 [date not given] (Ledger D, p. 18, noted on 7 Feb 1785, "By balance due you when we settled your account with Moses Ruth's Estate … £0.9.11")

Cook, Alexander (clockmaker), was treated by Dr. John Archer in Mar 1788 (Ledger F, p. 365)

Cook, Elisha, see William ----, q.v.

Cook, Jacob, see Mrs. Cook, q.v.

Cook, John (clockmaker), in Abingdon, was treated by Dr. John Archer in Aug 1787 (Ledger F, p. 351) [John Cook was a Revolutionary War veteran.]

Cook, Mrs., widow of Robert Cook, near Bald Friar [ferry landing on the Susquehanna River], was visited by Dr. John Archer who treated her and son Jacob in 1791 (Ledger F, p. 263)

Cook, Robert, see Mrs. Cook, q.v.

Cooke, Samuel, Belle Aire [Bel Air], was treated by Dr. John Archer in 1798 (Ledger I, which is missing, was abstracted by Dr. George W. Archer circa 1890; his notes are in the Archives of the Historical Society of Harford County file "Archer, G. W. Coll. – Ledgers and Day Books")

Cookston, Samuel, was prescribed medicine by Dr. Robert H. Archer twice in Mar 1801 (Rx Book, 1796-1801, pp. 41, 47)

Cooley, James, see John Cooley, q.v.

Cooley, John [c1755-1807], was visited by Dr. John Archer who inoculated him in 1777 and treated him in Nov 1780 and Mar 1781 and a child in Nov 1782 (Ledger C, p. 87; Ledger D, p. 105) [continued in Ledger G, which is missing]; "Capt. John Cooly" was visited by Dr. John Archer who treated "fil. Jacobus" [son James] in 1799 (Ledger I, which is missing, was abstracted by Dr. George W. Archer circa 1890; his notes are in the Archives of the Historical Society of Harford County folder "Archer, G. W. Coll. – Ledgers and Day Books") [John Cooley was a private in the Revolutionary War and apparently was styled "captain" some time after the war.]

Cooley, Mary, was treated by Dr. John Archer in April and May 1773 (Ledger B, p. 66, misspelled her name as Coolly)

Cooley, Richard, near James Clendennin's, was visited by Dr. John Archer who treated him and a child in 1791 (Ledger F, p. 334, misspelled their names as Cooly and Clendenon)

Cooper, Abram (Negro), was treated by Dr. Robert H. Archer after 1822 [no dates or details given] (Dr. Archer's "Alphabet to Ledger H" is his booklet [filed in the Archives of the Historical Society of Harford County] that contains his index to Ledger H [which is missing] for his patients in Baltimore before 1822 and Harford County after 1822, according to a notation by Dr. George W. Archer.); Abram's child died on 2 May 1846 ("True Book, 1845, 46, 47" filed in Archives of Historical Society of Harford County folder "Archer, Dr. Robert H., 1775-1857, Day Book, 1845-47"); Abraham Cooper (colored) was visited by Dr. Matthew J. Allen who treated his children [no names were given] and his wife, a child and daughter, all in March 1848 (p. 76) [The following statement was written on a separate page dated 24 Nov 1853 that was inserted in the back of Dr. Allen's ledger. The letter, addressed to Major Bond, was signed by I. Day and stated "I have just returned after 3 days ride to look up the Drs. of Dr. Allen and the following is the result." It mentioned several patients, including this one: "Negro Abram Cooper was absent, but his wife says he wants to pay part. I left word for him to call & pay you."]

Cooper, Alexander [1746-1815], was visited by Dr. John Archer who treated his child in Aug 1781 and his mother in Mar 1783 (Ledger D, p. 68) [account continued in Ledger E, which is missing]; Alexander Cooper, at Peach Bottom [on the Susquehanna River], was treated by Dr. John Archer in 1803 (Ledger F, p. 233)

Cooper, Calvin, see Mrs. Cooper, q.v.

Cooper, Henry, was visited by Dr. John Archer who inoculated sons William and Nathaniel in Mar 1776 (Ledger C, p. 34)

Cooper, Henry, Jr., was visited by Dr. John Archer who treated him and son Philip at various times between 1796 and 1802 (Ledger I, which is missing, was abstracted by Dr. George W. Archer circa 1890; his notes are in the Archives of the Historical Society of Harford County folder "Archer, G. W. Coll. – Ledgers and Day Books")

Cooper, Henry, Sr., was visited by Dr. James Archer who treated Nat's hand (opened it and dressed it several times in Oct and Nov 1806) and also treated his [Henry's] daughter in 1806 (p. 6)

Cooper, Jim, see Nat Cooper, q.v.

Cooper, John, was treated by Dr. Robert H. Archer in Baltimore before 1822 [no dates or details were given] (Dr. Archer's "Alphabet to Ledger H" is his booklet [filed in the Archives of the Historical Society of Harford County] that contains his index to Ledger H [which is missing] for his patients in Baltimore before 1822 and Harford County after 1822, according to a notation by Dr. George W. Archer.)

Cooper, John, near Peach Bottom [on the Susquehanna River], was visited by Dr. John Archer who treated him and his wife in 1791 (Ledger F, p. 23) [continued in Ledger H, which is missing]

Cooper, Matilda, see Nat Cooper, q.v.

Cooper, Mrs., widow of Calvin, was visited by Dr. John Archer who treated her and a child in Aug 1790 (Ledger F, p. 369) [account continued in Ledger G, which is missing]

Cooper, Nat (Negro), was mentioned in Dr. Robert H. Archer's ledger in Nov 1827, noting "to cash to wife to buy son Jim a suit of clothes" that cost $3.50; also mentioned his wife on 1 Aug 1828 and prescribed medicine for Nat on 17 Aug 1830 (pp. 255, 288; Rx book, 1825-1851, p. 101; Ledger F, p. 107, noted Archer hired Nat's daughter Matilda from 1 Jun 1824 to 25 Dec 1826)

Cooper, Nathaniel, see Henry Cooper, q.v.

Cooper, Nicholas, was treated by Dr. John Archer in Feb 1799 (Ledger F, p. 185) [account continued in Ledger K, which is missing]

Cooper, Philip, see Henry Cooper, Jr., q.v.

Cooper, Stephen T., see Mrs. Poole, q.v.

Cooper, William, see Henry Cooper, q.v.

Copeland, Frances (widow), was treated by Dr. John Archer in 1787 (Ledger F, p. 169, stated she "intermarried Greenbury Dorsey" and mentioned son George Copeland; and p. 159 in 1786 had listed her as "Mrs. Frances Copeland, of George")

Copeland, George, see Frances Copeland, q.v.

Copeland, Hitty or Hetty, see John Copeland, q.v.

Copeland, John, was visited by Dr. John Archer who treated him in Jul 1778, Mar 1781, Feb and Mar 1783 and May 1788 and him and his daughters Phebe and Hitty (or Hetty) Copeland and Miss Sally Gallion in 1789; John was also prescribed medicine by Dr. Archer on 18 Aug and 24 Aug 1802 (Ledger C, p. 115; Ledger F, pp. 131, 211; Rx Book, 1802-1804, pp. 15, 16) [accounts continued in Ledgers E and G, which are missing] [John Copeland was a Revolutionary War veteran.]; see Thomas Hinks, q.v.

Copeland, Phebe, see John Copeland, q.v.

Copper, Samuel, was treated by Dr. Robert H. Archer in Baltimore before 1822 [no dates or details were given] (Dr. Archer's "Alphabet to Ledger H" is his booklet [filed in the Archives of the Historical Society of Harford County] that contains his index to Ledger H [which is missing] for his patients in Baltimore before 1822 and Harford County after 1822, according to a notation by Dr. George W. Archer.)

Corbett, John, was prescribed medicine for his child on 24 Aug 1802 by Dr. Robert H. Archer (Rx Book, 1802-1804, p. 16)

Corbett, Samuel, near J. Ashmead's, was treated by Dr. John Archer in Nov and Dec 1777 and Jan 1778 and in 1790 when he also mentioned James Wilson (Ledger C, p. 86, spelled his name Corbit and noted "debt forgiven by order of testator;" Ledger F, p. 141, spelled his name Corbet) [Samuel Corbet or Corbett was a Revolutionary War veteran.]

Corbin, see Bennett Love, q.v.

Corbin, John, was visited by Dr. John Archer who treated him and his daughters Sally and Lydia at various times between 1796 and 1800 (Ledger I, which is missing, was abstracted by Dr. George W. Archer circa 1890; his notes are in the Archives of the Historical Society of Harford County folder "Archer, G. W. Coll. – Ledgers and Day Books")

Cord, Ashberry, was treated by Dr. John Archer in July 1775 (Ledger B, p. 56, misspelled his name as Ashbery Chord) [Ashberry Cord was a Revolutionary War veteran.]

Cord, Roger, was treated by Dr. John Archer in October 1786 (Ledger F, p. 87, misspelled his name as Rodger Chord)

Coskery, Barney, was treated by Dr. John Archer in 1786 (Ledger F, p. 42, spelled his name Coskey)

Cosley, John, was visited by Dr. John Archer who treated him in Jul 1779 and a child in Jul 1782 and inoculated John in Jan 1783 (Ledger C, p. 93, mentioned William Martin's note)

Cosley, Thomas, on Gunpowder Neck, was treated by Dr. John Archer in Dec 1781 and Jan and Feb 1782 (Ledger D, p. 112, spelled his name Cosly and noted "debt forgiven as before")

Couden, Joseph, was visited by Dr. Robert H. Archer who treated a child in Mar 1822, Negro Jupiter in Jul 1822, his [Joseph] wife in Jul 1822 and in Apr 1827 in consultation with Dr. John Archer and several times in June 1827 (pp. 223, 232, and p. 231 noted "ferriage" [i. e., ferry over the Susquehanna River to Cecil County], and Ledger F., p. 35, spelled his name Coudon) [Joseph Couden was a War of 1812 veteran.]

Coudon, Mr., see Lydia Taylor, q.v.

Coulston, Mrs., in Baltimore, was treated by Dr. John Archer in 1796 and his ledger noted "1803, ren^d. Mrs. Coulston who says look to Jno. Stump, Cecil" [County] for £2.2 (Ledger I, which is missing, was abstracted by Dr. George W. Archer circa 1890; his notes are in the Archives of the Historical Society of Harford County folder "Archer, G. W. Coll. – Ledgers and Day Books")

Coultrough, William, was treated by Dr. John Archer in 1786 (Ledger F, p. 112)

Councilman, George, was treated by Dr. Robert H. Archer in Baltimore before 1822 [no dates or details were given] (Dr. Archer's "Alphabet to Ledger H" is his booklet [filed in the Archives of the Historical Society of Harford County] that contains his index to Ledger H [which is missing] for his patients in Baltimore before 1822 and Harford County after 1822, according to a notation by Dr. George W. Archer.)

Courson, Jos. (Jas.?), was treated by Dr. Robert H. Archer after 1822 [no dates or details were given] (Dr. Archer's "Alphabet to Ledger H" is his booklet [filed in the Archives of the Historical Society of Harford County] that contains his index to Ledger H [which is missing] for his patients in Baltimore City before 1822 and in Harford County after 1822, according to a notation by Dr. George W. Archer.)

Courtney, Edward, see Cyrus Osborn, q.v.

Courtney, George [1781-1841], was visited by Dr. Robert H. Archer who treated his wife on 3 Sep 1822, in consultation with Dr. J. (sic) Archer and Dr. Worthington, and then treated him 20 more times through 24 Nov 1822 (pp. 16, 23; Ledger F, p. 72, spelled his name Courtnay) [George Washington Courtney was a War of 1812 veteran.]

Courtney, Jonas, see Cyrus Osborn, q.v.

Courtney, Michael, was treated by Dr. John Archer in May and Aug 1790 (Ledger F, pp. 300, 312; p. 301 spelled his name Courtnay)

Cousins or Duzan (sic), Robert, was treated by Dr. John Archer in Oct-Nov 1774 (Ledger B, p. 54)

Covenhoven, George, was treated by Dr. John Archer in Jan 1786 (Ledger F, p. 49)

Cowen, John, was mentioned in Dr. Robert H. Archer's ledger in a non-medical matter in Dec 1823 (Ledger F, p. 75)

Cowen, John, at Samuel Howell's, was visited by Dr. John Archer who treated him and a child in Jan 1777 (Ledger C, p. 81, spelled his name Cowin and noted "debt forgiven by order of testator") [John Cowen was a Revolutionary War veteran.]

Cowen, Thomas, was visited by Dr. James Archer who treated his wife fourteen times in Apr 1806 (p. 7, spelled his name Cowan) [Thomas Cowen was a Revolutionary War veteran.]

Cowen, William (schoolmaster), at Samuel Webster's Tanr (sic), was treated by Dr. John Archer in 1788 (Ledger F, p. 146, spelled his name Cowin)

Cowenevans, Hetty, daughter of Mrs. Barkley, was treated by Dr. John Archer in Sep and Oct 1779 and Feb 1783 (Ledger D, p. 17, noted "debt forgiven as before")

Cox, see David Davis, q.v.

Cox, Edward, see Isabella Cox, q.v.

Cox, Herman, was treated by Dr. Thomas Archer at times before Dec 1804 as noted in a complaint filed by the doctor who stated, in part, that "as a physician … [he had] performed and bestowed in and about the visiting of prescribing and furnishing and physic to and for the said Herman … labouring and languishing under divers diseases, maladies and disorders ..." and he had not been paid for his services. (Court Records File 39.24.4C at the Historical Society of Harford County)

Cox, Isabella, was visited at various times in 1826 and 1827 by Dr. Alonzo Preston who also treated daughter Sarah Ann several times in 1826 and M. E. (sic) and Edward in 1827; one entry stated on 4 May 1827 that $1.33½ paid "by Mr. Finley's bill rec'd. by her" and that the entire bill of $13.95½ had been paid (p. 81)

Cox, Israel, was visited by Dr. John Archer who treated him and wife in 1787 and 1791 and son William in 1787 (Ledger F, pp. 2, 64) [account continued in Ledger H, which is missing]; Israel Cox, dec'd., appeared on a list of debts dated 26 Dec 1822 and titled "A List of Allen's Claims" that were due and payable to Dr. Richard N. Allen for services rendered [no dates were given] by to Cox (Document filed in Historical Society of Harford County Archives folder "R. N. Allen")

Cox, James, see John Cox, Jr., q.v.

Cox, James, was treated by Dr. Matthew J. Allen in 1823 in Calvert County (p. 7a)

Cox, Jeremiah, was visited by Dr. Matthew J. Allen who treated him and a child in 1823 in Calvert County (p. 6a)

Cox, John, in Barrens [an area in the northwest part of the county near Pennsylvania], was visited by Dr. John Archer who treated his wife in Oct 1779, him in Dec 1779, his wife in Jan 1782, him in Sep 1782 and Jul 1783 and him and his daughter Mary in 1788, and Mary in 1790 (Ledger D, p. 33; Ledger F, pp. 22, 41)

Cox, John, see William Moore, Daniel Long and John Cox, Jr., q.v.

Cox, John, Jr., was visited by Dr. John Archer who treated his children John, Martha and James in 1795 (Ledger I, which is missing, was abstracted by Dr. George W. Archer circa 1890; his notes are in Archives of the Historical Society of Harford County file "Archer, G. W. Coll. - Ledgers and Day Books")

Cox, Martha, see John Cox, Jr., q.v.

Cox, Mary, see John Cox, q.v.

Cox, Miss, see Ruthen Garretson, q.v.

Cox, Mitchail, see William Cox, Jr., q.v.

Cox, Mr., was visited by Dr. Robert H. Archer who treated his wife "in partu" [in childbirth] on 29 May 1827 (p. 230)

Cox, Mrs., see Negro Jacob, q.v.

Cox, Samuel, was visited by Dr. Robert H. Archer who rendered obstetrical services to his wife on 22 Oct 1822 in consultation with Dr. Coale (p. 31; Ledger F, p. 110); see William Cox, q.v.

Cox, Sarah Ann, see Isabella Cox, q.v.

Cox, William, see Israel Cox and William Cox, Jr., q.v.

Cox, William, was visited by Dr. John Archer who treated him and son Samuel at various times in 1795 and 1796 (Ledger I, which is missing, was abstracted by Dr. George W. Archer circa 1890; his notes are in the Archives of the Historical Society of Harford County file "Archer, G. W. Coll. – Ledgers and Day Books")

Cox, William, was visited by Dr. James Archer who treated his wife four times in Jul 1806 (p. 8)

Cox, William, was treated by Dr. Robert H. Archer in May and June 1823 and in Apr and May 1828 (pp. 77, 272, 277; Ledger F, p. 12)

Cox, William, Jr., was visited by Dr. John Archer who treated a negro in Feb 1776, a negro in Sep 1779, his [William's] wife in Jun 1781, him and son William in Oct 1781, Negro Jacob in Aug 1782, a child in Jul 1783, him [William, Jr.] in Oct 1784, "Mitchail" in Feb 1785, his [William, Jr.'s] wife in May 1785, him in Oct 1785 and him and an infant in Sep 1789 (Ledger C, p. 39; Ledger D, pp. 13, 22, noted account was continued in Ledger F, p. 38, but then omitted the Jr.) [account continued in Ledger G, which is missing]

Cox, William, Sr., was visited by Dr. John Archer who treated his daughter Rachel in Aug 1781 and him in Sep 1781 and Apr 1782 (Ledger D, p. 68, noted "debt forgiven as before")

Crabbs, Mrs. was prescribed medicine by Dr. Robert H. Archer on 20 Aug 1803 and 23 Aug 1803 (Rx Book, 1802-1804, p. 54)

Craig, Alexander, was visited on 18 Sep 1821 by Dr. Robert H. Archer who treated him, his son Philip and daughter Nancy, and also mentioned L. H. Evans on 10 Apr 1838 (Ledger F, p. 21)

Craig, Nancy, see Alexander Craig, q.v.

Craig, Philip, see Alexander Craig, q.v.

Crandal, ---- [blank], was treated by Dr. Robert H. Archer in Oct 1821 (Ledger F, p. 19)

Craswell, see Creswell and Criswell, q.v.

Craswell, John, "trans fluis" ["across the water," meaning across the Susquehanna River in Cecil County], was visited by Dr. John Archer who treated him, his wife and a child named Linton in 1790 (Ledger F, p. 162) [account continued in Ledger H, which is missing]

Craswell, Linton, see John Craswell, q.v. [account continued in Ledger H, which is missing]

Craswell, Molly, Miss, was treated by Dr. John Archer in 1787 (Ledger F, p. 233, and indicated "this to be carried to Jas. Eagan's account")

Craswell, Robert, son of William, was visited by Dr. John Archer who treated him and his wife in Apr 1787, Feb 1790 and May 1792 (Ledger F, pp. 251, 319) [account continued in Ledger H, which is missing] [Robert Craswell or Criswell was a Revolutionary War veteran.]

Crawford, Alexander (schoolmaster), was visited by Dr. John Archer who treated him in Mar 1776 and Aug 1778 and his wife in Jul 1779 (Ledger C, p. 36)

Crawford, Alexander, at Cooptown, was visited by Dr. John Archer who treated him and his wife in 1792 (Ledger F, p. 132); see Mrs. Crawford, q.v.

Crawford, Cassy, see Robert Crawford, q.v.

Crawford, James, was visited by Dr. John Archer who treated a child in Jun 1780, him, his wife and a child at times between Jan and Sep 1790, and him in Oct and Nov 1790 (Ledger D, p. 72, spelled his name Crafford and noted "debt forgiven as before;" Ledger F, pp. 63, 125, 166)

Crawford, John, see Robert Crawford, q.v.

Crawford, John, was prescribed medicine for his child by Dr. Robert H. Archer on 18 Oct 1799 and 5 Nov 1802 and 16 Sep 1803 (Rx Book, 1796-1801, p. 25, Rx Book, 1802-1804, pp. 22, 56)

Crawford, Mordecai, Jr., was treated by Dr. John Archer in Sep 1786 (Ledger F, p. 57) [Mordecai Crawford was a Revolutionary War veteran.]

Crawford, Mrs., of Cooptown, widow of Alexander Crawford and daughter of G. Bradford, was treated by Dr. John Archer at times in 1786, 1788, 1789 and 1792 (Ledger F, pp. 52, 86, 132)

Crawford, Parker, see Robert Crawford, q.v.

Crawford, Peggy, see Robert Crawford, q.v.

Crawford, Robert (blacksmith), was visited by Dr. John Archer who treated him and children Cassy, John, Peggy and Parker in 1794 (Ledger I, which is missing, was abstracted by Dr. George W. Archer circa 1890; his notes are in the Archives of the Historical Society of Harford County folder "Archer, G. W. Coll. – Ledgers and Day Books")

Crawford, Seaborn, was treated by Dr. John Archer in Mar 1790 (Ledger F, p. 262) [account continued in Ledger G, which is missing]

Creagh, Mr., at Cooptown, was treated by Dr. John Archer in May 1786 (Ledger F, p. 283)

Creagh, Pierse, was treated by Dr. John Archer in Jun 1795 (Ledger F, p. 86) [account continued in Ledger I, which is missing]

Creighton, John, was treated by Dr. John Archer in Dec 1772 (Ledger B, p. 32)

Creswell, see Criswell and Craswell, q.v.

Creswell, Janey, see David Dickson, q.v.

Creswell, John, see Mrs. Creswell, q.v.

Creswell, Mrs., widow of John, at P. Deposit [i. e., Port Deposit in Cecil County], was treated by Dr. Robert H. Archer in Sep 1822 in consultation with Dr. J. Archer and Dr. Allen (pp. 23, 24; Ledger F, p. 89)

Cretin, Andrew, see Patrick Cretin, q.v.

Cretin, Antoinette, see John Cretin, q.v.

Cretin, Caroline, see John Cretin, q.v.

Cretin, Jacob, see John Cretin, q.v.

Cretin, James, was treated by Dr. John Archer in Sep 1777, Sep 1781, Mar 1784 and Sep and Oct 1785 (Ledger C, p. 53, noted "debt forgiven by order of testator;" Ledger D, p. 72) [account continued in Ledger H. which is missing] [James Cretin was a Revolutionary War veteran.]

Cretin, John, was visited by Dr. John Archer who treated him at various times between Aug 1772 and Jun 1775, Jimmy and his [John's] sister in Aug 1772, his wife in Aug 1772 and May 1773, a negro in Oct 1773, Negro Heny in Dec 1773, a negro child in May 1774, him in Aug 1777, Feb 1778, Sep and Dec 1779. a negro in Jul 1779, "Patrict McCrill" [i.e., Patrick McCrail or McGrill] in Sep 1779, him [John] at times between Apr and Nov 1780, in Mar 1781 (dressing a wound) and Aug 1781, a negro in Sep 1781, Nancy Flanigan in Nov 1781 (tooth extraction), a negro in Jun 1782 and him [John] in Oct and Dec 1782 and Jan and Sep 1783 (Ledger B, p. 15; Ledger C, p. 59; Ledger D, p. 63, listed him as John Creiton, Sr.) [account continued in Ledger E, which is missing]; see Elizabeth Hardy, Peter Hunter, Samuel Forwood, and Philip ---, q.v.

Cretin, John, Jr., was visited by Dr. John Archer who treated him in Jul 1781 and a negro "per order of your mother" in Feb 1783, inoculated his daughters Caroline, Matilda and Antoinette Creatin *(sic)* in 1795 and treated him and his wife in 1796 (Ledger D, p. 14; Ledger F, p. 281)

Cretin, Matilda, see John Cretin, q.v.

Cretin, Mrs., widow of John, was treated by Dr. John Archer in Feb 1788 (Ledger F, p. 156) [account continued in Ledger G, which is missing]

Cretin, Patrick, was visited by Dr. John Archer who treated him in Aug 1773, Jun and Jul 1774, Mar, Jun and Nov 1775, Feb 1778, Sep 1779, Aug and Nov 1780, and Apr 1784, Nat [Negro?] in Sep 1785, his [Patrick's] wife in Dec 1785, Nat in Feb 1786, his wife in Aug 1786 and him, his wife and sons Andrew and Jacob in 1799 (Ledger B, p. 25; Ledger C, p. 17; Ledger D, p. 26, spelled his name Creiton) [account continued in Ledger E, which is missing]; Ledger F, p. 20) [Patrick Cretin was a Revolutionary War veteran.]

Creton, Jas., see Moses Allen, q.v.

Criswell, see Craswell and Creswell, q.v.

Criswell, James, was treated by Dr. John Archer in Nov 1773 and Jan 1774 and Apr 1788 (Ledger B, p. 56; Ledger F, p. 167)

Criswell, Levi, was visited by Dr. Matthew J. Allen who treated his sister eighteen times between 24 May 1848 and 6 Oct 1848 (pp. 83, 89)

Criswell, Mr., was prescribed medicine by Dr. Robert H. Archer on 5 Nov 1802 (Rx Book, 1802-1804, p. 24)

Criswell, Mrs. (widow), was visited by Dr. John Archer who treated her and a child in Aug 1791 (Ledger F, p. 368); see ---- Lester, q.v.

Criswell, Robert, Sr., was treated by Dr. John Archer in May 1791 (Ledger F, p. 268) [Robert Criswell was a Revolutionary War veteran.]; see Robert Curswell, q.v.

Criswell, William, was visited by Dr. John Archer who treated him in 1772 [no details were given] and his wife in Nov 1774 (Ledger B, p. 14); see William Curswell, q.v.

Crockett, Benjamin, at Hickory, was treated by Dr. John Archer in 1796 (Ledger I, which is missing, was abstracted by Dr. George W. Archer circa 1890; his notes are in Archives of the Historical Society of Harford County folder "Archer, G. W. Coll. – Ledgers and Day Books")

Crockett, Samuel, "at Susquehanna," was treated by Dr. John Archer in May 1780 and noted "trans fluis" [i.e., "across the water" meaning across the Susquehanna River] (Ledger D, p. 64, noted "debt forgiven as before"); see Samuel Webb, William Webb and William McMath, q.v.

Crockett, Samuel was treated by Dr. John Archer in Oct and Nov 1781 (Ledger D, p. 83, noted "debt forgiven as before")

Cromwell, Betsey, Miss, was prescribed medicine by Dr. Robert H. Archer on 2 Sep 1802 and 28 Jun 1803 (Rx Book, 1802-1804, pp. 17, 46)

Cromwell, Mrs., was treated by Dr. Robert H. Archer in Baltimore before 1822 [no dates or details were given] (Dr. Archer's "Alphabet to Ledger H" is his booklet [filed in the Archives of the Historical Society of Harford County] that contains his index to Ledger H [which is missing] for his patients in Baltimore before 1822 and Harford County after 1822, according to a notation by Dr. George W. Archer.)

Crooks, Henry, was visited by Dr. John Archer who treated him and wife in Dec 1777 and him in Dec 1778 (Ledger C, p. 81, spelled his name Krooks and noted "debt forgiven by order of testator") [Henry Crooks was a Revolutionary War veteran.]

Crooks, Widow, was treated by Dr. John Archer in Oct 1777 and Feb 1778 (Ledger C, p. 60, noted "debt forgiven by order of testator")

Crooks, William, near Broad Creek, was visited by Dr. John Archer who treated him and his wife in Jul 1774 and him in Dec 1776 (Ledger B, p. 97, spelled his name Krooks; Ledger C, p. 73, noted "debt forgiven by order of testator") [William Crooks and William Crooks, Jr. were both Revolutionary War veterans.]

Crosby, Mr., was treated by Dr. Robert H. Archer in Baltimore before 1822 [no dates or details were given] (Dr. Archer's "Alphabet to Ledger H" is his booklet [filed in the Archives of the Historical Society of Harford County] that contains his index to Ledger H [which is missing] for his patients in Baltimore before 1822 and Harford County after 1822, according to a notation by Dr. George W. Archer.)

Cross, John, was treated by Dr. Robert H. Archer in Baltimore before 1822 [no dates or details were given] (Dr. Archer's "Alphabet to Ledger H" is his booklet [filed in the Archives of the Historical Society of Harford County] that contains his index to Ledger H [which is missing] for his patients in Baltimore before 1822 and Harford County after 1822, according to a notation by Dr. George W. Archer.)

Crossin, Nicholas, was visited by Dr. John Archer who treated Polly in Oct 1780 and Feb 1781 and him in Aug 1781 and Feb, Mar and May 1784 (Ledger D, p. 103, spelled his name Crosin and noted "debt forgiven as before," stated "transfer from Ledger C, fol. 76," and spelled his name Kroesen); see Nicholas Kroesen, q.v.

Crossin, Richard, was treated by Dr. John Archer in July 1780, Jan and Apr 1781, and Apr and Aug 1783 (Ledger D, p. 75) [continued in Ledger E, which is missing]; see Richard Kroesen, q.v.

Crosson, John, appeared on a list of debts dated 26 Dec 1822 and titled "A List of Allen's Claims" that were due and payable to Dr. Richard N. Allen for services rendered [no dates given] to said Crosson (Document filed in Historical Society of Harford County Archives folder "R. N. Allen")

Crouch, James (stage driver), Harford Town, was visited by Dr. John Archer who treated his family in 1797 (Ledger I, which is missing, was abstracted by Dr. George W. Archer circa 1890; his notes are in the Archives of the Historical Society of Harford County file "Archer, G. W. Coll. – Ledgers and Day Books")

Crouch, William, was treated by Dr. Robert H. Archer in Baltimore before 1822 [no dates or details were given] (Dr. Archer's "Alphabet to Ledger H" is his booklet [filed in the Archives of the Historical Society of Harford County] that contains his index to Ledger H [which is missing] for his patients in Baltimore before 1822 and Harford County after 1822, according to a notation by Dr. George W. Archer.)

Cuddy, Henry, was treated by Dr. John Archer in Sep 1775 (Ledger B, p. 83)

Cuddy, Jacob, see Charles Ogle, q.v.

Cuddy, Jas., at the Canal, was treated by Dr. John Archer on 7 Dec 1788 (Ledger F, p. 100, noted he was "poor and dead," but did not give the date of death)

Cuddy, John, was visited by Dr. John Archer who treated him in Sep 1777, his wife in Jan 1778 and him in May 1782 (Ledger C, p. 63, noted "debt forgiven by order of testator;" Ledger D, p. 7, noted "debt forgiven as before")

Cultrough, William, was visited by Dr. John Archer who treated his wife in Dec 1781 and Jun 1782 and him in Mar, Apr and May 1783 (Ledger D, p. 101) [account continued in Ledger E, which is missing]

Culver, Benjamin, was visited by Dr. John Archer who treated him in Mar 1774, circa 1776 [no date given] and Jun 1782, his wife in Sep 1782 and him in Jan 1784 and Dec 1792 (Ledger B, p. 88; Ledger C, p. 69; Ledger F, p. 183) [account continued in Ledger G, which is missing] [Benjamin Culver was a Revolutionary War veteran.]

Culver, Elizabeth, was treated by Dr. John Archer in Apr 1775 (Ledger B, p. 24)

Culver, Robert, was visited by Dr. John Archer who treated him in Feb 1777, him and a child in Mar 1778, him in Apr 1780, his wife in Oct 1780, and him in Apr 1781, Oct 1782 and Feb 1790 (Ledger C, p. 32; Ledger F, p. 249, noted bill was paid by William Luckie in June 1804) [Robert Culver was a Revolutionary War veteran.]; see James Evans, q.v.

Culver, Widow, was treated by Dr. John Archer in Nov 1776 (Ledger C, p. 60)

Cumberland Forge, see Frederick Fraley (Frailey), q.v.

Cuming, P., see John Evans, q.v.

Cummins, John, was treated by Dr. John Archer in Apr and Jul 1780 (Ledger D, p. 23, spelled his name Cummens, noted he paid £0.3.9 in cash and then noted "debt forgiven as before")

Cummins, Paul (dish turner), was visited by Dr. John Archer who treated a child in July 1775, him in Dec 1776 and Jan 1777, his wife in Aug 1777, him in Aug 1778 and Aug 1779, a child in Jul 1780, his wife in Aug 1780, him in Sep 1781, his wife in Oct 1784 and him and his wife in Sep 1788 (Ledger B, p. 66; Ledger C, p. 58, noted "paid by making a small ladle and 6 small wooden bowls," and p. 103; Ledger D, p. 73, noted "debt forgiven as before;" Ledger F, p. 56, noted he was "poor and dead," but did not give the date of death) [Paul Cummins was a Revolutionary War veteran.]

Cummins, Philip, was visited by Dr. John Archer who treated him in Jun 1781, his wife in Aug 1781 (sewed and dressed a wound), a child in Oct 1781, him in Nov and Dec 1781 and a girl (tooth extraction) in Jul 1783 (Ledger D, p. 36, also noted "debt forgiven as before") [Philip Cumming, possibly Cummings or Cummins, was a Revolutionary War veteran.]

Cunningham, Hopher, was treated by Dr. John Archer in Sep 1787 (Ledger F, p. 373)

Cunningham, James, "son-in-law to Perryman," was visited by Dr. John Archer who treated him and his wife in Mar 1789 (Ledger F, p. 82)

Cunningham, Joseph, appeared on a list of debts dated 26 Dec 1822 and titled "A List of Allen's Claims" that were due and payable to Dr. Richard N. Allen for services rendered [no dates were given] by him to said Cunningham (Document filed in Historical Society of Harford County Archives folder "R. N. Allen")

Cunningham, Mortimer, was visited by Dr. Matthew J. Allen who treated a child in Jul, Sep and Oct 1848 (p. 89)

Cunningham, Mr., "in Barrens near Mr. Slemmons's" [area in the northwest part of the county near Pennsylvania], was treated by Dr. John Archer in July 1782 (Ledger D, p. 26, noted "debt forgiven as before")

Cunningham, Walter, was visited by Dr. Alonzo Preston who treated his wife at various times in 1827 and 1828 (p. 23)

Curl(?), John (millwright), Rock Run, was treated by Dr. John Archer in 1797 (Ledger I, which is missing, was abstracted by Dr. George W. Archer circa 1890; his notes are in the Archives of the Historical Society of Harford County folder "Archer, G. W. Coll. – Ledgers and Day Books")

Currier, Jonathan, was visited by Dr. John Archer, Jr. who treated him in Mar 1813 and Aug 1821, and his wife in Oct 1820 (p. 44)

Currier, R., see Ann Wyatt, q.v.

Currier, Victor, was visited by Dr. John Archer, Jr. who treated him in Jun 1818 and his wife and an infant in May 1821; he was also treated by Dr. Robert H. Archer in Oct 1821 (Dr. John Archer, p. 9; Dr. Robert Archer, Ledger F, p. 14)

Currier, William, was treated by Dr. John Archer, Jr. in Dec 1817 (p. 9)

Curry, Amos, was treated by Dr. Matthew J. Allen in Jun 1845 (p. 48, spelled his name Currie)

Curry, Arthur, was visited by Dr. Alonzo Preston who treated him in 1824 and a child in 1825 (p. 22, spelled his name Currey)

Curry, Barney, was treated by Dr. John Archer in May 1782 (Ledger D, p. 37, noted "debt forgiven as before")

Curry, John, was visited by Dr. John Archer who treated him in Jan 1777, his wife in Sep 1777 and his wife and a child in 1791 (Ledger C, p. 82; Ledger F, p. 359) [John Curry was a Revolutionary War veteran.]

Curry, John [1780-1832], was visited by Dr. Robert H. Archer who treated his wife and prescribed medicine for her in Jul 1825 (pp. 141, 145; Rx Book, 1825-1851, p. 81) [John Curry was a War of 1812 veteran.]

Curry, Martha C., was treated by Dr. Matthew J. Allen in Jun 1847 (p. 55, spelled her name Currie)

Curry, Matthew, was treated by Dr. John Archer in Sep 1786 (Ledger F, p. 52)

Curry, Samuel, was treated by Dr. Robert H. Archer several times in May and June 1823 (pp. 75, 76, 77; Ledger F, p. 163)

Curry, William, "near Old Fields," was treated by Dr. John Archer circa 1786 [no dates were given] (Ledger F, p. 188)

Curry, William, was visited by Dr. Matthew J. Allen who treated his daughter in Aug 1844 (p. 40) [William Curry was a War of 1812 veteran.]

Curswell, see Creswell and Criswell, q.v.

Curswell, James, was treated by Dr. John Archer in Sep 1780 (Ledger D, p. 96, noted "debt forgiven as before")

Curswell, Robert, was visited by Dr. John Archer who treated him in Oct and Nov 1780 and Miss Blackburn in Jul 1781 (Ledger D, p. 102, "transferred to Ledger F, fol. 268" where it spelled his name Criswell) [Robert Carswell or Curswell was a Revolutionary War veteran.]; see Robert Criswell, q.v.

Curswell, William, was visited by Dr. John Archer who treated him in May 1781, son Robert in Dec 1781 and Jul 1783 and him in Oct 1783 [Ledger D, p. 21, noted "debt forgiven as before"]

Dale, James, was prescribed medicine for his wife by Dr. Robert H. Archer on 21 Mar 1803, for a negro on 9 Apr 1803, for him [James] on 25 Jul 1803, noting it was "to be sent to his store to go into the country the first opportunity," for him on 12 Aug 1803 and for him and for a child circa Dec 1804 (Rx Book, 1802-1804, pp. 37, 39, 51, 52, 69, 72)

Dallam, Ann, Mrs. (widow), was visited by Dr. John Archer who treated her in Nov 1776 and Jan 1777, an infant in May 1778, Elizabeth Webster in Sep 1778, and her [Ann] in Feb, Mar, Apr and Nov 1780 (Ledger C, p. 62, showed account in name of "Mrs. Ann Dallam, widow, or Bennet Matthews"); see Bennett Matthews and Mrs. Dallam (widow), q.v.

Dallam, Dr., see Nicholas Baker, q.v.

Dallam, Eliza, see Josias William Dallam, q.v.

Dallam, Elizabeth, see Margaret Dallam, q.v.

Dallam, Fanny, see John Dallam, q.v.

Dallam, Francis, was visited by Dr. John Archer who treated him in Sep 1780, his wife in Feb 1783 and a negro in Oct 1783 (Ledger D, p. 95, noted the £5 bill, including interest, was paid in full in cash by Jos. Wm. Dallam on 1 May 1787); see Josias William Dallam, q.v.

Dallam, John, was visited by Dr. John Archer who treated him in Aug 1781, his wife in Dec 1781, inoculated three of his children, Samuel, Fanny and Peggy, in Jan 1781 and treated him [John] in Aug 1789 (Ledger D, p. 66; Ledger F, p. 248) [account continued in Ledger G, which is missing]; John Dallam was also treated by Dr. Thomas Archer at times before Dec 1804 as noted in a complaint filed by the doctor who stated, in part, that " as a physician … [he had] performed and bestowed in and about the visiting of prescribing and furnishing and physic to and for the said John … labouring and languishing under divers diseases, maladies and disorders ..." and he had not yet been paid for his services. (Court Records File 39.24.4C at the Historical Society of Harford County) [John Dallam was a Revolutionary War veteran.]

Dallam, John, was visited by Dr. Matthew J. Allen who treated him for herpes in Nov 1847, and treated Caroline [Negro?] in Mar and Apr 1848, him [John] in May 1848, Caroline's child in Jun 1848 and "N. Elizth." [Negro Elizabeth] (tooth extraction) in Aug 1848 (p. 69)

Dallam, Jos., see John Brown and John Wilds, q.v.

Dallam, Josias William [1747-1820], was visited by Dr. John Archer who treated him, a child and Miss Patty Smith in Jul 1779, him in May 1780, him and his wife in Sep 1781, son William and Miss Fanny Henderson in Oct 1781, him in Nov 1781 and Aug and Sep 1782, his wife in Nov 1782, son Richard in Aug 1783, him [Josias Wm.] in Mar 1784, and him, his wife, daughter Eliza, and sons Middlemore, Richard and Francis in 1787 and 1788 (Ledger D, p. 3, spelled his name Dellam) [account continued in Ledger E, which is missing]; Ledger F, pp. 177, 357, 358); see John Kimberry, Michael McCoy, Francis Dallam and Widow Thorn, q.v.

Dallam, Margaret, was visited by Dr. John Archer who treated her and daughter Elizabeth in Oct 1789 (Ledger F, p. 269) [account continued in Ledger G, which is missing]

Dallam, Margaret, "widow Jr.," was visited by Dr. John Archer who treated her in Nov 1776, a child in May 1779 and her in Jul 1779, Aug 1781 and Feb 1783 (Ledger C, p. 125, noted "debt forgiven by order of testator")

Dallam, Middlemore, see Josias William Dallam, q.v.

Dallam, Mrs. (widow), was visited by Dr. John Archer who treated her in Mar, May and Jul 1781, a negro in Sep 1781, inoculated four children, Fanny, Betsy, Cassy and Winston and Negro Linus and Negro Bet in Jan 1782, and treated Mrs. Dallam in Apr 1782 (Ledger D, p. 125, noted "debt forgiven as before") [account continued in Ledger E, which is missing; Dr. Archer also noted a credit transferred from page 1 and mentioned Capt. B. Matthews]; see Bennett Matthews, q.v.

Dallam, Peggy, see John Dallam, q.v.

Dallam, Richard, see Josias William Dallam, q.v.

Dallam, Richard [c1714-1805], was visited by Dr. John Archer who treated him eleven times between 17 Sep 1773 and 15 Jan 1775, a negro in May 1774, his [Richard's] children, a negro in Jan 1777 and inoculated 13 of his [Richard's] family in May 1777; treated a negro in May 1778 and Jun 1779, Negro Sharper in Feb 1780, him [Richard] in Mar and Oct 1781, Judie in Apr 1782, a negro in May 1782, him [Richard] in Jul 1782 and Jan 1783, an "African at Cattail" in Jul 1783, him [Richard] in Aug 1783, a child at Parker Lee's in Aug 1783, his son William in consultation with Dr. Henderson in Aug 1783, and him [Richard] in Jun 1787 (Ledger B, p. 57; Ledger C, p. 84, misspelled his name Dellam [account continued in Ledger E, which is missing]; Ledger F, p. 225, "colonel" was written in a different handwriting by his name); Richard Dallam was also treated by Dr. Thomas Archer at times before Dec 1804 as noted in a complaint filed by the doctor who stated, in part, that " as a physician … [he had] performed and bestowed in and about the visiting of prescribing and furnishing and physic to and for the said Richard … labouring and languishing under divers diseases, maladies and disorders ..." and he had not been paid. (Court Records File 39.24.4C at the Historical Society of Harford County) [Richard Dallam was a Revolutionary War veteran and a signer of the Bush Declaration on March 22, 1775.]

Dallam, Richard [1788-1870], was visited by Dr. Robert H. Archer who treated his wife in Jan, Feb, Mar and Apr 1823, an infant in Mar 1823, him in Aug and Sep 1823, his wife in Aug and Nov 1833, Feb 1834, Jul 1835, Apr 1842, Mar and Apr 1844 and at various times in 1845 (pp. 48, 51, 52, 53, 57, 68, 93; Ledger F, pp. 136, 163); Richard Dallam was treated by Dr. Robert H. Archer in Baltimore before 1822 [no dates or details were given] (Dr. Archer's "Alphabet to Ledger H" is his booklet [filed in the Archives of the Historical Society of Harford County] that contains his index to Ledger H [which is missing] for his patients in Baltimore before 1822 and Harford County after 1822, according to a notation by Dr. George W. Archer.) [Richard Dallam was a War of 1812 veteran.]

Dallam, Samuel, see John Dallam, q.v.

Dallam, Vincent, was treated by Dr. Robert H. Archer in Baltimore before 1822 [no dates or details were given] (Dr. Archer's "Alphabet to Ledger H" is his booklet [filed in the Archives of the Historical Society of Harford County] that contains his index to Ledger H [which is missing] for his patients in Baltimore before 1822 and Harford County after 1822, according to a notation by Dr. George W. Archer.)

Dallam, W. H., see James Monks, William Welch, John Ward, George Preston and John Waters, q.v.

Dallam, William, in Baltimore, was visited by Dr. Robert H. Archer who treated his niece Miss Hopkins in Sep 1825 in consultation with Dr. Worthington (p. 155; Ledger F, p. 145)

Dallam, William, see Richard Dallam and Carvil Treadway, q.v.

Dallam, William M., see Paca Smith and Garrett Garrettson, q.v.

Dallam, William S., was treated by Dr. Thomas Archer at times before Dec 1804 as noted in a complaint filed by the doctor who stated, in part, he "performed and bestowed in and about the visiting of and furnishing and prescribing physic to and for the said William labouring and languishing under divers diseases, maladies and disorders ..." (Court Records File 39.24.4C at the Historical Society of Harford County)

Dallam, Winston, was treated by Dr. John Archer in June 1777 and in April and May 1778 (Ledger C, p. 21, misspelled his name Dellam and noted "debt forgiven by order of testator") [Winston Smith Dallam was a Revolutionary War veteran.]

Dalrumple, James A. D., see James Buckmaster, q.v.

Dalrymple, Thomas, was treated by Dr. Matthew J. Allen in 1823 in Calvert County (p. 10a)

Dane, Dr., see R. N. and M. J. Allen, q.v.

Dane, ----, died in 1830: An inquisition taken at Bush Town on 6 Dec 1830 determined that "a man named Dane came to his death on last night by intoxication and exposure to the inclemency of the weather." (Document filed in the Archives of the Historical Society of Harford County folder "Inquisitions – Unknown Persons")

Darmond, Jno., "German taylor in Belle Aire" [tailor in Bel Air], was treated by Dr. John Archer in Feb 1789 (Ledger F, p. 275)

Daugherty, "Charles, not Cornelius" *(sic)*, settled his £5 medical bill due Dr. John Archer on 26 Apr 1773, but no dates of treatment were recorded in the ledger (Ledger B, p. 95)

Daugherty, Charles, was visited by Dr. James Archer who treated him three times in 1806 [no dates were given, but the bill was sent to him on 27 Oct 1806 for inflammation of the lungs] (p. 9)

Daugherty, Hugh, was visited by Dr. John Archer who treated his daughter Kitty in May 1773 (Ledger B, p. 86)

Daugherty, James, appeared on a list of debts dated 26 Dec 1822 and titled "A List of Allen's Claims" that were due and payable to Dr. Richard N. Allen for services rendered [no dates were given] by him to said Daugherty (Document filed in Historical Society of Harford County Archives folder "R. N. Allen"); James was visited by Dr. Alonzo Preston who treated his wife four times in Jan 1825; the $8 medical bill was paid in part in May 1826 with 70¢ worth of butter and the balance was "settled by note" on 7 Dec 1830 (p. 15)

Daugherty, Kitty, see Hugh Daugherty, q.v.

Daugherty, Samuel, was visited by Dr. John Archer who treated him before 1772 [no dates or details were given] and at various times between Aug 1773 and Jun 1775, and in Feb 1780 and Jan 1782, and treated Negro Dick in Mar 1774, a negro in Sep 1782 and Jan 1784, and a negro child in Feb 1784 (Ledger B, p. 16; Ledger D, p. 48)

Daugherty, Samuel, was treated by Dr. John Archer from 1794 to 1800 (Ledger I, which is missing, was abstracted by Dr. George W. Archer circa 1890; his notes are in the Archives of the Historical Society of Harford County folder "Archer, G. W. Coll. – Ledgers and Day Books")

Davidge, Dr., see George Morrison, q.v.

Davidson, Elizabeth, see George Davidson, q.v.

Davidson, Frances, see George Davidson, q.v.

Davidson, George, was visited by Dr. John Archer, Jr. who treated an infant in Aug 1815, his daughter Elizabeth in Sep 1815, his wife in Oct 1816, daughter Sarah in Dec 1816, daughter Frances in Feb 1819 and negroes Dick, William, Maria and Amy; George was visited by Dr. Robert H. Archer who treated his sons James and William in Sep 1821, a child in Mar 1822 and Jun 1824 and daughters Margaret and Sarah in Jul 1824 (Dr. John Archer, p. 18; Dr. Robert H. Archer, pp. 111-113, Ledger F, pp. 7, 36); see Nancy Thomas, q.v.

Davidson, James, see Nancy Thomas and George Davidson, q.v.

Davidson, John, was treated by Dr. John Archer in Oct 1777 (Ledger C, p. 83)

Davidson, Margaret, see George Davidson, q.v.

Davidson, Sarah, see Nancy Thomas and George Davidson, q.v.

Davidson, William, see George Davidson, q.v.

Davis, Captain, was prescribed medicine for his daughter by Dr. Robert Archer on 11 Mar 1801 (Rx Book, 1796-1801, p. 43)

Davis, Daniel, near Samuel Forwood's, was treated by Dr. John Archer in 1786 (Ledger F, p. 108)

Davis, David, near Cox's Mill, was treated by Dr. John Archer in Aug 1786 (Ledger F, p. 27)

Davis, Dr., was consulted by Dr. John Archer in 1787 and 1788 (Ledger F, pp. 128, 214)

Davis, Elijah, was treated by Dr. John Archer in Feb 1786 (Ledger F, p. 98)

Davis, Elijah (doctor), see Dr. Davis and Negro Polydore, q.v.

Davis, Eliza, see Joseph Davis, q.v.

Davis, Ellen, see Reuben H. Davis, q.v.

Davis, Fanny, was treated by Dr. John Archer in Aug 1782 (Ledger D, p. 67, noted "debt forgiven as before")

Davis, Harriet, see Reuben H. Davis, q.v.

Davis, James G., was visited by Dr. Alonzo Preston who treated him at various times between 1823 and 1825 [no dates or details were given] and treated an unnamed black girl in 1825 (p. 29) [James G. Davis was a War of 1812 veteran.]

Davis, Joseph (blacksmith), was visited by Dr. John Archer who treated him in Aug and Nov 1772, at times from May to July 1773 and Feb 1774, treated him and his wife and inoculated his apprentice in Dec 1775, treated his daughter and a negro in Oct 1779, him [Joseph] in Dec 1779, a child in Dec 1780 and Jul 1781, inoculated 5 of his family in 1782, treated him and a child in Apr 1783, his wife in May 1783 and a child in

Sep 1783 (Ledger B, p. 18, spelled his name Davies, but p. 21 spelled his name Davis; Ledger C, p. 9, was continued in Ledger D, p. 39, but this ledger did not note that he was a blacksmith)

Davis, Joseph, was visited by Dr. John Archer who treated his daughter Eliza in 1788 and him in July 1790 (Ledger F, p. 130) [continued in Ledger H, which is missing]; see Mary Miller, q.v.

Davis, Joseph, Sr., was visited by Dr. Robert H. Archer who treated him and a negro boy in Apr 1826, his [Joseph's] wife in Jan and Feb 1827 and Nov 1828, him in Sep 1827 and his daughter and a negro in May 1829 (pp. 180, 213, 214, 245, 246, 300; Ledger F, p. 12)

Davis, Mary, see Reuben H. Davis, q.v.

Davis, Moses &ca *(sic)*, was treated by Dr. Robert H. Archer in Baltimore before 1822 [no dates or details were given] (Dr. Archer's "Alphabet to Ledger H" is his booklet [filed in the Archives of the Historical Society of Harford County] that contains his index to Ledger H [which is missing] for his patients in Baltimore before 1822 and Harford County after 1822, according to a notation by Dr. George W. Archer.)

Davis, Mr., "brother-in-law to Riggs," was treated by Dr. Robert H. Archer after 1822 [no dates or details were given] (Dr. Archer's "Alphabet to Ledger H" is his booklet [filed in the Archives of the Historical Society of Harford County] that contains his index to Ledger H [which is missing] for his patients in Baltimore before 1822 and Harford County after 1822, according to a notation by Dr. George W. Archer.)

Davis, Mrs. (widow), was treated by Dr. Robert H. Archer in Baltimore before 1822 [no dates or details were given] (Dr. Archer's "Alphabet to Ledger H" is his booklet [filed in the Archives of the Historical Society of Harford County] that contains his index to Ledger H [which is missing] for his patients in Baltimore before 1822 and Harford County after 1822, according to a notation by Dr. George W. Archer.)

Davis, Reuben H. (reverend) [and principal of Bel Air Academy], was visited by Dr. Robert H. Archer who treated his wife in Nov 1822 and a child in Dec 1822 and was visited by Dr. Alonzo Preston who treated John Ward several times in Apr 1826, Master Brison in May 1826, Richards Jr. *(sic)* and a black woman in June 1826, Master Poor in Jul 1826, Master Poke and a black woman in Aug 1826, a black child and Master Wilkins in Nov 1826, a black child and W. Finley in Jan 1827, C. Levering, Master Beal in June and July 1827, a black boy named Charles in Aug and Sep 1827 and Oct 1828, George Finley in 1827, "a young man" in Sep 1827, a black child and a servant (both not named) in Apr 1828 and an unnamed child in May 1828; visited by Dr. Robert H. Archer who treated daughter Harriet in May 1826, daughter Mary in Jun 1826, a negro in July 1827, L. Richards in Oct 1827, daughter Ellen in June 1828, and Diffenderfer *(sic)* and Defender *(sic)* in Sep 1828 (Dr. Preston, pp. 73, 92; Dr. Archer, pp. 39, 40, 41, 180, 184, 185, 190, 240, 249, 280, 295; Dr. Archer, Ledger F, p. 41)

Davis, William, was treated by Dr. John Archer in Jun 1782 and Aug 1783 (Ledger D, p. 90)

Dawes, Elisha, at Josiah Lee's, was treated by Dr. John Archer in Apr 1778, Dec 1779 and Sep 1783 (Ledger C, p. 106, spelled his name Daws and noted "paid by a guinea rec'd. of Henry Waters" on 4 Nov 1789 and the balance of the "debt forgiven by order of testator") [Elisha Dawes might actually be Elijah Dawes who was a Revolutionary War veteran who died circa 1788.]

Dawes, Mordecai, near Winter's Run, was treated in Sep 1786 by Dr. John Archer (Ledger F, p. 67, misspelled his name Doz)

Dawes, William, appeared on a list of debts dated 26 Dec 1822 and titled "A List of Allen's Claims" that were due and payable to Dr. Richard N. Allen for services rendered [no dates] by him to said Dawes (Document filed in Historical Society of Harford County Archives folder "R. N. Allen")

Dawson, Jesse (blacksmith), was treated by Dr. John Archer in Jun 1790 (Ledger F, p. 231) [account continued in Ledger G, which is missing]

Day, Dr., was consulted by Dr. John Archer in 1790 (Ledger F, p. 378)

Day, I. (Ishmael), see William Paca, William Preston, Moses Preston, James Moffitt, Prush Bond, George Haughey, Hughy Haughey, Robert Cantling, Abram Cooper, Robert Boarman, Thomas Grier, Andrew Redding, George Wilgis and Jacob James q.v.

Day, John, at Edward Hanson's, was treated by Dr. John Archer in Apr 1788 (Ledger F, p. 158)

Day, Joshua, son-in-law to Edward Hanson, was treated by Dr. John Archer in Apr 1788 and Nov 1789 (Ledger F, pp. 256, 260) [account continued in Ledger K, which is missing]

Deacon, Francis, "near the church," was treated by Dr. John Archer in Feb 1773 (Ledger B, p. 10, noted as "dead and insolvent," but gave no date of death)

Dead, Emmory (colored), was treated by Dr. Matthew J. Allen in May 1844 (p. 33, noted "good for nothing" and was not clear whether Emmory was dead or if his name was Emmory Dead)

Dean, Nathan, was treated by Dr. Alonzo Preston in 1825 (p. 42)

Deaver, also see Dever, q.v.

Deaver, Aquila [1756-c1830], was treated by Dr. John Archer in Aug 1795 (Ledger F, p. 325, stated his security was James Deaver) [Aquila Deaver was a Revolutionary War veteran.]

Deaver, Andrew, see John Clark, q.v.

Deaver, David, on Deer Creek, was visited by Dr. John Archer who treated him and his wife in 1798 and 1799 (Ledger I, which is missing, was abstracted by Dr. George W. Archer circa 1890; his notes are in the Archives of the Historical Society of Harford County folder "Archer, G. W. Coll. – Ledgers and Day Books") [David Deaver was a Revolutionary War veteran.]

Deaver, James, was visited by Dr. John Archer who treated him and his wife in Jul 1793 (Ledger F, p. 324) [account continued in Ledger H, which is missing] [One of two men named James Deaver who were Revolutionary War veterans.]; see Aquila Deaver, q.v.

Deaver, James, "in the [or York?] Barrens, philosopher, wolf-catcher and Jim-boy" *(sic)*, was visited by Dr. John Archer who treated him and his family at times between 1796 and 1800 (Ledger I, which is missing, was abstracted by Dr. George W. Archer circa 1890; his notes are in the Archives of the Historical Society of Harford County folder "Archer, G. W. Coll. – Ledgers and Day Books") [Two men named James Deaver were Revolutionary War veterans.]

Deaver, Polly, was inoculated by Dr. John Archer in Feb 1782 (Ledger D, p. 96, noted "debt forgiven as before")

Deaver, Stephen, was treated by Dr. Robert H. Archer in Baltimore before 1822 [no dates or details were given] (Dr. Archer's "Alphabet to Ledger H" is his booklet [filed in the Archives of the Historical Society of Harford County] that contains his index to Ledger H [which is missing] for his patients in Baltimore before 1822 and Harford County after 1822, according to a notation by Dr. George W. Archer.)

Debruler, James, near Isaac Webster's, was visited by Dr. John Archer who treated his wife in Oct 1777 (Ledger C, p. 97, noted "debt forgiven by order of testator")

Dedricks, Rev. Mr., see Ignatius Matthews, q.v.

Defender, see Reuben H. Davis, q.v.

Deladehat, Monsr., at Abingdon, was treated by Dr. John Archer in 1795 (Ledger I, which is missing, was abstracted by Dr. George W. Archer circa 1890; his notes are in Archives of the Historical Society of Harford County file "Archer, G. W. Coll. - Ledgers and Day Books")

Delcher, Christian, was treated by Dr. Robert H. Archer in Baltimore before 1822 [no dates or details were given] (Dr. Archer's "Alphabet to Ledger H" is his booklet [filed in the Archives of the Historical Society of Harford County] that contains his index to Ledger H [which is missing] for his patients in Baltimore before 1822 and Harford County after 1822, according to a notation by Dr. George W. Archer.)

Delehat, Miss, was prescribed medicine by Dr. Robert H. Archer on 23 Jun 1799 (Rx Book, 1796-1801, p. 22)

Deling, George, had an account in Dr. John Archer's ledger before 1772 [no details from the previous ledger except he owed £0.17.6] and no other entries were made in this ledger (Ledger B, p. 21)

Dellam, Mrs., see Bennett Matthews, q.v.

Dempsey Luke, was treated by Dr. Robert H. Archer in Baltimore before 1822 [no dates or details were given] (Dr. Archer's "Alphabet to Ledger H" is his booklet [filed in the Archives of the Historical Society of Harford County] that contains his index to Ledger H [which is missing] for his patients in Baltimore City before 1822 and in Harford County after 1822, according to a notation by Dr. George W. Archer.)

Deniston, James, was treated by Dr. John Archer before 1772 [no details given] (Ledger B, p. 20)

Dennison, Barbara, see William Dennison, q.v.

Dennison, Gideon, was treated by Dr. John Archer at various times between 1797 and 1799 (Ledger I, which is missing, was abstracted by Dr. George W. Archer circa 1890 and spelled his name Denison; Dr. George W. Archer's notes are in the Archives of the Historical Society of Harford County file "Archer, G. W. Coll. – Ledgers and Day Books")

Dennison, James, at Samuel Wilson's, was treated by Dr. John Archer in Jul 1787 (Ledger F, p. 179)

Dennison, Marcus (grocer), in Baltimore, was mentioned in Dr. Robert H. Archer's medical ledger in a non-medical matter in Oct 1826 and Jun 1827 (pp. 207, 234, spelled his name Denison)

Dennison, William, was visited by Dr. John Archer, Jr. who treated him, his wife and a child in Jul 1817, his wife in Jan 1821 and daughter Barbara in Jun 1821; also noted that his son William was "hired" by Dr. Archer in Jul 1818 (p. 37)

Denny, Michael, was treated by Dr. John Archer in Sep 1778, Oct 1780 and Nov 1780 and Aug 1781 (Ledger C, p. 120) [account continued in Ledger G, which is missing]

Denny, Mrs., widow of Simon, was treated by Dr. John Archer in Oct 1791 (Ledger F, p. 178)

Denny, Simon, was visited by Dr. John Archer who inoculated 8 of his family in Feb 1776 (Ledger C, p. 29, noted the bill was paid "for a cow and twenty shillings ready money"); see Mrs. Denny and George Brown, q.v.

Dermot, James, was treated by Dr. John Archer in Aug 1781 (Ledger D, p. 66, noted "debt forgiven as before")

Develin, Mr., was prescribed medicine by Dr. Robert H. Archer on 17 Sep 1803 (Rx Book, 1802-1804, p. 56)

Dever, see Frances Osborn and also see Deaver, q.v.

Dever, Hugh [1752-1787], was treated by Dr. John Archer in Jul 1780, Apr 1781, Jun and Aug 1782, and Aug 1783 (Ledger D, p. 79) [account continued in Ledger G, which is missing] [Hugh Dever was a Revolutionary War veteran.]

Dever, Hugh, was visited by Dr. James Archer who treated him and his family fourteen times during Aug and Sep 1806 and also noted "particu. on account of son Robert, in consultation with Dr. Bryarly" (p. 10); see Benjamin Bayless, q.v.

Dever, Mrs., "near X roads," sister of Col. William Smith, was treated by Dr. Robert H. Archer in Aug 1826 and in July 1827 (pp. 197, 238, 239, 240)

Dever, Robert, was visited by Dr. Robert H. Archer who treated a child in Oct 1822 and a child in Aug 1827 (pp. 31, 242; Ledger F, p. 112); see Hugh Dever, q.v.

Devin, Catherine, was treated by Dr. John Archer in June 1786 (Ledger F, p. 331)

Devin, Hugh, near James Rigbie's place, was visited by Dr. John Archer who treated his children [no names were given] in Aug 1781 (Ledger D, p. 57, noted "debt forgiven as before")

Devoe, Hugh (blacksmith), near Hickory Tavern, was treated by Dr. John Archer in 1794 [no dates were given] for apoplexy [stroke] (Ledger I, which is missing, was abstracted by Dr. George W. Archer circa 1890; his notes are in the Archives of the Historical Society of Harford County folder "Archer, G. W. Coll. – Ledgers and Day Books")

Devoe, John, "O Town" [Old Town], was treated by Dr. Robert H. Archer in Baltimore before 1822 [no dates or details were given] (Dr. Archer's "Alphabet to Ledger H" is his booklet [filed in the Archives of the Historical Society of Harford County] that contains his index to Ledger H [which is missing] for his patients in Baltimore City before 1822 and in Harford County after 1822, according to a notation by Dr. George W. Archer.)

Dew, Mrs. (widow), was treated by Dr. Robert H. Archer in Baltimore before 1822 [no dates or details were given] (Dr. Archer's "Alphabet to Ledger H" is his booklet [filed in the Archives of the Historical Society of Harford County] that contains his index to Ledger H [which is missing] for his patients in Baltimore City before 1822 and in Harford County after 1822, according to a notation by Dr. George W. Archer.)

Dewitt, Mr., was prescribed medicine for his child by Dr. Robert H. Archer on 25 Aug 1802 and 14 Dec 1804 (Rx Book, 1802-1804, pp. 16, 66)

Dewitt, Thomas, was prescribed medicine by Dr. Robert H. Archer on 27 Dec 1802 (Rx Book, 1802-1804, p. 28)

Dick, David, Dr., see Thaddeus Jewett, q.v.

Dick, James, was treated by Dr. Matthew J. Allen in Jun 1845 (p. 49, noted that he paid $1.00 of the $1.25 bill "by cash" on 8 Dec 1852)

Dickson, Benjamin, was treated by Dr. John Archer in May 1778 and Nov 1781 (Ledger C, p. 58, noted "debt forgiven by order of testator"); see Samuel Willet, q.v.

Dickson, David, was visited by Dr. John Archer who treated him in Feb and Jun 1773, his wife in Jul and Sep 1773, him in Jul 1774, his wife in Nov 1774, an infant in Feb 1775, his wife in Mar 1775, him in Apr and Sep 1775; mentioned "assumption for Janey Creswell" in Mar 1777 and treated him [David] 15 times between 15 Apr 1778 and 29 Oct 1778 (Ledger B, p. 11; Ledger C, p. 85) [David Dickson was a Revolutionary War veteran.]

Dickson, James, see Samuel Willet, q.v.

Dickson, Jane (widow), was visited by Dr. John Archer who treated a child in 1781 [exact date was not given] (Ledger D, p. 52, noted "debt forgiven")

Dickson, John, see Sally Dickson, q.v.

Dickson, Maurice or Morris, see Sally Dickson, q.v.

Dickson, Mrs., see Polly Moore, q.v.

Dickson, Peter, see Peter Dixon, q.v.

Dickson, Sally, daughter of Maurice or Morris Dickson, on Bush River Neck, was treated by Dr. John Archer in Nov 1788 (Ledger F, p. 285, stated John Dickson was security; 1776 Census)

Didier, Mr., was prescribed medicine for his child by Dr. Robert H. Archer on 31 Jul 1796 (Rx Book, 1796-1801, p. 7)

Diemer, John, was visited by Dr. John Archer who treated his mother and wife in Feb 1774 in consultation with Dr. Annan, him in Nov 1779 and Apr 1782, him and his wife in May 1782, his wife in Jun 1782, a negro (dressed a wound) in Jun 1782, and him [John] in Jun 1790 (Ledger B, p. 61; Ledger D, p. 37 [account continued in Ledger E, which is missing]; Ledger F, p. 30) [John Diemer was a Revolutionary War veteran.]

Diffenderfer, see Reuben H. Davis, q.v.

Dill, Hannah, Miss, at Ring Factory [on Winters Run, west of Bel Air], was treated by Dr. Matthew J. Allen in Dec 1847 (tooth extraction) (p. 70)

Dillon, George, was visited by Dr. John Archer who treated his wife in Jun 1778, him in Feb and Nov 1779 and Sep 1780, and him and a child in Jun 1788 (Ledger C, p. 114, noted "debt forgiven by order of testator;" Ledger F, p. 360, spelled his name Dillan)

Dimsey, Patrick, at Widow Smith's Mill, was treated by Dr. John Archer in Sep 1788 (Ledger F, p. 281)

Dinen, Judett, Miss, was treated by Dr. Robert H. Archer after 1822 [no dates or details were given] (Dr. Archer's "Alphabet to Ledger H" is his booklet [filed in the Archives of the Historical Society of Harford County] that contains his index to Ledger H [which is missing] for his patients in Baltimore before 1822 and Harford County after 1822, according to a notation by Dr. George W. Archer.)

Dines, Mrs. (widow), was treated by Dr. John Archer in May 1783 and Dec 1786 (Ledger D, p. 2, noted "debt forgiven as before;" Ledger F, p. 170); see James Hughes, q.v.

Dinsmore, Jos.(?), was treated by Dr. John Archer, Jr. in Dec 1816 (p. 11)

Diver, Joseph, was treated by Dr. John Archer in Sep 1787 (Ledger F, p. 10)

Divers, Holland, was visited by Dr. Matthew J. Allen who treated his wife in Feb 1844 (p. 32)

Divers, W. Holland, was visited by Dr. Robert H. Archer who treated his wife "in partu" [in childbirth] on the night of 31 Aug 1828 (p. 295)

Divin, John, was treated by Dr. John Archer in 1787 (Ledger F, p. 198)

Divin, Michael (weaver), was visited by Dr. John Archer who treated him and a child in Feb 1789 (Ledger F, p. 307)

Divis, William, was visited by Dr. John Archer who treated him and his wife and a child in Mar 1793 (Ledger F, p. 343)

Dixon, see Dickson, q.v.

Dixon, ---- [blank], was treated by Dr. Robert H. Archer in Baltimore before 1822 [no dates or details were given] (Dr. Archer's "Alphabet to Ledger H" is his booklet [filed in the Archives of the Historical Society of Harford County] that contains his index to Ledger H [which is missing] for his patients in Baltimore before 1822 and Harford County after 1822, according to a notation by Dr. George W. Archer.)

Dixon, Peter, "in the Neck near Phillips," was treated by Dr. John Archer in May 1779 (Ledger C, p. 107, noted "debt forgiven by order of testator")

Dobbins, James, was treated by Dr. John Archer in July 1779 (Ledger C, p. 126, noted "debt forgiven by order of testator")

Dockson, Jacob, was visited by Dr. Matthew J. Allen who treated his wife and son in Feb 1844 and rendered obstetrical services to his wife on 31 Jul 1845 (p. 31, noted $5 paid "by cash per Mr. Wann" and "son Kinsey's acct. fr. Fol. 42")

Dockson, Kinsey, was treated by Dr. Matthew J. Allen in Jan 1845 (p. 42); see Jacob Dockson, q.v.

Doherty, Samuel, was prescribed medicine for his wife by Dr. Robert Archer on 22 May 1796 (Rx Book, 1796-1801, p. 5)

Dohorty, Samuel, was treated by Dr. John Archer in Oct 1789 (Ledger F, p. 312) [account continued in Ledger H, which is missing]

Donahoo, Daniel, was visited by Dr. John Archer who treated his wife and also inoculated him in Sep 1779 (Ledger D, p. 11, misspelled his name as Donahow) [Daniel Donahoo was a War of 1812 veteran.]

Donahoo, John [1786-1858] (mason), was treated by Dr. John Archer, Jr. in Aug 1815 (p. 20)

Donn, Capt., in Havre de Grace, was visited by Dr. John Archer who treated him and his family [no names were given] in 1797 (Ledger I, which is missing, was abstracted by Dr. George W. Archer circa 1890; his notes are in the Archives of the Historical Society of Harford County folder "Archer, G. W. Coll. – Ledgers and Day Books")

Donn, Mary Ann, see Jackson & Fox, q.v.

Donovan, see Dunnavin and Dunovan, q.v.

Donovan, Thomas, was treated by Dr. John Archer in Apr 1787 (Ledger F, p. 261)

Doran, Hugh, near Samuel Ashmead's, was treated by Dr. John Archer in Apr 1778 (Ledger C, p. 107, misspelled his name Dorand and noted "debt forgiven by order of testator")

Dorney, John, was treated by Dr. Robert H. Archer in Baltimore before 1822 [no dates or details were given] (Dr. Archer's "Alphabet to Ledger H" is his booklet [filed in the Archives of the Historical Society of Harford County] that contains his index to Ledger H [which is missing] for his patients in Baltimore before 1822 and Harford County after 1822, according to a notation by Dr. George W. Archer.)

Dorney, William, was treated by Dr. Robert H. Archer in Baltimore before 1822 [no dates or details were given] (Dr. Archer's "Alphabet to Ledger H" is his booklet [filed in the Archives of the Historical Society of Harford County] that contains his index to Ledger H [which is missing] for his patients in Baltimore before 1822 and Harford County after 1822, according to a notation by Dr. George W. Archer.)

Dorsey, Caleb, see John Ireland, q.v.

Dorsey, Charlotte, see Sarah Dorsey, q.v.

Dorsey, Col., see Walter Farnandis, q.v.

Dorsey, Dr., see Aaron Allen and William W. Lawrence, q.v.

Dorsey, Edward, of Greenberry, see William Luster, q.v.

Dorsey, Frisby, was treated by Dr. John Archer in Mar 1790 (Ledger F, p. 318) [account continued in Ledger H, which is missing] [Frisby Dorsey was a Revolutionary War veteran.]

Dorsey, Greenberry [1729-1789], was treated by Dr. John Archer in Jul 1788 (Ledger F, p. 152, misspelled his name Greenbury) [account continued in Ledger G, which is missing] [Greenberry Dorsey was a Revolutionary War veteran and a signer of the Bush Declaration on March 22, 1775.]; see Frances Copeland, q.v.

Dorsey, Harry (lawyer), Bel Air, was visited by Dr. John Archer who treated him at times between 1794 and 1798 [no dates were given] (Ledger I, which is missing, was abstracted by Dr. George W. Archer circa 1890; his notes are in the Archives of the Historical Society of Harford County folder "Archer, G. W. Coll. – Ledgers and Day Books")

Dorsey, Henry [c1770-1846], was visited by Dr. Alonzo Preston who treated him at times between 1823 and 1827 [no details were given], his wife and James in 1825, his children and family at times between 1825 and 1827, Water Fernandis [Walter Farnandis] twenty times in 1826 and 1827, a black woman and a black boy in 1827 (pp. 30, 90, noting the bill totaled $24.83: "This account to be credited with $10 paid in the winter of 1828-9 as recollected by Mrs. Preston, 11 June 1829" and it was initialed by "W.B.B., admr." [referring to Dr. William B. Bond] and the remainder of the bill was paid in full on 21 Jul 1830. [Henry Dorsey was a War of 1812 veteran.]

Dorsey, John H. [1754-1826], was visited by Dr. Richard Sappington who treated his wife in Feb 1801 (Document filed in Historical Society of Harford County Archives folder "Sappington, Dr. Richard – Accounts, 1783-1830") [John Hammond Dorsey was a Revolutionary War veteran.]

Dorsey, Mr., see Christianna Lancaster and Christianna McKenney, q.v.

Dorsey, Mrs., see James Metcalf, q.v.

Dorsey, Sarah, Mrs., was visited by Dr. Matthew J. Allen who treated Charlotte nine times in Feb and Mar 1848 (p. 74)

Dorsey, Samuel, in Baltimore, son-in-law to Mrs. Preston, was visited by Dr. John Archer who treated him and his family in 1797 (Ledger I, which is missing, was abstracted by Dr. George W. Archer circa 1890; his notes are in the Archives of the Historical Society of Harford County folder "Archer, G. W. Coll. – Ledgers and Day Books"); he was also treated by Dr. Robert H. Archer in Baltimore before 1822 [no dates or details were given] (Dr. Archer's "Alphabet to Ledger H" is his booklet [filed in the Archives of the Historical Society of Harford County] that contains his index to Ledger H [which is missing] for his patients in Baltimore City before 1822 and in Harford County after 1822, according to a notation by Dr. George W. Archer.)

Dorsey, Stephen H. [1758-1825], was treated by Dr. John Archer in Mar 1786 (Ledger F, p. 30) [Stephen Dorsey was a Revolutionary War veteran.]

Dorsey, Thomas, see Robert Sanders (Saunders), q.v.

54

Dorsey, Walter, was visited by Dr. Matthew J. Allen who treated him and Mrs. Dorsey in 1832 in Calvert County (p. 23); see Cyrus Osborn, q.v.

Downey, John, was treated by Dr. John Archer in Aug 1789 (Ledger F, p. 171) [John Downey was a Revolutionary War veteran.]

Downey, Richard, was treated by Dr. John Archer in Sep 1773 (Ledger B, p. 74)

Downfield, George, was treated by Dr. Matthew J. Allen in Mar 1845 (tooth extraction) (p. 47)

Downing, Samuel, was treated by Dr. John Archer in July 1787 (Ledger F, p. 348)

Downing, William, was visited by Dr. John Archer who treated a child in Dec 1779 and Jul 1780, his wife in Dec 1780, Mar and Sep 1785 and in 1786, and him in 1791 (Ledger D, p. 38, noted "debt forgiven as before" and "gone to the western country," but did not give the date of departure; Ledger F, p. 115) [William Downing was a War of 1812 veteran.]

Downs, Henry, was prescribed medicine by Dr. Robert H. Archer on 26 Nov 1802 (Rx Book, 1802-1804, p. 26)

Downs, Samuel, near Upper Cross Roads, was treated by Dr. John Archer in 1788 (Ledger F, p. 239)

Downs, Thomas, was treated by Dr. John Archer in Nov 1785 (Ledger D, p. 35, noted "debt forgiven as before")

Downs, William, was treated by Dr. John Archer in 1789 (Ledger F, p. 114) [account continued in Ledger G, which is missing] [William Downs was a Revolutionary War veteran.]

Doyne, Robert, was treated by Dr. Robert H. Archer in Baltimore before 1822 [no dates or details were given] (Dr. Archer's "Alphabet to Ledger H" is his booklet [filed in the Archives of the Historical Society of Harford County] that contains his index to Ledger H [which is missing] for his patients in Baltimore before 1822 and Harford County after 1822, according to a notation by Dr. George W. Archer.)

Drew, Anthony, see Henry Drew, q.v.

Drew, George, was visited by Dr. John Archer who treated him and his wife in 1787 (Ledger F, p. 58) [George Drew was a Revolutionary War veteran.]; see James Resin, q.v.

Drew, Henry, was treated by Dr. John Archer in 1787 (Ledger F, p. 183, stated his security was Anthony Drew)

Drummond, Thomas, was treated by Dr. John Archer in Oct 1780 (Ledger D, p. 98, noted "debt forgiven as before")

Dryden, Michel (sic), was treated by Dr. Robert H. Archer in Baltimore before 1822 [no dates or details were given] (Dr. Archer's "Alphabet to Ledger H" is his booklet [filed in the Archives of the Historical Society of Harford County] that contains his index to Ledger H [which is missing] for his patients in Baltimore before 1822 and in Harford County after 1822, according to a notation by Dr. George W. Archer.)

Dryden, Mr., was prescribed medicine by Dr. Robert H. Archer on 7 Jul 1803 (Rx Book, 1802-1804, p. 48)

Dryden, Mylly, was prescribed medicine "for Boy" by Dr. Robert H. Archer on 8 Jul 1803 and medicine ("strengthening pills") for her sister [name not given] on 13 Sep 1803, medicine for a child on 13 Oct 1804 and medicine for herself [Mylly] on 17 Oct 1804 and also circa Dec 1804 (Rx Book, 1802-1804, pp. 49, 55, 58, 59, 75)

Dubree, Joseph, "at D. Lee's Mill, L. Falls" [i.e., David Lee's Jerusalem Mill on Little Gunpowder River], was treated by Dr. John Archer in Jan 1786 (Ledger F, p. 51)

Dubroceur, Monsr., Frenchman, at Mr. Husbands', was treated by Dr. John Archer in 1796 (Ledger I, which is missing, was abstracted by Dr. George W. Archer circa 1890; his notes are in Archives of Historical Society of Harford County folder "Archer, G. W. Coll. – Ledgers and Day Books")

Duff, Miss, was prescribed medicine by Dr. Robert H. Archer on 21 Sep 1828 (Rx Book, 1825-1851, p. 92)

Duff, Thomas, was visited by Dr. Matthew J. Allen who treated a child in Aug 1844, his wife in Jun 1847, a child in Jul 1847, his wife and child in Aug 1847 and children (teeth extractions) in Jun 1848 (pp. 38, 54; p. 88 spelled his name Duft) [Thomas Duff was a Revolutionary War veteran.]

Duit, Nancy, was treated by Dr. John Archer in 1786 (Ledger F, p. 116)

Duly, William, was treated by Dr. Robert T. Allen in Mar and Sep 1822 (Document filed in Historical Society of Harford County Archives folder "R. N. Allen") [William Duly was a Revolutionary War veteran.]

Dun, William, see William Hopkins, Jr., q.v.

Duncan, Major, was treated by Dr. Robert H. Archer in Baltimore before 1822 [no dates or details were given] (Dr. Archer's "Alphabet to Ledger H" is his booklet [filed in the Archives of the Historical Society of Harford County] that contains his index to Ledger H [which is missing] for his patients in Baltimore before 1822 and Harford County after 1822, according to a notation by Dr. George W. Archer.)

Dungan, Thomas, was treated by Dr. John Archer in May 1782 (Ledger D, p. 34, noted the "debt forgiven as before")

Dungin, Benjamin, near Quaker Meeting House, was treated by Dr. John Archer in 1798 (Ledger I, which is missing, was abstracted by Dr. George W. Archer circa 1890; his notes are in the Archives of the Historical Society of Harford County file "Archer, G. W. Coll. – Ledgers and Day Books")

Dunn, Diggins, see John Dunn, q.v.

Dunn, John (saddler), was visited by Dr. John Archer who treated a child in Feb 1782, son Diggins in 1788 and him [John] in 1794 (Ledger C, p. 86; Ledger F, p. 257)

Dunnavin, Daniel, was visited by Dr. John Archer who treated him in Jul and Aug 1778; he also inoculated daughter Rachel in 1777 (Ledger C, p. 83; spelled his name Dunnavan); see William Judd and John Sullivan, q.v.

Dunnavin, John, was inoculated by Dr. John Archer in 1777 [no exact date] (Ledger C, p. 83, spelled his name Dunnavan and noted "debt forgiven by order of testator")

Dunnavin, Philip, was treated by Dr. John Archer in Aug 1787 (Ledger F, p. 349, spelled his name Dunavin)

Dunnavin, William, was visited by Dr. John Archer who treated him and a child in Sep 1786 (Ledger F, p. 59)

Dunning, James (schoolmaster), was treated by Dr. John Archer in 1794 and 1795 (Ledger I, which is missing, was abstracted by Dr. George W. Archer circa 1890; his notes are in the Archives of the Historical Society of Harford County folder "Archer, G. W. Coll. – Ledgers and Day Books")

Dunovan, John, was treated by Dr. Robert H. Archer in Baltimore before 1822 [no dates or details were given] (Dr. Archer's "Alphabet to Ledger H" is his booklet [filed in the Archives of the Historical Society of Harford County] that contains his index to Ledger H [which is missing] for his patients in Baltimore before 1822 and Harford County after 1822, according to a notation by Dr. George W. Archer.)

Durbin, Francis, was treated by Dr. John Archer before 1772 [no dates or details were given] and in Feb 1773 (Ledger B, p. 19) [Francis Durbin was a War of 1812 veteran.]

Durbin, Mary, was treated by Dr. John Archer in Oct 1773 (Ledger B, p. 10)

Durbin, Mrs., widow of Thomas, was treated by Dr. John Archer in Oct 1788 (Ledger F, p. 341) [account continued in Ledger G, which is missing]

Durbin, Thomas, see John Wood and Mrs. Durbin, q.v.

Durbin, William, was treated by Dr. John Archer in Dec 1776 (Ledger C, p. 66, noted "debt forgiven by order of testator")

Durham, ----, see James Ratican (Ratigan), q.v.

Durham, Ann, Mrs., was visited by Dr. John Archer who treated her daughter Charlotte in 1797 (Ledger I, which is missing, was abstracted by Dr. George W. Archer circa 1890; his notes are in the Archives of the Historical Society of Harford County folder "Archer, G. W. Coll. – Ledgers and Day Books")

Durham, Aquila, was visited by Dr. John Archer who treated him in Jul 1776 and Jan 1777 and his mother in Apr 1782 and Jan 1783 (Ledger C, p. 52, noted "debt forgiven by order of testator") [Aquila Durham was a Revolutionary War veteran.]; see Mrs. Durham, q.v.

Durham, Aquila (doctor), was treated by Dr. John Archer in Nov 1796 and May 1797 (Ledger I, which is missing, was abstracted by Dr. George W. Archer circa 1890 and noted the debt was "forgiven;" Dr. George W. Archer's notes are in Archives of the Historical Society of Harford County folder "Archer, G. W. Coll. – Ledgers and Day Books")

Durham, Charlotte, see Ann Durham, q.v.

Durham, Mrs., widow of Samuel, was visited by Dr. John Archer who treated her and son Aquila in 1788 and daughters Susan and Nelly in 1789 (Ledger F, pp. 7, 173)

Durham, Nelly, see Mrs. Durham, q.v.

Durham, Samuel, was treated by Dr. John Archer in Nov 1786 and Samuel, son of Samuel, was treated in Sep 1791 (Ledger F, pp. 61, 175) [Samuel Durham was a Revolutionary War veteran.]; see Mrs. Durham, q.v.

Durham, Susan, see Mrs. Durham, q.v.

Durham, Thomas, was prescribed medicine for a negro by Dr. Robert H. Archer on 8 Aug 1802 and for Thomas' child on 8 May 1803 (Rx Book, 1802-1804, pp. 8, 42); see Daniel Smithson, q.v.

Duzan or Cousins (sic), Robert, was treated by Dr. John Archer in Oct-Nov 1774 (Ledger B, p. 54)

Duzan, Alexander, was treated by Dr. John Archer in July 1791 (Ledger F, p. 43, stated Alexander moved to Kentucky [no date of departure was given] and his brother John paid his medical bill in 1793); see John Duzan, q.v.

Duzan, Jacob, in Bush River Neck, was treated by Dr. John Archer in 1787 (Ledger F, p. 38) [Jacob Duzan or Duzans was a Revolutionary War veteran.]

Duzan, John, was treated by Dr. John Archer in 1791 (Ledger F, p. 98, stated he paid his bill and his brother Alexander's bill in 1793 and moved to Kentucky); see Alexander Duzan, q.v.

Dyer, William, see William Karr, q.v.

Eagen (Eagens), James, in York Co., was treated by Dr. John Archer in Aug 1791 (Ledger F, p. 276); see Molly Craswell, q.v.

Earnest, George, was treated by Dr. Robert H. Archer in Sep 1815 (Ledger F, p. 12)

Eden, Richard &ca *(sic)*, was treated by Dr. Robert H. Archer in Baltimore before 1822 [no dates or details were given] (Dr. Archer's "Alphabet to Ledger H" is his booklet [filed in the Archives of the Historical Society of Harford County] that contains his index to Ledger H [which is missing] for his patients in Baltimore before 1822 and Harford County after 1822, according to a notation by Dr. George W. Archer.)

Eden, William, near Abingdon, was visited by Dr. John Archer who treated him, his wife and a child in 1789 (Ledger F, p. 147) [account continued in Ledger G, which is missing]

Eddy, William, see Vincent Richardson, q.v.

Edwards, James, was treated by Dr. Robert H. Archer in Baltimore before 1822 [no dates or details were given] (Dr. Archer's "Alphabet to Ledger H" is his booklet [filed in the Archives of the Historical Society of Harford County] that contains his index to Ledger H [which is missing] for his patients in Baltimore before 1822 and Harford County after 1822, according to a notation by Dr. George W. Archer.)

Edwards, John, was treated by Dr. Robert H. Archer in Baltimore before 1822 [no dates or details were given] (Dr. Archer's "Alphabet to Ledger H" is his booklet [filed in the Archives of the Historical Society of Harford County] that contains his index to Ledger H [which is missing] for his patients in Baltimore before 1822 and Harford County after 1822, according to a notation by Dr. George W. Archer.)

Edwards, Joseph, at Ring Factory [on Winters Run, west of Bel Air], was treated by Dr. Matthew J. Allen for a head wound in Sep 1847 (p. 65)

Edy, William, see Bazil Buckingham, q.v.

Ellet, Mr., was prescribed medicine for his sister by Dr. Robert H. Archer on 24 Jan 1801 (Rx Book, 1796-1801, p. 28)

Ellice, Ellice, see Alexander Murray, q.v.

Elliot, Edward, see Sucky Waldron, q.v.

Elliot, John, see John Gregg & Co., q.v.

Elliot, Sally, see Harford County for Pensioners, q.v.

Elliott, James, was treated by Dr. John Archer in Jul, Aug and Oct 1780 (Ledger D, p. 83, spelled his name Ellot)

Elliott, Mrs. (widow), above Trapp [i. e. Trappe, an area south of Dublin, west of Darlington, near Trappe Church], was visited by Dr. John Archer who treated her and a grandchild in 1795 (Ledger F, p. 346, spelled her name Elliot)

Elliott, Robert [1742-1820s], was visit by Dr. Alonzo Preston who treated his wife in 1825 and him in 1826 (p. 34, spelled his name Elliot) [Robert Elliott or Elliot was a War of 1812 veteran.]

Elliott, Samuel, near James Clendennin's, was visited by Dr. John Archer who treated him and his wife in 1791 (Ledger F, p. 377, listed the names as Elliot and Clendennon) [Samuel Elliott (1757-1841) and Samuel Elliott (1748-1795) were both Revolutionary War veterans.]

Elliott, Thomas [1749-1820s], was inoculated by Dr. John Archer in Jan 1776 (Ledger C, p. 6) [Thomas Elliott was a Revolutionary War veteran.]

Elliott, Thomas, "at Wia. *(sic)* near Trap" [i. e., Trappe, an area west of Darlington, near Trappe Church], was treated by Dr. John Archer in July 1787 (Ledger F, p. 354, spelled his name Elliot)

Elliott, Widow, see John Fleharty and Mrs. Elliott, q.v.

Ellis, Catherine, Miss, was visited by Dr. James Archer who treated her five times in July and Aug 1805 with "various medicines and bleedings" as treatment for "pneumonicula" (p. 11)

Ellis, John (farmer), "on Lord's Gift," was visited by Dr. John Archer who treated an infant, aunt Margaret Gardner, and Monohon *(sic)* in Jan 1775 (Ledger B, p. 22)

Ellis, John (tailor), was visited by Dr. John Archer who treated him and son Samuel, Joseph and William at various times between 1796 and 1801 (Ledger I, which is missing, was abstracted by Dr. George W. Archer circa 1890; his notes are in the Archives of the Historical Society of Harford County folder "Archer, G. W. Coll. – Ledgers and Day Books")

Ellis, John, was visited by Dr. John Archer who treated him, his wife and a child in 1789 (Ledger F, p. 142) [account continued in Ledger G, which is missing]

Ellis, Joseph, see John Ellis (tailor), q.v.

Ellis, Samuel, see John Ellis (tailor), q.v.

Ellis, William, see John Ellis (tailor), q.v.

Emmerson, James, was prescribed medicine for his child on 2 Jul 1803 by Dr. Robert H. Archer (Rx Book, 1802-1804, p. 46)

Emmory, John, was listed in Dr. Matthew J. Allen's ledger in a non-medical matter in 1844 (p. 39)

Empy, Sarah (negro), was treated by Dr. Robert H. Archer in Baltimore before 1822 [no dates or details were given] (Dr. Archer's "Alphabet to Ledger H" is his booklet [filed in the Archives of the Historical Society of Harford County] that contains his index to Ledger H [which is missing] for his patients in Baltimore before 1822 and Harford County after 1822, according to a notation by Dr. George W. Archer.)

England, John, see Aquila Preston, q.v.

English gentleman *(sic)*, was prescribed medicine by Dr. Robert H. Archer on 17 Nov 1804 (Rx Book, 1802-1804, p. 61)

Enlows, James [1756-1822], "near White Hall" [actually lived near White House in Fallston], was visited by Dr. John Archer who treated him and son Thomas at various times between 1797 and 1801 (Ledger I, which is missing, was abstracted by Dr. George W. Archer circa 1890; his notes are in the Archives of the Historical Society of Harford County folder "Archer, G. W. Coll. – Ledgers and Day Books" spelled his name Enlow)

Ennis, Thomas, was treated by Dr. Robert H. Archer in Baltimore before 1822 [no dates or details were given] (Dr. Archer's "Alphabet to Ledger H" is his booklet [filed in the Archives of the Historical Society of Harford County] that contains his index to Ledger H [which is missing] for his patients in Baltimore before 1822 and Harford County after 1822, according to a notation by Dr. George W. Archer.)

Ensor, William, "near the X Roads," was visited by Dr. John Archer who treated a son in Jan 1776, his wife and a negro man in Oct 1777, him [William] in Mar 1778 and Feb 1780, a son in Jan 1780, his wife in Dec 1781 and Sep and Oct 1782, and inoculated 9 of his family (Ledger C, pp. 7-8; Ledger D, p. 47, noted on 15 Sep 1785 "By an order on Jos. Gallion for £7.1.9 which when paid shall be credited")

Erskine, Cornelius, was treated by Dr. John Archer in Sep 1781 (Ledger D, p. 70, noted the "debt forgiven as before")

Erwin, James, was treated by Dr. John Archer in Jul and Aug 1781 (Ledger D, p. 32, noted the "debt forgiven as before")

Erwin, Mrs., was prescribed medicine by Dr. Robert H. Archer circa Dec 1804 [exact date not given] (Rx Book, 1802-1804, p. 70)

Evans, ---- [blank] (tailor), "at X Roads," was visited by Dr. Robert H. Archer who treated a child in June 1826 and his wife in June 1827 (Ledger F, p. 99)

Evans, Amos (plasterer), was treated by Dr. John Archer at various times between 1797 and 1799 (Ledger I, which is missing, was abstracted by Dr. George W. Archer circa 1890; his notes are in the Archives of the Historical Society of Harford County folder "Archer, G. W. Coll. – Ledgers and Day Books")

Evans, Evan, was visited by Dr. Alonzo Preston who treated his wife "in partu" [in childbirth] on 25 Dec 1824, a child on 2 Jan 1826, his family [names not given] in 1826 and a child in 1827 (p. 6) [Evan Evans was a War of 1812 veteran.]

Evans, James, on Robert Culver's place, was treated by Dr. John Archer in 1788 (Ledger F, p. 301)

Evans, James, was treated by Dr. John Archer, Jr. in Jan 1817; the account mentioned Robert Evans, executor, in Nov 1817 and James Evans in Jan 1818 (p. 16); see Lloyd Bailey, q.v.

Evans, James, of James, was visited by Dr. John Archer, Jr. who treated his wife and child in Jan 1817, son John in Apr 1817, a child in Feb 1818, his wife in May 1818 and Apr 1819, and him [James] in Jul 1818; also mentioned Thomas Patten paid in Jan 1818 and Lloyd Bailey paid in Dec 1819 (p. 68)

Evans, John, see James Evans, of James, q.v.

Evans, John, at John Forwood's, was treated by Dr. John Archer in Oct 1786 (Ledger F, p. 117, spelled his name Evins) [John Evans was a War of 1812 veteran.]

Evans, John, "directed to P. Cuming, son-in-law," was treated by Dr. John Archer in Dec 1777 (Ledger C, p. 80)

Evans, John, on Hopkins' place, was visited by Dr. Robert H. Archer who treated his child in June 1824, his wife in Apr 1839, and vaccinated three children [names not given] on 8 Jan 1834 (p. 115; Ledger F, p. 102)

Evans, John (plasterer), was mentioned by Dr. Robert H. Archer in a non-medical matter in May 1823 (Ledger F, p. 27)

58

Evans, John (tailor), was visited by Dr. Robert H. Archer who prescribed medicine for a child on 21 Jun 1826 and also treated a child in June 1827 and his wife in Oct and Nov 1828 (pp. 235, 299, 300 [John Evans was a War of 1812 veteran.]

Evans, L. H., was mentioned in a non-medical matter when he received $84.00 from Dr. Robert H. Archer "for tranters[?] sold R. Road Co." circa 1820s [no date and no page number – information was written on the inside of the back cover of medical Ledger F]; see Alexander Craig, q.v.

Evans, Mary, Mrs., was treated by Dr. Matthew J. Allen in Aug 1844 and Feb 1845 (p. 37)

Evans, Robert, see James Evans, q.v.

Evans, Robert, Jr., was treated by Dr. John Archer, Jr. in Jan 1816 (p. 3)

Evans, Sally, see Thomas Huggins, q.v.

Evatt, see Evitt, q.v.

Evatt, John, was visited by Dr. Robert H. Archer who treated his wife in Jul 1832, Nov 1833 and Jul 1834 (Ledger F, p. 85) [John Evatt was a War of 1812 veteran.]

Evatt, Margaret (widow), was treated by Dr. John Archer at various times between 1794 and 1802 [no dates were given] (Ledger I, which is missing, was abstracted by Dr. George W. Archer circa 1890; his notes are in the Archives of the Historical Society of Harford County folder "Archer, G. W. Coll. – Ledgers and Day Books")

Evatt, Mr., at Dublin, was treated by Dr. Robert H. Archer in Sep 1822 (p. 21)

Evatt, William, on Hughes & Adlam's place, was treated by Dr. John Archer between 1794 and 1801 (Ledger I, which is missing, was abstracted by Dr. George W. Archer circa 1890; his notes are in the Archives of the Historical Society of Harford County folder "Archer, G. W. Coll. – Ledgers and Day Books"); see William Evitt, q.v.

Everest, Benjamin (1750-1820), was visited by Dr. John Archer who treated him and his wife and a child in 1790 (Ledger F, p. 34)

Everest, Joseph, son of Joseph, was visited by Dr. John Archer who treated him, wife and infant in 1796 (Ledger F, p. 227)

Everest, Thomas, at Gravelly, was treated by Dr. John Archer in Apr 1786 (Ledger F, p. 227)

Everet, see Thomas Gilbert, q.v.

Everist, Benjamin, see Thomas Whord, q.v.

Everist, James, was visited by Dr. Matthew J. Allen who rendered obstetrical services to his wife on 16 Mar 1845 (p. 46, noted the $10 medical bill was "by cash paid Mr. Greme in full")

Everist, Joseph, was visited by Dr. John Archer who treated his wife in 1786 and 1791 and him in Sep 1793 and also mentioned Jacob Greenfield in Nov 1799 (Ledger F, p. 140) [Joseph Everist or Everest was a Revolutionary War veteran.]

Evitt, Alexander, was treated by Dr. John Archer in Feb 1781 (Ledger D, p. 123, spelled his name Evett and noted "debt forgiven as before")

Evitt, James, was visited by Dr. John Archer who treated his wife in Sep 1781 (Ledger D, p. 75, noted "debt forgiven as before")

Evitt, Richard, was visited by Dr. John Archer who treated his wife in Oct and Nov 1781 and him in Jan 1787 (Ledger D, p. 92, noted "debt forgiven as before;" Ledger F, p. 170, spelled his name Evit) [Richard Evatt was a War of 1812 veteran.]

Evitt, William, near Susquehanna, was visited by Dr. John Archer who treated him in Oct 1773, a cousin in May 1774, a maid in Jan 1775, his wife in Apr and May 1775, him in Oct 1778, him and his wife in Sep 1779, his wife in May 1780 (tooth extraction), him in Jun 1780, his wife in Jan 1781 and him in Mar and Oct 1781, Feb and Apr 1782, Mar and Apr 1783 and Aug 1792 (Ledger B, p. 10; Ledger C, p. 27; Ledger D, pp. 73, 123 [account continued in Ledger E, which is missing]; Ledger F, p. 268, spelled his name Evit) [continued in Ledger G, which is missing] [William Evitt was a Revolutionary War veteran.]; see William Evatt, q.v.

Ewen, George, was visited by Dr. John Archer who treated him in Mar, May and Jun 1781, his wife in Jul 1781 and him in Aug and Oct 1781 and Aug 1783 (Ledger D, p. 127, noted "debt forgiven as before")

Ewing, ----, see Mathew Judd, q.v.

Ewing, Alexander, appeared in Dr. John Archer's ledger in 1772, but no entries were made in this account, and he was treated by Dr. Archer in Apr 1788 (Ledger B, p. 22; Ledger F, pp. 162, 166)

Ewing, Gilbert, see William Ewing (farmer), q.v.

Ewing, James, was inoculated by Dr. John Archer in Jan 1782 (Ledger C, p. 57, noted "debt forgiven by order of testator") [James Ewing was a Revolutionary War veteran.]

Ewing, James, was visited by Dr. John Archer who treated him and child in 1802 (Ledger F, p. 19)

Ewing, Jane, was treated by Dr. John Archer in Jan 1786 (Ledger F, p. 85)

Ewing, John, see William Ewing, q.v.

Ewing, Mr. (fence maker), was treated by Dr. Robert H. Archer in Jul 1822 (p. 12)

Ewing, Samuel, was treated by Dr. Robert H. Archer in Sep 1815 (Ledger F, p. 5) [Samuel Ewing was a War of 1812 veteran.]

Ewing, Thomas, in Baltimore Town, was visited by Dr. John Archer who treated him before 1772 [no dates or details were given], a servant in Sep 1772, and him [Thomas] in Mar and Jun 1773 and May 1774 (Ledger B, p. 25)

Ewing, William, was visited by Dr. Robert H. Archer who treated him before 4 Oct 1822 [date paid] and a child in May 1826; William and Mrs. Ewing were mentioned in Mar 1827 by Dr. Robert H. Archer in a non-medical matter and mentioned son John at that time; William Ewing & Co. also had an account with Dr. Archer in Aug 1822 (pp. 26, 187, 217-225; Ledger F, pp. 62, 92)

Ewing, William (farmer), was mentioned in non-medical matters in Dr. Robert H. Archer's ledger between Apr 1823 and Jun 1824, and mentioned Gilbert [son?] in Aug 1823 (Ledger F, p. 161)

Fany Jehu, see Negro Patience, q.v.

Farcher, Dr., was consulted by Dr. John Archer in 1792 (Ledger F, p. 128)

Farmer, Hannah, see Richard Farmer, q.v.

Farmer, John, was visited by Dr. John Archer who treated his children in Sep 1777, his wife and son in Jan 1778, a child (stepdaughter) in Feb 1778, him [John] in Aug 1778, an infant in Apr 1781 and his wife in Mar 1782; also mentioned William Miller in 1778 (Ledger C, p. 98) [account continued in Ledger E, which is missing] [John Farmer was a Revolutionary War veteran.]

Farmer, Richard [1766-1838], was visited by Dr. Robert H. Archer who treated him on 7 May 1823, his wife on 20 Sep 1825 (and prescribed medicine), daughter Hannah in Oct 1825 and son [not named] in Mar 1827 (pp. 157, 158, 164, 219; Ledger F, p. 21; Rx Book, 1825-1851, p. 84)

Farnandis, Henry, was treated by Dr. Matthew J. Allen in Jun 1848 (p. 84, noted that the bill was paid in cash in full in Oct 1852)

Farnandis, Mr., was prescribed medicine for a negro by Dr. Robert H. Archer on 14 Dec 1803 (Rx Book, 1802-1804, p. 66)

Farnandis, Walter [1782-1856], was visited by Dr. Robert H. Archer who treated his child in Aug 1826 and also mentioned Col. Dorsey (p. 198); see Henry Dorsey, q.v.

Fenigin, Mrs. (widow), was treated by Dr. John Archer in May 1781 and June 1783 (Ledger D, p. 17, noted "debt forgiven as before")

Ferguson, Andrew (tailor), was visited by Dr. John Archer who treated a child in Feb 1773, his wife in Mar 1773, him in Nov 1773, his wife in Mar 1777, him in Sep 1777 and Aug and Dec 1779, and him and his wife in Jun 1786 (Ledger B, p. 29; Ledger C, p. 41, noted "13 Jan 1779, paid by work done which was by taking advantage of the times as he only made a suit of cloaths for two of my children & I had to pay him 20 Continental Dollars as a balance;" Ledger F, p. 318) [Andrew Ferguson was a Revolutionary War veteran.]

Ferguson, H., see Thomas Huggins, q.v.

Ferrell, Mrs., was treated by Dr. John Archer, Jr. in 1816 (p. 42)

Ferril, ---- [blank], near H. Seales, was treated by Dr. Robert H. Archer in Baltimore before 1822 [no dates or details were given] (Dr. Archer's "Alphabet to Ledger H" is his booklet [filed in the Archives of the Historical Society of Harford County] that contains his index to Ledger H [which is missing] for his patients in Baltimore before 1822 and Harford County after 1822, according to a notation by Dr. George W. Archer.)

Ferril (Fervil?), George, see James Clendenin, q.v.

Fettorman, George, was treated by Dr. John Archer in Dec 1786 (Ledger F, p. 184)

Fields, Joseph, "by Mr. Garrett's," was visited by Dr. John Archer who treated him, his wife and child in Apr 1780 and him in May 1780 (Ledger D, p. 63, noted "debt forgiven as before") [Joseph Fields was a Revolutionary War veteran.]

Fife, Mr., was prescribed medicine for his wife by Dr. Robert H. Archer on 19 Nov 1804 and 5 Dec 1804 (Rx Book, 1802-1804, pp. 61, 66)

Finagan, Elizabeth, see Vincent Richardson, q.v.

Finagan, Isabel, alias Smith, was treated by Dr. John Archer in Dec 1772 (Ledger B, p. 4, noted she was "poor")

Fink, Allen, was visited by Dr. Matthew J. Allen who treated him and his wife in Jul 1847 (p. 60)

Finley, Alexander, now living at William Coale's, was treated by Dr. John Archer in 1797 (Ledger I, which is missing, was abstracted by Dr. George W. Archer circa 1890; his notes are in Archives of the Historical Society of Harford County file "Archer, G. W. Coll. - Ledgers and Day Books")

Finley, George, see Reuben H. Davis, q.v.

Finley, Mr., see Isabella Cox, q.v.

Finley, W., see Reuben H. Davis, q.v.

Finney, Dr., see ---- Strickland, q.v.

Finney, Ebenezer, see William Finney, q.v.

Finney, John, see William Finney, q.v.

Finney, John, son of Manassah, was treated by Dr. John Archer in July 1773 (Ledger B, p. 56, spelled his name Finny and noted he was poor); see John Stevenson, q.v.

Finney, Manassah, was treated by Dr. John Archer in Feb 1788 (Ledger F, p. 68, spelled name Finny); see John Finney, q.v.

Finney, Mrs., and Mrs. Magaw, were named together on the same account and both were prescribed medicine by Dr. Robert H. Archer on 13 Oct 1841 (Rx Book, 1825-1851, p. 117)

Finney, Susan, see William Finney, q.v.

Finney, William [1788-1873] (reverend), was visited by Dr. Robert H. Archer who treated his wife "in partu" [in childbirth] during the night of 3 Sep 1823 and mentioned Mrs. Miller; he also treated his mother-in-law and his son in Mar 1824, a child in Jul and Aug 1824, daughter Susan several times between Sep and Dec 1826 and in Mar 1828, a child in Oct 1827, and sons Eben: [Ebenezer] and John in Oct 1828 (pp. 91, 101, 114, 116, 207, 208, 209, 251, 268, 269, 296, 298, 299; Ledger F, pp. 65. 103); see Daniel Coale, q.v.

Fisher, ----, see Benjamin Fleetwood, q.v.

Fisher, Alexander, was treated by Dr. John Archer in Apr 1788 (Ledger F, p. 293)

Fisher, George, see William Fisher, q.v.

Fisher, J---- [illegible], son of J., was treated by Dr. John Archer in Dec 1790 (Ledger F, p. 202)

Fisher, James, was visited by Dr. John Archer who treated him in Apr and Aug 1780, a daughter in Sep 1781, him in Aug and Sep 1782, his wife and child in Feb 1783, and him in Aug 1791 (Ledger D, p. 57; Ledger F, p. 255) [account continued in Ledger H, which is missing]; see Margaret Connoly," q.v.

Fisher, John, appeared on a list of debts dated 26 Dec 1822 and titled "A List of Allen's Claims" that were due and payable to Dr. Richard N. Allen for services rendered [no dates were given] by him to said Fisher (Document filed in Historical Society of Harford County Archives folder "R. N. Allen"); see Thomas Huggins & Co., q.v.

Fisher, Robert, see William Fisher, q.v.

Fisher, Thomas, was visited by Dr. Robert H. Archer who treated him and a child in Oct 1822 and Apr 1824 and his brother-in-law's child [no names were given] in Aug 1824 (pp. 30, 102, 103, 104; Ledger F, p. 108)

Fisher, William, was treated by Dr. John Archer in Feb 1777 (Ledger C, p. 86)

Fisher, William, Sr., was treated by Dr. John Archer in Mar 1779 (Ledger C, p. 127, noted "debt forgiven by order of testator")

Fisher, William (captain), was treated by Dr. John Archer in Mar, Apr and Jun 1781 (Ledger D, p. 2, noted "debt forgiven as before") [William Fisher was a Revolutionary War veteran.]

Fisher, William, near Dublin, was visited by Dr. Robert H. Archer in Sep 1822 who treated his nephew George Stubbins in Nov 1822 and Apr-May 1823, his brother-in-law's child [name not given, but most probably George Stubbins] in May 1823 and Aug 1824, his [William's] wife in Dec 1824, and his brother Robert Fisher in Oct 1825 (pp. 22, 36, 70, 71, 115, 162; Ledger F, p. 87) [William Fisher and Robert Fisher were both War of 1812 veterans.]

Fitz, Mr., "O Town" [Old Town], was treated by Dr. Robert H. Archer in Baltimore before 1822 [no dates or details were given] (Dr. Archer's "Alphabet to Ledger H" is his booklet [filed in the Archives of the Historical Society of Harford County] that contains his index to Ledger H [which is missing] for his patients in Baltimore before 1822 and Harford County after 1822, according to a notation by Dr. George W. Archer.)

Fitzgerald, ---- [blank] (carpenter), Bel Air, was treated by Dr. John Archer at times between 1795 and 1797 [no dates were given] (Ledger I, which is missing, was abstracted by Dr. George W. Archer circa 1890; his notes are in the Archives of the Historical Society of Harford County folder "Archer, G. W. Coll. – Ledgers and

Day Books"); Mr. ---- Fitzgerald was visited by Dr. Robert H. Archer who treated him and his wife on 23 Aug 1824 and the doctor noted he had "Died Pauper," but did not give the date of death (p. 118); see Simon Fitzgerald, q.v.

Fitzgerald, Simon [1753-c1822] (tailor), Bel Air, was treated by Dr. John Archer in 1795 and 1796 (Ledger I, which is missing, was abstracted by Dr. George W. Archer circa 1890; his notes are in the Archives of the Historical Society of Harford County folder "Archer, G. W. Coll. – Ledgers and Day Books"); he appeared on a list of debts dated 26 Dec 1822 and titled "A List of Allen's Claims" that were due and payable to Dr. Richard N. Allen for services rendered [no dates were given] to said Fitzgerald (Document filed in Historical Society of Harford County Archives folder "R. N. Allen") [Simon Fitzgerald was a Revolutionary War veteran.]

Fitzgerald, William, was treated by Dr. John Archer, Jr. in Nov 1818 (Ledger F, p. 11)

Flagan, E., see ---- McDannal, q.v.

Flaharty, Thomas, near Hickory, was treated by Dr. John Archer in 1795 (Ledger I, which is missing, was abstracted by Dr. George W. Archer circa 1890; his notes are in Archives of the Historical Society of Harford County file "Archer, G. W. Coll. – Ledgers and Day Books")

Flanagan, see William Beatty, q.v.

Flanagan, Ann, was treated by Dr. John Archer in Aug 1790 (Ledger F, p. 307)

Flanagan, Archa.(?), see Edward Flanagan, q.v.

Flanagan, Carol, see Edward Flanagan, q.v.

Flanagan, Edward, was visited by Dr. John Archer who treated him in Mar 1781, him and a negro in May 1781, him in Jun 1781, a negro in Oct and Nov 1781, him [Edward] in Dec 1781, a negro in Apr 1782, a child in May 1782, a negro in May and Jul 1782, him Nov and Dec 1782 and Mar 1783, Negro Spinner in Mar 1783, his [Edward's] daughter Sophia in 1787, daughter Carol in 1789 and him in 1792 (Ledger D, p. 127 [account continued in Ledger E, which is missing]; Ledger F, p. 275) [Edward Flanigan (sic) also had an account in Ledger I which is missing, but it was abstracted by Dr. George W. Archer circa 1890 who noted "inoculated your children, Maria, John and Archa.(?), and a negro, in Feb 1795" and also treated "children Neachy(?) and Nelly"] (Archives of the Historical Society of Harford County folder "Archer, G. W. Coll. – Ledgers and Day Books"); Mrs. Flannagan, widow, was visited by Dr. Archer who treated children Nache(?), Nelly, Maria and Sophia in 1797 and noted "she afterwards married Mr. Welsh." (Ledger I, which is missing, was abstracted by Dr. George W. Archer circa 1890; his notes are in the Archives of the Historical Society of Harford County file "Archer, G. W. Coll. – Ledgers and Day Books"); see James Cain, q.v.

Flanagan, John, near R. Amoss', was treated by Dr. John Archer in 1786 (Ledger F, p. 208)

Flanagan, John, see Edward Flanagan, q.v.

Flanagan, Mary (widow), was visited by Dr. John Archer who treated her before 1772 [no dates or details were given], her maid in Sept 1772 and her [Mary] in Dec 1776 (Ledger B, p. 23, spelled her name Flannagan; Ledger C, p. 74)

Flanagan, Maria, see Edward Flanagan, q.v.

Flanagan (Flannagan), Mrs., see Edward Flanagan, q.v.

Flanagan (Flanigan), Nancy, see John Cretin, q.v.

Flanagan, Neachy(?), see Edward Flanagan, q.v.

Flanagan, Nelly, see Edward Flanagan, q.v.

Flanagan, Sophia, see Edward Flanagan, q.v.

Flanagan, Widow, was treated by Dr. Robert H. Archer in Baltimore before 1822 [no dates or details were given] (Dr. Archer's "Alphabet to Ledger H" is his booklet [filed in the Archives of the Historical Society of Harford County] that contains his index to Ledger H [which is missing] for his patients in Baltimore before 1822 and Harford County after 1822, according to a notation by Dr. George W. Archer.)

Flanagan, William, was treated by Dr. Robert H. Archer in Baltimore before 1822 [no dates or details were given] (Dr. Archer's "Alphabet to Ledger H" is his booklet [filed in the Archives of the Historical Society of Harford County] that contains his index to Ledger H [which is missing] for his patients in Baltimore before 1822 and Harford County after 1822, according to a notation by Dr. George W. Archer.)

Fleetwood, Benjamin, was visited by Dr. John Archer in 1774 who treated a domestic named Fisher and inoculated Mrs. Fleetwood and 2 daughters in Dec 1774 (Ledger B, p. 96)

Fleharty, John, grandson of Widow Elliott, was treated by Dr. John Archer at Samuel Lee's Quarter in Sep 1790 (Ledger F, p. 370)

Flet (LeFlet?), Peter, "X Roads," was visited by Dr. John Archer who treated him and his family at various times between 1796 and 1799 (Ledger I, which is missing, was abstracted by Dr. George W. Archer circa 1890; his notes are in the Archives of the Historical Society of Harford County folder "Archer, G. W. Coll. – Ledgers and Day Books")

Flinn, Mrs., at Forge, was treated by Dr. Matthew J. Allen in Jun 1847 (p. 55)

Flowers, John, appeared on a list of debts dated 26 Dec 1822 and titled "A List of Allen's Claims" that were due and payable to Dr. Richard N. Allen for services rendered [no dates] by him to said Flours (Document filed in Historical Society of Harford County Archives folder "R. N. Allen" misspelled his name as Flours)

Floyd, Alexander, was treated by Dr. Robert H. Archer in Baltimore before 1822 [no dates or details were given] (Dr. Archer's "Alphabet to Ledger H" is his booklet [filed in the Archives of the Historical Society of Harford County] that contains his index to Ledger H [which is missing] for his patients in Baltimore before 1822 and Harford County after 1822, according to a notation by Dr. George W. Archer.)

Foard, Charles, see Bob Howard, q.v.

Ford, ---- [blank] (shoemaker) at Bald Friar [ferry landing on the Susquehanna River], was visited by Dr. John Archer who inoculated 2 of his family in 1777 (Ledger C, p. 73, noted "debt forgiven by order of testator")

Ford, ---- [blank] (trunk maker), was treated by Dr. Robert H. Archer in Baltimore before 1822 [no dates or details were given] (Dr. Archer's "Alphabet to Ledger H" is his booklet [filed in the Archives of the Historical Society of Harford County] that contains his index to Ledger H [which is missing] for his patients in Baltimore before 1822 and Harford County after 1822, according to a notation by Dr. George W. Archer.)

Ford, Charles, was treated by Dr. John Archer, Jr. in June 1816 (p. 52)

Ford, James, son-in-law of Enoch West, was visited by Dr. John Archer who inoculated 3 of his family in 1779 (Ledger C, p. 122, noted the bill was paid by Micajah Mitchell on 20 Jun 1785) [Two men named James Ford were Revolutionary War veterans.]

Ford, John Peake, was treated by Dr. Robert H. Archer in Baltimore before 1822 [no dates or details were given] (Dr. Archer's "Alphabet to Ledger H" is his booklet [filed in the Archives of the Historical Society of Harford County] that contains his index to Ledger H [which is missing] for his patients in Baltimore before 1822 and Harford County after 1822, according to a notation by Dr. George W. Archer.)

Fordacre, ---- [blank], was visited by Dr. Matthew J. Allen who treated him and his wife in 1823 in Calvert County (p. 12a)

Forsyth, Samuel, near Dublin, was visited by Dr. John Archer who treated his family in 1798 (Ledger I, which is missing, was abstracted by Dr. George W. Archer circa 1890; his notes are in the Archives of the Historical Society of Harford County folder "Archer, G. W. Coll. – Ledgers and Day Books")

Forsythe, ---- [blank], was treated by Dr. Robert H. Archer in Oct 1822 (Ledger F, p. 191)

Forwood, see William Carr, q.v.

Forwood, Dr., see Thomas Green, George Morrison, Otho Scott, Howell Mitchell and Joseph Parker and John Kean, q.v. [Forwood was often misspelled Forward in Dr. Robert H. Archer's ledger.]

Forwood, Ed., was treated by Dr. Robert H. Archer after 1822 [no dates or details were given] (Dr. Archer's "Alphabet to Ledger H" is his booklet [filed in the Archives of the Historical Society of Harford County] that contains his index to Ledger H [which is missing] for his patients in Baltimore City before 1822 and in Harford County after 1822, according to a notation by Dr. George W. Archer.)

Forwood, Hannah, was treated by Dr. John Archer in Jul 1781 (Ledger C, p. 109, noted her account was transferred "to Mathew Conklin's account in Ledger E," which is missing)

Forwood, Jacob, was visited by Dr. John Archer who treated his maid in 1777 [her name and the exact date were not given] and him [Jacob] in Mar 1778, Sep 1782 and Feb 1783 (Ledger C, p. 100) [account continued in Ledger E, which is missing] [Jacob Forwood was a Revolutionary War veteran.]; see John Forwood, of Jacob, q.v.

Forwood, John, Sr. [1761-1840] (nailer), was visited by Dr. John Archer who treated him in 1790 and him, his wife and a child in 1803 (Ledger F, pp. 60, 77); see Garrett Garrettson, Henry Thomas, John Evans and Samuel Webb, q.v.

Forwood, John, was visited by Dr. John Archer who treated him four times in Jan 1775, his wife in May 1775, his wife, his brother Joseph Forwood in Mar 1780, Charles Burkins in Mar 1780 and him [John] in Sep 1780 and Jan 1783 (Ledger B, p. 90; Ledger C, p. 51)

Forwood, John, of Jacob, was visited by Dr. Richard Sappington who treated him and his son in Sep 1806, him in May 1807, his wife "at Capt. Loney's" on 17 May 1806, "from Garrettson's" on 18 May 1806 and twice more in May 1806 and again in Jun, Aug and Sep 1806, son William in Sep 1806, his [John's] wife 40 times between 2 Mar 1809 and 24 Nov 1809; visited by Dr. William Sappington who treated him in May 1812, a son in Sep 1812, him in Feb 1813, son William in Sep, Oct and Dec 1813, a negro man in Oct 1813, Negro Pol in Dec 1813 and Jan 1814, John's sons (including William) in Jan 1814, him [John] in Feb and May 1814, Negro Sal in May 1814, him [John], sons Thomas and William and Negro Cas in Aug 1814, him [John] in Oct 1814, his wife in Dec 1814 and Jan and Feb 1815, him [John], son Thomas, a negro man and Negro Sam in Feb 1815, him [John], his wife, "negro Barney at Sappington's," "negro Sam at Sappington's," Negro Welton, Negro Sam, a negro boy, "negroes at your house and at William Brooks," negroes Sophia, Cam and Bill, and "son Thomas from Sappington's" in Mar 1815, negroes Bill, Andrew and Neoma in Mar and Apr 1815, him [John], his wife, son Thomas, and family [no names were given] in Apr 1815, and negro(?) Mane(?) in May 1815; Abraham Jarrett, a Justice of the Peace, on 18 Aug 1815, certified his account to be a true copy from the books of Drs. Richard and William Sappington; and, Dr. William Sappington received $200 in partial payment from Joseph Brownley, one of the administrators of John Forwood, of Jacob, dec., on 21 Dec 1815; another account was presented with "errors excepted" by John W. Sappington and it was sworn to be accurate by Dr. Richard Sappington and verified on 6 Mar 1817 by Z. O. Bond, Justice of the Peace, as being a just and true copy of the account in the doctor's medical book (Documents filed in Historical Society of Harford County Archives folder "Sappington, Dr. Richard – Accounts, 1783-1830" [which referred to him only as John Forwood] and folder "Sappington, Dr. William" [which referred to him as John Forwood, of Jacob, deceased]

Forwood, John, of William, was visited by Dr. John Archer who treated his wife and child in 1787 and treated him [John] at Samuel Forwood's (Ledger F, p. 374)

Forwood, John [1789-c1842], was visited by Dr. Robert H. Archer who treated his son John in Aug 1827 (p. 245) [John Forwood was a War of 1812 veteran.]

Forwood, Joseph, was visited by Dr. John Archer who treated him in Sep and Oct 1773, Apr 1774 and Apr 1776, an infant in Nov 1777, and him [Joseph] in Jan and Apr 1778 (Ledger B, p. 87; Ledger C, p. 109); see John Forwood, q.v.

Forwood, Samuel, was visited by Dr. John Archer who inoculated his son and daughter in Mar 1776 and treated him in Feb 1780, Apr and Dec 1781, Mar 1782 and Jan and Feb 1783, his daughter in Aug 1787, and him and his wife in Aug 1791 (Ledger C, p. 34; Ledger D, p. 8, stated bill was paid in part by John Cretin's note on 3 Feb 1784 [account continued in Ledger E, which is missing]; Ledger F, p. 58, 112) [account continued in Ledger H, which missing]; see John Forwood, Daniel Davis, George Lewis, Rosannah Shields and George Riely, q.v.

Forwood, Thomas, see John Forwood, of Jacob, q.v.

Forwood, William, see John Forwood, of Jacob, and John Forwood, of William, q.v.

Fosset, Jonathan, was visited by Dr. John Archer who treated him in Nov and Dec 1780 and Jan 1781 and "widdow Fosset" in Feb 1781, and noted "Henry Vansickle and Archibald Beatty promised to pay me to the amount of £5 if I would attend J. Fosset." (Ledger D, p. 107, noted "debt forgiven as before")

Foster, Henry, near the Black Horse on York Road, was visited by Dr. John Archer who treated a child in May 1785 (Ledger D, p. 28, noted "debt forgiven as before")

Foster, Mrs. (widow), was treated by Dr. John Archer in March 1786 (Ledger F, p. 154)

Foster, Robert (weaver), was visited by Dr. John Archer who treated him and his wife in 1789 (Ledger F, p. 45) [account continued in Ledger G, which is missing]

Fout, John, "Still at Mr. Morgan's," was visited by Dr. John Archer who treated him in May 1782 and Jul 1783, him, his wife, a child and an infant in Sep 1783 (Ledger D, p. 45, noted the "debt forgiven as before")

Foxcroft, Elisa or Eliza, Mrs., was treated by Dr. Matthew J. Allen in Feb 1844 (p. 31, noted the bill was paid "by cash in full" in Sep 1852)

Fox & Jackson, had an account that mentioned a wife [name not given, but probably Peggy Jackson] was treated by Dr. Robert H. Archer in Sep 1821 (Ledger F, p. 22); see Jackson & Fox, q.v.

Fox, Mrs., see William Goslee, q.v.

Fox, P., see Peggy Jackson and Jackson & Fox, q.v.

Foy, Harry, was visited by Dr. Alonzo Preston who treated him and a child at times in 1825 and 1826, his wife "in partu" [in childbirth] on 2 Apr 1826, and John Foy in Nov 1826 (p. 44) [Harry or Henry Foy was a War of 1812 veteran.]

Foy, John, see Harry Foy, q.v.

Foy, Mary, was treated by Dr. John Archer in Dec 1781 (Ledger D, p. 103, noted "debt forgiven as before")

Francis, Peter, appeared on a list of debts dated 26 Dec 1822 and titled "A List of Allen's Claims" that were due and payable to Dr. Richard N. Allen for services rendered [no dates were given] by him to said Francis (Document filed in Historical Society of Harford County Archives folder "R. N. Allen")

Fraizer, Mr., at James Ramsey's, was treated by Dr. John Archer in Jul 1787 (Ledger F, p. 324)

Fraley (Frailey), Frederick (blacksmith), was visited by Dr. John Archer who treated him in Jul 1777, an infant in May 1778, his wife in Jul 1779, him in Mar 1780, Mar 1781 and May 1782, his wife in Oct 1782, him in Aug 1785 and a child in Sep 1785; also mentioned "an order on Cumberland Forge" (Ledger C, p. 27; Ledger D, p. 55)

Frazier, M., see Adam Jameson, q.v.

Freeman, William, at Port Deposit [Cecil County], was visited by Dr. John Archer, Jr. who treated him and his wife in March 1817 and his wife in June 1819 (p. 73)

French, Jacob, Estate of, was mentioned in Dr. Matthew J. Allen's ledger in Calvert County in 1832 (p. 20); see John French, q.v.

French, John, was visited by Dr. Matthew J. Allen in Calvert County who treated him and Jacob French in 1823 (p. 18); see R. N. Allen and M. J. Allen, q.v.

Frisby, see Phrisby, q.v.

Frisby, Peregrine, was treated by Dr. John Archer in Dec 1780 and Jan 1781 (Ledger D, p. 110, noted "debt forgiven as before")

Fryar, Isaac, was visited by Dr. John Archer who treated him in Dec 1778, his wife in Jan 1779 and him in Aug 1781 and May 1782 (Ledger C, p. 126, noted "debt forgiven by order of testator")

Fullerton, John, was visited by Dr. James Archer who treated his wife by "dysecting an unguis from your wife's eye & sundry medicines" on 30 Apr 1806 (p. 12) ["unguis" is a fingernail or toenail]

Fulton, Elizabeth, was treated by Dr. John Archer in June and Aug 1779 (Ledger C, p. 71, noted "debt forgiven by order of testator")

Fulton, Betsy, see Jenny Harris, q.v.

Fulton, James, was visited by Dr. Matthew J. Allen who treated Susan in Oct 1847, Mary in Jan 1848, Susan in Feb, Mar and Apr 1848, Mary in Apr 1848, Sue in Jun 1848 and his wife in Jul and Aug 1848 (pp. 67, 85, 89, mentioned Jos. W. and E. Reynolds); see Edward Reynolds, q.v.

Fulton, Jenny, see Jenny Harris, q.v.

Fulton, Mary, see James Fulton, q.v.

Fulton, Samuel, near Slate Ridge, was visited by Dr. John Archer who inoculated his children in 1775 (Ledger C, p. 1)

Fulton, Susan, see James Fulton, q.v.

Gaa, John, see Mrs. Gaa, q.v.

Gaa, Mrs., "of Robert," at Bush River Neck, was visited by Dr. John Archer who treated her and son John in 1788 (Ledger F, p. 203) [account continued in Ledger G, which is missing]

Gaa, Robert, see Mrs. Gaa, q.v.

Galaspy, Samuel, was treated by Dr. John Archer in Aug 1780 (Ledger D, p. 84, noted "debt forgiven as before")

Gale, ---- [blank], at the mouth of Rumney [Creek]on Henry Vansickle's race, was visited by Dr. John Archer who treated him or her and an infant in 1787 (Ledger F, p. 13)

Gale, Ann, Mrs., was visited by Dr. John Archer, Jr. who treated daughter Susan in Sep 1816, daughter Sally in Jan 1817 and negroes Ben, Fanie, Harriet, John, Dorsey, Lloyd and Juda in 1817 (pp. 40, 81)

Gale, Anna Maria, see George Gale and Margaret Gale, q.v.

Gale, George (esquire), at Damascus [Cecil Co.], was visited by Dr. John Archer at various times between 1795 and 1797 and treated children Nancy, Sally, Leah, Henrietta, Levin, George, Anna Maria and Peggy; in Dec 1797 he visited Peggy and treated her daily for 8 weeks and treated him [George] for 2 weeks during this same time (Ledger I, which is missing, was abstracted by Dr. George W. Archer circa 1890; his notes are in the Archives of the Historical Society of Harford County file "Archer, G. W. Coll. – Ledgers and Day Books"); George was visited Dr. Robert H. Archer who treated him at various times in 1817 and 1818, and negroes Fanny, Rebecca, Nicholas, John, Beck, Nelson, Georgeanne, Jinny, Sally and Ben in 1821, sister Nancy in Sep 1821, sisters Harriet and George Anna in Sep 1822, sister Sally in Nov and Dec 1822 and Apr and May 1824, Negro Ben in Feb 1823, Negro Sal in Feb 1823, sister George Anna in Jan 1824, sister Leah in May 1824, sister Harriet in Mar 1827 "in consultation with Dr. J. Archer, including ferriage" [which meant they ferried across the Susquehanna River], again in consultation with Dr. J. Archer and Dr. Broughton in Apr and June 1827, and treated his sister [unnamed] and included "ferriage" in Feb 1828 (pp. 17, 20, 38, 41, 53, 96, 107, 217, 222, 232, 261; Ledger F, pp. 23, 141) [George Gale was a Revolutionary War veteran]; see Chamberlaine & Gale and Henry Lawrence and Henry Holliday, q.v.

Gale, George Anna, see George Gale, q.v.

Gale, Harriet, see George Gale, q.v.

Gale, Henrietta, see George Gale, q.v.

Gale, Henry, see Margaret Gale, q.v.

Gale, James, at Mrs. Copeland's, was treated by Dr. John Archer in Apr 1788 (Ledger F, p. 189)

Gale, James, was visited by Dr. John Archer who treated a child in 1788 and him [James] in Mar 1789 (Ledger F, p. 117, noted that the account was paid by William Hollis on 17 Feb 1797)

Gale, John, see William Gale, q.v.

Gale, Leah, see George Gale and Margaret Gale, q.v.

Gale, Levin (Leven), was visited by Dr. John Archer, Jr. who treated him, his wife and negroes Charlotte, Ben, Richard and Bob in 1815; Dr. Robert H. Archer treated negroes Perry and Robert in 1822 (Dr. John Archer, Jr.'s Ledger, p. 6; Dr. Robert H. Archer's Ledger F, p. 30); see Margaret Gale, George Gale, and John Gregg & Co., q.v.

Gale, Lyttleton, was treated by Dr. John Archer, Jr. in Oct 18-- [illegible] and mentioned "L. Gale's executor" in May 1828 and Mrs. Margaret Gale in Nov 1835 (p. 23)

Gale, Margaret, Mrs., was visited by Dr. John Archer, Jr. who treated son Leven in Sep 1815, daughter Anna Maria in Jul 1816, daughter Susan in Sep 1816, son Robert in Dec 1816, daughter Leah in Aug 1817 and negroes Jack, Jude, Tom, Crecy, Jenny and Betty between 1815 and 1817; Dr. Robert H. Archer treated Margaret and son Henry and Negro Tom in 1821 [bottom part of the page in Ledger F was cut out of book] (Dr. John Archer, Jr.'s Ledger, pp. 21 77; Dr. Robert H. Archer's Ledger F, p. 24); see Lyttleton Gale, q.v.

Gale, Nancy, see George Gale, q.v.

Gale, Robert, see Margaret Gale, q.v.

Gale, Sally, see George Gale and Ann Gale, q.v.

Gale, Susan, see Ann Gale and Margaret Gale, q.v.

Gale, William, near Bush [Bush Town, or Harford Town, near Abingdon], was visited by Dr. John Archer who treated him twelve times between Sep 1774 and May 1775, son Johan: [John] in May 1775, him [William] in Jul 1776 and Oct and Nov 1779, his wife in Aug 1780 and him in Sep, Oct and Nov 1780 and Jan 1781 (Ledger B, p. 92; Ledger C, pp. 55, 95, noted "debt forgiven by order of testator") [William Gale was a Revolutionary War veteran.]

Gallion, Elizabeth, of James, was treated by Dr. John Archer in August 1790 (Ledger F, p. 262)

Gallion, Gregory, was treated by Dr. John Archer in April 1790 (Ledger F, p. 232) [Gregory Gallion was a Revolutionary War veteran.]

Gallion, James, was treated by Dr. John Archer in Feb 1774 in consultation with Dr. Annan (Ledger B, p. 104)

Gallion, James, "R. Congress," was visited by Dr. John Archer who treated him and his daughter in Sep 1786 (Ledger F, p. 55); see Elizabeth Gallion, q.v.

Gallion, James, Sr., was visited by Dr. John Archer who treated his daughter and son in Jun 1773, his daughter in Sep 1773 and Patty in May 1774 (Ledger B, p. 100)

Gallion, John, was visited by Dr. John Archer who treated his child in Nov 1774 and him in Feb 1775 (Ledger B, p. 100) [John Gallion was a Revolutionary War veteran.]; see Joseph Gallion, q.v.

Gallion, Joseph, was visited by Dr. John Archer who treated his wife in Apr 1778, him and son John in Sep 1781, inoculated two of his family in 1782 and treated him and son John in Apr 1790 (Ledger C, p. 63; Ledger D, p. 17; Ledger F, p. 50) [account continued in Ledger G, which is missing]; see William Ensor and George Walker, q.v.

Gallion, Nancy, was treated by Dr. John Archer in 1786 (Ledger F, p. 86)

Gallion, Nathan (or Nathaniel), was visited by Dr. John Archer who treated him in Jan 1775, his wife and Bob in Feb 1775, him in Aug 1778 and Jun 1779, his wife in Sep 1779, him in Oct 1779, Mar, Apr and Aug 1781, Mar, Jul, Aug and Sep 1783, a child in Aug 1783 and him, his wife and child in Mar 1789 (Ledger B, p. 100, listed him as Nathaniel; Ledger C, p. 118, and Ledger F, p. 146, both listed his name as Nathan) [accounts continued in Ledgers E and H, which are missing] [Nathan Gallion was a Revolutionary War veteran.]; see John Wilson (carpenter), q.v.

Gallion, Patty, was treated by Dr. John Archer twice circa Feb 1775(?) [illegible] (Ledger B, p. 60); see Phebe Gallion, q.v.

Gallion, Phebe, "widow senr." *(sic)*, was visited by Dr. John Archer who treated Patty in Jan 1777, granddaughter Pheby in Mar 1781, and Phebe herself at various times between Apr 1782 and Mar 1784 and in Dec 1787 (Ledger C, p. 1; Ledger F, p. 299)

Gallion, Sally, see John Copeland, q.v.

Gallion, Samuel, was visited by Dr. John Archer who treated him and his wife in Nov 1774 (Ledger B, p. 100); Samuel Gallion, near Benjamin Herbert's, was treated by Dr. John Archer in May 1789 (Ledger F, p. 299) [Samuel Gallion was a Revolutionary War veteran.]

Gallispie, Thomas [name possibly James Thomas Gillespie?], was visited by Dr. Alonzo Preston who treated him and his daughter in 1825 (p. 19)

Galloway, Absalom, was visited by Dr. John Archer who treated him and his family in 1797 (Ledger I, which is missing, was abstracted by Dr. George W. Archer circa 1890; his notes are in the Archives of the Historical Society of Harford County folder "Archer, G. W. Coll. – Ledgers and Day Books")

Gallup, Joseph, was treated by Dr. Robert H. Archer in Baltimore before 1822 [no dates or details were given] (Dr. Archer's "Alphabet to Ledger H" is his booklet [filed in the Archives of the Historical Society of Harford County] that contains his index to Ledger H [which is missing] for his patients in Baltimore before 1822 and Harford County after 1822, according to a notation by Dr. George W. Archer.)

Gardner, Margaret, see John Ellis, q.v.

Gardner, William, at Joseph Hopkins', was treated by Dr. John Archer in Nov 1787 (Ledger F, p. 66, indicated he was poor)

Garland, Francis, was treated by Dr. John Archer in Jan, Feb and Mar 1781 and in Jun and Aug 1781 for a puncture (Ledger D, pp. 28, 115, noted "debt forgiven as before") [Francis Garland was a Revolutionary War veteran.]

Garretson, see Garrettson, q.v.

Garretson, James, was visited by Dr. John Archer who treated him in Oct 1786 and him and a child in Sep 1789 (Ledger F, pp. 100, 245)

Garretson, John, was treated by Dr. John Archer in Jul 1773 (Ledger B, p. 89)

Garretson, Rachiel, Miss, see Ruthen Garretson, q.v.

Garretson, Ruthen [1764-1830], at B. Neck [probably Bush River Neck], was treated by Dr. John Archer in Jan 1791 (Ledger F, p. 354); Ruthen was visited by Dr. William M. Dallam who treated his wife in Jul 1807 and Jun and Oct 1810, Miss Rachiel in Oct 1810, him in Feb and Oct 1813, Luther Norris in Jan 1814, a negro in Feb 1814, his [Ruthen's] wife in Jun, Oct, Nov and Dec 1814, Negro Jack in May 1810, Apr 1811 and Feb 1815, him [Ruthen] in Feb, Apr and May 1815, negroes in Mar and Apr 1815, Miss Cox in Apr 1815, Miss Rachiel in Nov 1815, negroes in Sep 1815, Mar 1816 and Sep 1816, his wife in Feb 1816, him in Sep 1823 [treated by Dr. Richard Sappington], Miss Cox in Jul 1825 [treated by Dr. Jacob A. Preston who was paid in full in 1829] and Ruthen and his family through 1828 [no names and treatment dates were listed in Dr. William M. Dallam's bill] (Documents filed in Historical Society of Harford County Archives folder titled "Medical Bills – Dr. William M. Dallam" and "Sappington, Dr. Richard – Accounts, 1783-1830" and folder titled "Preston, Jacob A."); see Garrett Garrettson, q.v.

Garretson, Widdow *(sic)*, was treated by Dr. John Archer in Jan 1779 (Ledger D, p. 40, noted "debt forgiven as before")

Garrett, Amos (esquire), was visited by Dr. John Archer who treated him in Oct 1780, a negro in Sep 1781, him [Amos] in Oct 1781, him and a negro in Jan 1782, a negro man and woman in Jul 1782 and [negro] Duke in Feb 1783 and him [Amos] in Sep 1786 (Ledger D, pp. 79, 102, noted "debt forgiven as before" [account continued in Ledger E, which is missing]; Ledger F, p. 81)

Garrett, Mr., see Joseph Fields, q.v.

Garrett, Thomas (mulatto), on Rumsey's place, was treated by Dr. John Archer in Aug 1791 (Ledger F, p. 315)

Garrett, William, was treated by Dr. John Archer in March 1786 (Ledger F, p. 198, spelled his name Garret and indicated his security was Francis Clark)

Garrettson, see John Forwood and also see Garretson, q.v.

Garrettson, Aquila, was treated by Dr. John Archer in Aug 1789 (Ledger F, p. 237)

Garrettson, Fanny, Miss, was treated by Dr. John Archer in Jan 1787 (Ledger F, p. 163)

Garrettson, Garrett, was visited by Dr. William M. Dallam who treated him in Feb 1807 and him and a child in Jan, Feb and May 1808; Garrett died before 17 Dec 1808 when Abraham Jarrett, Register of Wills, noted on the £7.2.6 bill that "this amount will pass when paid." Jacob Forwood, Justice of the Peace, noted on 8 Dec 1808 that he had examined the book from which the above account was taken and found it a true copy and the doctor's books were yearly proved. Dr. Dallam noted on the bill, on 2 Jan 1810, "Received of Mr. Ruthen Garrettson the sum of two pounds eighteen shillings & six nine pence in part of the within account." On 7 Mar 1810, he noted "Received the within account in full." (Document filed in Historical Society of Harford County Archives folder titled "Medical Bills – Dr. William M. Dallam")

Garrettson, Molly, Miss, at Josias Hall's, was treated by Dr. John Archer in 1788 (Ledger F, p. 64)

Garrettson, Patty, Miss, was treated by Dr. John Archer in Mar 1787 (Ledger F, p. 182, stated she "married W. Jos. Hall," but the date of marriage was not given)

Garrettson, Ruthen, see Ruthen Garretson, q.v.

Garrish, Francis, was prescribed medicine for his wife by Dr. Robert H. Archer on 13 Mar 1801 (Rx Book, 1796-1801, p. 46); Francis Garish was treated by Dr. Archer in Baltimore before 1822 [no dates or details were given] (Dr. Archer's "Alphabet to Ledger H" is his booklet [filed in the Archives of the Historical Society of Harford County] that contains his index to Ledger H [which is missing] for his patients in Baltimore before 1822 and Harford County after 1822, according to a notation by Dr. George W. Archer.); see Mr. Gerish, q.v.

Gash, Mr., see Thomas Lancaster, q.v.

Gash, Thomas, was visited by Dr. John Archer who treated him in Sep 1773 and Jan 1775, a child in Sep 1777 and him in May and Sep 1779, Apr 1781, Jun 1786 and Jan 1791 and a child in Aug 1787 (Ledger B, p. 77; Ledger C, p. 101; Ledger F, pp. 143, 333, 369) [account continued in Ledger E, which is missing]; see Gilbert Thompson and James West, q.v.

Gates, Jacob, was visited by Dr. John Archer who treated an infant in Mar 1780, him [Jacob] in Apr 1780, Jul 1781 and Nov 1782 and child in Mar 1783 (Ledger D, p. 51) [account continued in Ledger E, which is missing]

Gawley, William, was treated by Dr. John Archer in Jan 1787 (Ledger F, p. 158)

Gay, Samuel, "Cecil" [Cecil County], was visited by Dr. John Archer who treated him and "Carolin:" in Sep 1779 (Ledger D, p. 21, noted "debt forgiven as before")

George, Sidney (esquire), was visited by Dr. John Archer who treated his wife "across the river" [across the Susquehanna in Cecil County] in 1796 and 1804 (Ledger I, which is missing, was abstracted by Dr. George W. Archer circa 1890; his notes are in Archives of the Historical Society of Harford County folder "Archer, G. W. Coll. – Ledgers and Day Books")

Gerish, Mr., was prescribed medicine for his wife by Dr. Robert H. Archer on 29 Dec 1799 (Rx Book, 1796-1801, p. 17); see Francis Garrish, q.v.

Giant, Isaac, was treated by Dr. John Archer in Jun 1786 (Ledger F, p. 322) [Isaac Giant was a Revolutionary War veteran.]

Gibbon, Thomas B., was treated by Dr. Matthew J. Allen in 1823 in Calvert County (p. 11b)

Gibbs, John, see Patty Brown, q.v.

Gibson, Ignatius, see John Lee Gibson, q.v.

Gibson, James, see Polly Gibson, q.v.

Gibson, John, was treated by Dr. Alonzo Preston in 1825 [no details were given] and 1827 (p. 59) [One John Gibson was a Revolutionary War veteran and one was a War of 1812 veteran.]

Gibson, John Lee (esquire), was visited by Dr. John Archer who treated him in Jan 1779, a negro in Sep 1779, him [John] in Jul 1780 and Dec 1780, Mr. Hudson in Feb 1781, an infant in Apr 1782, him [John] in May 1782, Thomas in Jan 1783, him [John] in Sep 1783, him, his wife and child in 1788, him in May 1789 and him and children William, Ignatius and John at times between 1794 and 1801 [no dates were given] (Ledger C, p. 27; Ledger D, p. 112 [account continued in Ledger E, which is missing]; Ledger F, pp. 89, 233) [account continued in Ledger G, which is missing]; Ledger I, which is missing, was abstracted by Dr. George W. Archer circa 1890; his notes are in the Archives of the Historical Society of Harford County folder "Archer, G. W. Coll. – Ledgers and Day Books"); see John Grindell, q.v.

Gibson, Polly, was visited by Dr. Robert H. Archer who treated her and sons Robert and James in 1821 (Ledger F, p. 1, noted "dead & I suppose insolvent," but no date of death was given)

Gibson, Robert, see Polly Gibson, q.v.

Gibson, Thomas, was treated by Dr. John Archer in Sep 1787 and Jan 1790 (Ledger F, p. 300, 355) [account continued in Ledger G, which is missing]; see John Lee Gibson, q.v.

Gibson, William, see John Lee Gibson, q.v.

Gilbert, Abram, see Parker Gilbert, q.v.

Gilbert, Aquila, see James Gilbert, q.v.

Gilbert, Betsy, see James Gilbert, q.v.

Gilbert, Billy, see James Gilbert, q.v.

Gilbert, E., see Peggy Morgan, q.v.

Gilbert, Charles, Sr. [1723-1798], was visited by Dr. John Archer who treated his wife in Oct and Nov 1781 and him in Sep 1791 (Ledger D, p. 90; Ledger F, p. 142); see Edward Thompson, q.v.

Gilbert, George T. [1811-1885], was visited by Dr. Matthew J. Allen who treated a child in Feb 1844, him and a child in Mar and May 1844, and a child in Jun 1844 (p. 32 stated the bill was "Settled by note," but gave no date) [Obituary gave full name as George Thomas Gilbert. The following statement was written on a separate page dated 24 Nov 1853 that was inserted in the back of Dr. Allen's ledger. The letter, addressed to Major Bond, was signed by I. Day and stated "I have just returned after 3 days ride to look up the Drs. of Dr. Allen and the following is the result." It mentioned several patients, including: "Geo. Gilbert will call in 2 weeks to pay you his note."]

Gilbert, Henry [1794-1856], was treated by Dr. Robert H. Archer after 1822 [no dates or details were given] (Dr. Archer's "Alphabet to Ledger H" is his booklet [filed in the Archives of the Historical Society of Harford County] that contains his index to Ledger H [which is missing] for his patients in Baltimore before 1822 and Harford County after 1822, according to a notation by Dr. George W. Archer.) [Henry Gilbert was a War of 1812 veteran.]

Gilbert, James [1760-1827], son of Michael, was visited by Dr. John Archer who treated him and children Billy, Betsy, Jimmy and Johnson in 1791 (Ledger F, p. 172) [continued in Ledger H, which is missing]; also inoculated his children William, James, Aquila and Johnson in 1795 and treated him [James, the father] between 1795 and 1800 (Ledger I, which is missing, was abstracted by Dr. George W. Archer circa 1890; his notes are in the Archives of the Historical Society of Harford County file "Archer, G. W. Coll. – Ledgers and Day Books")

Gilbert, Jarvis [1776-1840s], near Nicholas Baker's, was treated by Dr. John Archer in May 1801 and was visited by Dr. Robert H. Archer who treated his wife in Mar 1828 and Apr 1828 (pp. 267, 271, 272, spelled his name Jaarvis; Ledger F, p. 456, spelled his name Jervis and stated his account was paid by Stevenson Archer on 22 Feb 1809)

Gilbert, Jimmy, see James Gilbert, q.v.

Gilbert, Johnson, see James Gilbert, q.v.

Gilbert, Martin T. [1739-1797], was treated by Dr. John Archer in Apr 1788 (Ledger F, p. 195) [His full name was Martin Taylor Gilbert.]; also see Taylor Gilbert, q.v.

Gilbert, Micah [1734-1827], was visited by Dr. John Archer who treated his wife in May, Jul and Aug 1774, him and wife in Dec 1775, his wife in Aug 1776, him in Feb, Mar and Apr 1781 and Jan, Apr and May 1782, his wife in May 1782 and him in Dec 1780, Jan 1781 and Apr 1788 (Ledger B, p. 24, spelled his name Micha; Ledger C, p. 15; Ledger D, p. 114 [account continued in Ledger E, which is missing]; Ledger F, p. 259)

Gilbert, Michael, see James Gilbert, Parker Gilbert and Mrs. Gilbert, q.v.

Gilbert, Michael [1764-1828], was treated by Dr. Robert H. Archer in Mar 1828 (p. 268)

Gilbert, Michael, was visited by Dr. Matthew J. Allen who treated his wife in Mar 1848 and a negro girl Minerva three times in Jul 1848 (p. 75, noted "June 1st, 1850, settled by John B. McFadden by act. against M J. Allen")

Gilbert, Michael, Sr. [1707-1784], was treated by Dr. John Archer in Jan 1779, May and Aug 1782, and Jan and Feb 1784 (Ledger D, p. 37, noted the £4.2.6 bill was paid in cash on 9 Oct 1784)

Gilbert, Mr. (carpenter), near Boner's, was visited by Dr. Robert H. Archer who treated his wife in Apr 1827 (p. 223)

Gilbert, Mrs. widow of Michael Gilbert, was treated by Dr. John Archer in May 1789 (Ledger F, p. 65) [account continued in Ledger G, which is missing]

Gilbert, Parker [1740-c1803], was visited by Dr. John Archer who treated him in Aug, Sep and Nov 1778 and Jun and Jul 1783, and inoculated two of his children, Michael and Abram, in 1791 (Ledger C, p. 120, noted "debt forgiven by order of testator;" Ledger F, p. 220) [account continued in Ledger H, which is missing] [Parker Gilbert was a Revolutionary War veteran.]

Gilbert, Philip [c1742-1805], was treated by Dr. John Archer in Jun 1788 (Ledger F, p. 304) [account continued in Ledger G, which is missing]

Gilbert, Taylor, was treated by Dr. John Archer in May 1773 and inoculated 6 of his family in May 1777 (Ledger B, p. 102; Ledger C, p. 80, noted that he paid his $18 bill in cash on 26 Jan 1778); see Martin Taylor Gilbert, q.v.

Gilbert, Thomas, below Everet's Mill, was treated by Dr. John Archer in Sep 1786 (Ledger F, p. 23)

Gilbert, William, see James Gilbert, q.v.

Gilbert, William, was visited by Dr. Robert H. Archer who treated a child and a negro in Jul 1823 (pp. 84, 84a)

Gilbert, William, was treated by Dr. Matthew J. Allen in Jan and Mar 1844 (p. 30)

Gilcrease, Elizabeth, at James Clendenin's, was treated by Dr. John Archer in Jun 1787 (Ledger F, p. 318)

Giles, Aquila [major, 1757-1822], was visited by Dr. John Archer who treated him in Dec 1780 and Aug 1781, his wife "in labor" on 16 Sep 1781, Mrs. Giles and Negro Susan in Nov 1781, his wife in Dec 1781, him in May and Jul 1782, his child and a negro in Nov 1782, him in Jan and Feb 1783 and inoculated three negroes (Ledger D, p. 109) [account continued in Ledger E, which is missing] [Aquila Giles was a Revolutionary War veteran.]

Giles, Charles Henry [1798-1873], was treated by Dr. Robert H. Archer after 1822 [no dates or details were given] (Dr. Archer's "Alphabet to Ledger H" is his booklet [filed in the Archives of the Historical Society of Harford County] that contains his index to Ledger H [which is missing] for his patients in Baltimore City before 1822 and in Harford County after 1822, according to a notation by Dr. George W. Archer.)

Giles, Eliza, Miss, was treated by Dr. Robert H. Archer in Baltimore before 1822 [no dates or details were given] (Dr. Archer's "Alphabet to Ledger H" is his booklet [filed in the Archives of the Historical Society of Harford County] that contains his index to Ledger H [which is missing] for his patients in Baltimore before 1822 and Harford County after 1822, according to a notation by Dr. George W. Archer.); see Thomas Giles, q.v.

Giles, Jacob, see Thomas Giles, Negro Valentine and Negro Rachel, q.v.

Giles, Jacob, Jr. was treated by Dr. John Archer in Nov and Dec 1780, Aug 1781, and Jun and Jul 1782 (Ledger D, p. 104, noted the bill was paid in full by Mr. Clifford, of Philadelphia)

Giles, James (esquire), was visited by Dr. John Archer who treated an infant in Feb 1775 in consultation with Dr. Annon (Ledger B, p. 75) [James Giles was a Revolutionary War veteran.]

Giles, Johanna, Mrs. (widow), was treated by Dr. John Archer in 1792 and 1796 (Ledger F, p. 315, misspelled her name as Joanna) [account continued in Ledger H, which is missing] (Ledger I, which is missing, was abstracted by Dr. George W. Archer circa 1890 and her name was spelled correctly as Johanna; Dr. George W. Archer's notes are in the Archives of the Historical Society of Harford County folder "Archer, G. W. Coll. – Ledgers and Day Books")

Giles, John, see Thomas Giles, q.v.

Giles, Mr., see Mrs. Scott, q.v.

Giles, Mrs., see Richard Burling, q.v.

Giles, Sarah, see Thomas Giles, q.v.

Giles, Thomas [1754-1798], was visited by Dr. John Archer who treated him in Jan 1777, Dec 1780, Dec 1781 and Feb, Jun, Oct and Nov 1782, and him, his wife, sons Jacob and John and daughter Sarah in 1787, and him, his wife and son Jacob in 1790, and him and children Eliza, Jacob and John at various times between 1794 and 1798 (Ledger C, p. 80; Ledger D, p. 107 [account continued in Ledger E, which is missing]; Ledger F, pp. 17, 32, 70, 81, 82, 102, 355) [account continued in Ledger G, which is missing]; Ledger I, is also missing, but was abstracted by Dr. George W. Archer circa 1890 and his notes are in the Archives of the Historical Society of Harford County folder "Archer, G. W. Coll. – Ledgers and Day Books") [Thomas Giles was a Revolutionary War veteran.]; see Beckey ----, q.v.

Gill, Mr., at J. W. Williams', was treated by Dr. Robert H. Archer in Aug 1822 (p. 14)

Gillespie, Francis, see Thomas Huggins & Co., q.v.

Gillespie, James, was visited by Dr. John Archer, Jr. who treated him and his wife in Aug 1820 and his wife and Hagan(?) in July 1821 (p. 76); see Thomas Huggins, q.v.

Gillespie, James Thomas, see Thomas Gallispie, q.v.

Gillespie, Samuel, see Samuel Galaspy, q.v.

Gilmore, Charles (weaver), was visited by Dr. John Archer who treated him in Nov 1774, a child in Dec 1776 and his wife in Apr 1778 (Ledger B, p. 98; Ledger C, p. 69, noted "debt forgiven by order of testator")

Gilmore, John, was treated by Dr. John Archer in Nov 1787, Mar 1788 and Oct 1791 (Ledger F, pp. 207, 213, 218)

Gilmore, Mrs. (widow), was visited by Dr. John Archer who treated a grandchild in 1787 and her [Mrs. Gilmore] and daughter Nancy in Apr 1789 (Ledger F, p. 379)

Gilmore, Nancy, see Mrs. Gilmore, q.v.

Gilmore, Sally, was treated by Dr. John Archer in Oct 1791 (Ledger F, p. 136)

Gilmore, Widow, see Jane Clinging, q.v.

Gitchel, Increase, was treated by Dr. Robert H. Archer in Sep 1815 (Ledger F, p. 3)

Gittings, Griffith, see John Chamberlain, q.v.

Gittings, Miss, see Bennett Matthews, q.v.

Glanville, James, was visited by Dr. Matthew J. Allen who treated his wife and child [daughter?] in Jul 1847 (p. 59)

Glasgow, D., see James Pannell, q.v.

Glasgow, Dolly, Miss, was prescribed medicine by Dr. Robert H. Archer on 20 June 1832 (Rx Book, 1825-1851, p. 106)

Glasgow, Elizabeth, Mrs. [1788-1826, widow of Dr. James Glasgow, 1782-1823], was visited by Dr. Robert H. Archer who treated her in June 1824 and Aug 1825, son James in March 1825 and Feb 1826, and daughter Susan or Susanna in July and Aug 1825; also mentioned James Pannell and noted "debt cancelled, being against the widow of a deceased intimate friend and professional brother;" Elizabeth died before 29 Nov 1826 at which time Dr. Robert H. Archer was paid by her administrator (p. 125, 126, 147, 210; Ledger F, p. 98)

Glasgow, George, see James Pannell, q.v.

Glasgow, George R. [1822-1894], was treated by Dr. Robert H. Archer obviously some time after 1822 [no dates or details were given] (Dr. Archer's "Alphabet to Ledger H" is his booklet [filed in the Archives of the Historical Society of Harford County] that contains his index to Ledger H [which is missing] for his patients in Baltimore before 1822 and Harford County after 1822, according to a notation by Dr. George W. Archer.) [His full name was George Robert Glasgow.]

Glasgow, Hugh (merchant), at Slate Ridge, was treated by Dr. John Archer in 1798 and 1799 (Ledger I, which is missing, was abstracted by Dr. George W. Archer circa 1890; his notes are in the Archives of the Historical Society of Harford County folder "Archer, G. W. Coll. – Ledgers and Day Books")

Glasgow, James [1818-1887], was treated by Dr. Matthew J. Allen in Apr 1848 (p. 80, noted the bill was paid in Sep 1852)

Glasgow, James, Dr., see Elizabeth Glasgow, q.v.

Glasgow, Robert, of Cecil Co., was visited by Dr. John Archer who treated him at times in 1780, 1781 and 1782 and him and wife in 1787 and 1788 (Ledger D, p. 42, noted "Enquire of James Clendennin" and "debt forgiven as before;" Ledger F, pp. 46, 90, spelled his name Glascow)

Glasgow, Susan or Susanna, see Elizabeth Glasgow, q.v.

Glenn, David, was visited by Dr. John Archer who treated him in Aug and Nov 1780, inoculated his daughter Peggy in 1782, and treated him, his wife and a daughter in Mar 1783, his wife and a daughter in Jun 1783, him in Oct 1785 and him and daughter Jinny in May 1787 (Ledger D, pp. 87, 98, noted "debt forgiven as before;" Ledger F, p. 46, also spelled his name Glen)

Glenn, Peggy, see David Glenn, q.v.

Glenn, Jinny, see David Glenn, q.v.

Glenn, William, was treated by Dr. John Archer eight times between Apr 1773 and Dec 1776 (Ledger B, p. 67, spelled his name Glen)

Glover, Robert, "vulgo Black Bob," was treated by Dr. Robert H. Archer in Sep 1825 (Ledger F, p. 148) [Since "vulgo" means "spurious," he was illegitimate according to the doctor who also listed him once as Robert Gover, vulgo Black Bob] [continued in Ledger G, which is missing]

Goghagan, Ambrose, was visited by Dr. John Archer who treated him in Dec 1781, his sister in Oct and Dec 1782 and treated him six times in Feb 1783 (Ledger D, p. 101) [account continued in Ledger E, which is missing]

Golden, Betsy [Elizabeth], was treated by Dr. John Archer in May 1786 (Ledger F, p. 289); see Alexander Hanna and Andrew Wilson, q.v.

Goldsmith, Vincent, at William Smithson's, was visited by Dr. John Archer who treated his wife in Sep 1777 and him in Jun, Jul and Sep 1778 and Jan and Oct 1779; also mentioned Thomas Barnes (Ledger C, p. 76) [Vincent Goldsmith was a Revolutionary War veteran.]

Goodwin, Margaret, was visited by Dr. John Archer who treated her and a child in Aug 1791 (Ledger F, p. 93, spelled her name Goodwins) [account continued in Ledger H, which is missing]

Goodwin, Mr., was prescribed medicine for wife by Dr. Robert H. Archer on 19 Jun 1801 (Rx Book, 1796-1801, p. 53); he was treated by Dr. Archer in Baltimore before 1822 [no dates or details were given] (Dr. Archer's "Alphabet to Ledger H" is his booklet [filed in the Archives of the Historical Society of Harford County] that contains his index to Ledger H [which is missing] for his patients in Baltimore City before 1822 and in Harford County after 1822, according to a notation by Dr. George W. Archer.)

Goodwin, William, Jr., was prescribed medicine by Dr. Robert H. Archer on 4 Aug 1802 (Rx Book, 1802-1804, p. 7)

Gordon, Aaron, was visited by Dr. John Archer who treated him in Aug 1780, Aug 1781, Aug 1782, a child in Sep 1782, him in Oct 1782, an infant in 1786 and him in 1788 (Ledger D, p. 86, noted "debt forgiven as before") [account continued in Ledger E, which is missing]; (Ledger F, p. 372, spelled his name Aron) [account continued in Ledger G, which is missing]

Gordon, Charles, was visited by Dr. John Archer who treated him, his wife and children between 1794 and 1801 (Ledger I, which is missing, was abstracted by Dr. George W. Archer circa 1890; his notes are in the Archives of the Historical Society of Harford County folder "Archer, G. W. Coll. – Ledgers and Day Books")

Gordon, Elenor, was treated by Dr. John Archer in 1786 (Ledger F, p. 194); see Thomas Hall, q.v.

Gordon, James, near Slate Ridge, was visited by Dr. John Archer who treated a child in March 1779 (Ledger C, p. 127, noted that the "debt forgiven by order of testator") [James Gordon was a Revolutionary War veteran.]

Gordon, Robert, at Wiley's near J. McCandless, was treated by Dr. John Archer in Aug 1788 (Ledger F, p. 306) [Robert Gordon was a Revolutionary War veteran.]

Gordon, Robert, near John Sample's, was treated by Dr. John Archer in Dec 1785 (Ledger D, p. 23, noted "debt forgiven as before")

Gorrell, Abram (weaver), was treated by Dr. John Archer in Dec 1781 and Jul 1785 (Ledger D, p. 105, spelled his name Gorrel) [account continued in Ledger G, which is missing]

Gorrell, B., see Zadock Gorrell, q.v.

Gorrell, Bondfield, was mentioned by Dr. Robert H. Archer in a non-medical matter (purchased cider) in May 1827 (p. 226); see Zadock Gorrell, q.v.

Gorrell, Gershom or Greshom [1799-1822], at Dublin, was treated by Dr. Robert H. Archer in Sep and Nov 1822 (p. 36; Ledger F, p. 118)

Gorrell, J., see Rezin Gorrell, q.v.

Gorrell, Jacob, see William Gorrell, q.v.

Gorrell, James, was visited by Dr. John Archer, Jr. who treated him in Mar 1816, an infant in Jul 1817 and Richard Harris in Jun 1817 (p. 47)

Gorrell, John, was treated by Dr. Matthew J. Allen in Mar and Apr 1844 (p. 33, spelled his name Gorrall); see Lawson Gorrell, q.v.

Gorrell, Joseph, was visited by Dr. Robert H. Archer who treated an infant in Dec 1822 and Jun 1823, a nephew in May 1823, a child in Jun 1823, Mar 1824, May 1827 and Mar 1828, Richard Hopkins [his brother-in-law] in May 1824, and him [Joseph] and "Mahaley (since his wife)" *(sic)* in May 1827 (pp. 44, 82, 268; Ledger F, p. 150, and p. 132 spelled his name Gorrel); see Richard Hopkins, q.v.

Gorrell, Lawson, brother of John Gorell, was mentioned in Dr. Robert H. Archer's ledger in a non-medical matter in 1827 and 1828 and also mentioned their father (pp. 258, 259) [Lawson Gorrell was a War of 1812 veteran.]

Gorrell, Neeper, see Zadock Gorrell, q.v.

Gorrell, Oliver, was treated by Dr. John Archer before 1772 [no details were given] and in May 1775 (Ledger B, p. 25, spelled his name Gorrel); see Rezin Gorrell, q.v.

Gorrell, Rezin, was treated by Dr. John Archer, Jr. in 1818 and mentioned J. Gorrell; was visited by Dr. Robert H. Archer who treated his wife in Nov 1824, him and his son Oliver in July and Aug 1825, a child in Nov 1825, a son and a child in Apr 1827 and a child in Jun 1828; R. Gorrell was prescribed medicine for his child by Dr. Robert H. Archer on 18 Jun 1830 (Dr. John Archer, Jr., p. 54; Dr. Robert H. Archer, pp. 144, 145, 146,

147, 150, 167, 222, 282; Rx Book, 1825-1851, p. 101; Ledger F, p. 37) [Rezin or Reasin Gorrell was a War of 1812 veteran.]

Gorrell, William, was visited by Dr. John Archer who treated his wife in Aug 1781, his brother Jacob in Jan and Oct 1783, and him [William] in May 1787 (Ledger D, p. 64, and Ledger F, p. 309, both spelled his name Gorrel)

Gorrell, William, was visited by Dr. John Archer, Jr. who treated his wife and Betsy Ryan in Feb 1817, a child in Jul 1820 and William himself in Feb 1822 (p. 69, spelled his name Gorrel)

Gorrell, Zadock, was treated by Dr. Robert H. Archer in Mar 1824; mentioned Zadock, Bondfield and Neeper Gorrell in Jan 1827 and B. Gorrell in Apr 1829 (Ledger F, pp. 86, 89)

Gorsuch, see Negro ----, q.v.

Gorsuch, N., see Robert H. Archer, q.v.

Goslee, William, was treated by Dr. John Archer, Jr. in Nov 1815 and mentioned his sister Mrs. Fox and Mrs. Fox's child in Jan 1816 (p. 33)

Gough, Harry D. [1792-1867], was visited by Dr. Alonzo Preston who treated him at various times between 1823 and 1825 [no details were given], his wife in Dec 1825 and Aug 1828 and an unnamed black boy in Dec 1826; the total bill due was $14.00 and the doctor noted that Gough "says he has a receipt." (p. 63) [Harry Dorsey Gough was a War of 1812 veteran.]

Gover, Cassandra; was treated by Dr. John Archer in Jul 1779 (Ledger C, p. 113 noted "debt forgiven by order of testator"); see Samuel Gover, q.v.

Gover, Elizabeth (widow), was visited by Dr. John Archer who treated a negro in Dec 1776 and Jan 1777, her in Jan 1777, a negro in Feb 1777, her in Mar 1778 and June and July 1779, her daughter, a negro and Mrs. Bussey in Aug 1779, her and daughter and a negro in Sep 1779, Gideon in Apr 1780, her in Dec 1780, Jul 1781, Sep 1782 and Jan and May 1783 (Ledger C, pp. 82, 93, 113; Ledger D, p. 19) [continued in Ledger E, which is missing]; see Samuel Gover, q.v.

Gover, Ephraim, see Robert Gover and Samuel Gover, q.v.

Gover, Gerard, was visited by Dr. John Archer who treated him and his family at various times in 1797 and 1798 (Ledger I, which is missing, was abstracted by Dr. George W. Archer circa 1890; his notes are in the Archives of the Historical Society of Harford County folder "Archer, G. W. Coll. – Ledgers and Day Books"); Gerard was treated by Dr. Robert H. Archer in Baltimore City before 1822 [no dates or details were given] (Dr. Archer's "Alphabet to Ledger H" is his booklet [filed in the Archives of the Historical Society of Harford County] that contains his index to Ledger H [which is missing] for his patients in Baltimore City before 1822 and Harford County after 1822, according to a notation by Dr. George W. Archer.)

Gover, Gittings, was treated by Dr. John Archer in Jun and Jul 1779, May and Aug 1781 and Jul 1782 and at various times between 1797 and 1802 (Ledger C, p. 113, noted "debt forgiven by order of testator") (Ledger I, which is missing, was abstracted by Dr. George W. Archer circa 1890; his notes are in Archives of the Historical Society of Harford County file "Archer, G. W. Coll. – Ledgers and Day Books"); Gittings Gover was treated by Dr. Robert H. Archer in Baltimore before 1822 [no dates or details were given] (Dr. Archer's "Alphabet to Ledger H" is his booklet [filed in the Archives of the Historical Society of Harford County] that contains his index to Ledger H [which is missing] for his patients in Baltimore before 1822 and in Harford County after 1822, according to a notation by Dr. George W. Archer.)

Gover, James, see Robert Gover (miller), q.v.

Gover, Joseph, was treated by Dr. Robert H. Archer in Baltimore before 1822 [no dates or details were given] (Dr. Archer's "Alphabet to Ledger H" is his booklet [filed in the Archives of the Historical Society of Harford County] that contains his index to Ledger H [which is missing] for his patients in Baltimore before 1822 and Harford County after 1822, according to a notation by Dr. George W. Archer.)

Gover, Mr., see Abraham Jarrett, Augustus J. Greme and Richard Pool, q.v.

Gover, Mrs., widow of Philip, was treated by Dr. John Archer in Jul 1788 and Feb 1790 (Ledger F, pp. 165, 187, and the name "Elizabeth" was written in a different handwriting over her name); see Peggy Reese and Elizabeth Gover, q.v.

Gover, Peggy, see Samuel Gover, q.v.

Gover, Philip, was treated by Dr. John Archer in Jul 1789 (Ledger F, p. 267) [Philip Gover was a Revolutionary War veteran.]; see Mrs. Gover, Priscilla Gover and Moses Cannon, q.v.

Gover, Priscilla, "sister-in-law of P. Gover" [most probably Philip Gover], was treated by Dr. John Archer in Feb 1790 (Ledger F, p. 29)

Gover, Prissy, see Samuel Gover, q.v.

Gover, Robert, see Robert Glover, q.v.

Gover, Robert, of Ephraim, was treated by Dr. John Archer in Oct 1789 and he was visited many years later by Dr. Robert H. Archer who treated a negro in Jan 1823, his [Robert's] wife in Apr 1823 in consultation with Dr. Preston, him [Robert] in May 1823 and July 1825, Negro Angus in Jan 1834 and his [Robert's] wife in May 1838, and mentioned Negro Carvil in July 1843; also noted "payment assumed by his son-in-law Dr. Richard N. Allen." (Dr. John Archer, Ledger F, pp. 8, 137; Dr. Robert H. Archer, pp. 48, 66, 74) [continued in Ledger G, which is missing]

Gover, Robert (miller), was visited by Dr. Robert H. Archer who treated his son James thirteen times between 13 Oct 1827 and 3 Dec 1827 in consultation with Dr. Allen (pp. 250-256)

Gover, Robert, on Deer Creek, was treated by Dr. Robert H. Archer in July and Sep 1825 (pp. 141, 158, 159)

Gover, Samuel, was visited by Dr. John Archer who treated him and a negro boy in Dec 1776, him, a negro boy, a negro girl, Casey and sister Cass: [Cassandra] in Jan 1777, a negro man in Feb 1777, him [Samuel] and wife in Oct 1777, and also noted medicine charged to Elizabeth Gover (Ledger C, p. 64) [Samuel Gover was a Revolutionary War veteran.]

Gover, Samuel, of Ephraim, was visited by Dr. John Archer who treated him in Sep 1788 and him and daughters Peggy and Prissy at various times in 1797 and 1798 (Ledger F, p. 225; (Ledger I, which is missing, was abstracted by Dr. George W. Archer circa 1890; his notes are in the Archives of the Historical Society of Harford County folder "Archer, G. W. Coll. – Ledgers and Day Books"); see James Spence, q.v.

Grace, Aaron [c1734-c1788], was treated by Dr. John Archer in Sep 1786 (Ledger F, p. 238, spelled his first name Aron) [account continued in Ledger G, which is missing] [Aaron Grace was a Revolutionary War veteran.]

Grace, John, was treated by Dr. John Archer at various times between Sep 1777 and Aug 1779, in Aug, Sep and Oct 1780, his wife in Sep 1781, and his son Samuel in Dec 1781 (Ledger C, p. 3; Ledger D, p. 6, noted "debt forgiven as before")

Grace, Samuel, see John Grace, q.v.

Grafton, Aquila, was treated by Dr. John Archer in Nov 1787 (Ledger F, p. 76)

Grafton, Curtis, was visited by Dr. Matthew J. Allen who treated his wife in Jun and Aug 1847 and Jun, Jul and Sep 1848 (p. 54)

Grafton, Daniel, was treated by Dr. John Archer in Aug 1803 (Ledger F, p. 196)

Grafton, James, appeared on a list of debts dated 26 Dec 1822 and titled "A List of Allen's Claims" that were due and payable to Dr. Richard N. Allen for services rendered [no dates were given] by him to said Grafton (Document filed in Historical Society of Harford County Archives folder "R. N. Allen") [James Grafton was a War of 1812 veteran.]

Grafton, John, was visited by Dr. Alonzo Preston who treated Mary in 1826 and 1827, Maryam (sic) in 1826 and Rebecca in 1827 (p. 68, noted the bill was paid with 2½ bushels of chopped rye and 15 bushels of cut straw in 1826 and 114 lbs. of beef and 6½ bushels of oats in 1828)

Grafton, Mary, see John Grafton, q.v.

Grafton, Maryam, see John Grafton, q.v.

Grafton, Mrs. (widow), was treated by Dr. John Archer in July 1780 (Ledger D, p. 78, noted the bill was paid in full in cash by Alexander Thompson on 18 Jun 1788)

Grafton, Nathan [1826-1915], at Ashton's B.S.S. [i. e., John Ashton's blacksmith shop near Forest Hill where Grafton was a wheelwright], was treated by Dr. Matthew J. Allen in Apr 1848 (p. 81)

Grafton, William, was treated by Dr. John Archer in Oct 1788 (Ledger F, p. 102) [William Grafton was a Revolutionary War veteran.]; see David Thomas, q.v.

Grafton, William, was treated by Dr. Matthew J. Allen in Aug 1848 (p. 91) [William Grafton, of Aquila, and William Grafton, of Daniel (1786-1879), were both War of 1812 veterans]

Graham, Charles, see R. N. and M. J. Allen, q.v.

Graham, Richard (captain), was visited by Dr. Matthew J. Allen who treated him and his son Richard in 1823 in Calvert Co. (p. 5b); see James Mackall, q.v.

Graham, William (doctor), was treated by Dr. Matthew J. Allen in 1832 in Calvert County (p. 18)

Grahame, Charles, was treated by Dr. Matthew J. Allen in 1832 in Calvert County (p. 25, noted a payment was made with one buffalo skin worth $3.50)

Grant, John (stage driver), was treated by Dr. John Archer in 1795 (Ledger I, which is missing, was abstracted by Dr. George W. Archer circa 1890; his notes are in the Archives of the Historical Society of Harford County folder "Archer, G. W. Coll. – Ledgers and Day Books")

Grant, Mr., "near White House," was treated by Dr. Robert H. Archer in June 1826 and he was also prescribed medicine by Dr. Robert H. Archer on 14 May 1827, 18 May 1827 and 23 May 1829 (p. 190; Rx Book, 1825-1851, pp. 89, 90, 94)

Gray, Harry, see John Gray, q.v.

Gray, James, was treated by Dr. John Archer in Dec 1788 (Ledger F, p. 244)

Gray, John, at Bush Town, was visited by Dr. John Archer who treated him and sons Joseph and Harry between 1794 and 1795 (Ledger I, which is missing, was abstracted by Dr. George W. Archer circa 1890; his notes are in the Archives of the Historical Society of Harford County folder "Archer, G. W. Coll. – Ledgers and Day Books")

Gray, Joseph, see John Gray, q.v.

Gray, Joseph (negro), was prescribed medicine by Dr. Robert H. Archer circa Dec 1804 (Rx Book, 1802-1804, p. 67)

Gray, William, was treated by Dr. Matthew J. Allen in 1832 in Calvert County (p. 17)

Green, Andrew, was treated by Dr. John Archer in Jul 1778 and Mar 1783 (Ledger C, p. 115, noted "debt forgiven by order of testator")

Green, Benjamin [1730-1808], was visited by Dr. John Archer who treated him in Sep 1778 and Jan, Mar and Apr 1781, a negro in Sep 1781 and inoculated 7 of his family and son Benjamin in Dec 1781 (Ledger C, p. 70, noted part of the bill was paid on 15 Dec 1785 and part was paid on 5 Dec 1791); Benjamin Green, Sr., was visited by Archer who treated him and children Benjamin, Sally, Clement and Henry in 1796 (Ledger I, which is missing, was abstracted by Dr. George W. Archer circa 1890; his notes are in the Archives of the Historical Society of Harford County file "Archer, G. W. Coll. – Ledgers and Day Books") [Benjamin Green was a Revolutionary War veteran.]; see Edward Bevin, q.v.

Green, Bennett, was visited by Dr. John Archer who treated him and wife in 1792 (Ledger F, p. 24, spelled his name Bennit) [Bennett Green was a Revolutionary War veteran.]

Green, C., see Mrs. Wheeler, q.v.

Green, Clement, near Long Green, was visited by Dr. John Archer who treated him, his wife and "consobrin" [cousin] Henry in 1787 (Ledger F, p. 121, noted that Clement Green, Jr. paid off the account [over 18 years later] on 29 Nov 1805)

Green, Clement [c1790-1829], was visited by Dr. Alonzo Preston who treated him in 1824, Miss Ellen in 1827 and a black girl in 1828; Clement was visited by Dr. Robert H. Archer who treated him and his wife in Aug 1823, him in July 1825 and he was prescribed medicine on 1 Aug 1825 (Dr. Preston, p. 2; Dr. Archer, pp. 88, 145; Rx Book, 1825-1851, p. 82; Ledger F, p. 60, noted "died insolvent," but did not give a date of death) [Clement Green was a War of 1812 veteran.]; see Benjamin Green, q.v.

Green, Clement, Jr., see Clement Green, near Long Green, q.v.

Green, Edward, was treated by Dr. John Archer in Sep 1794 (Ledger F, p. 257)

Green, Elizabeth, was visited by Dr. Alonzo Preston who treated her at various times between 1824 and 1827, daughter Sarah (also called Sally) in 1825 and son John in 1825, 1826 and 1827 (p. 41, noted that a $1 part of the medical bill was paid "by ½ cord oak wood by John" in August 1826)

Green, Ellen, Miss, see Clement Green, q.v.

Green, Harriet (colored), was visited by Dr. Matthew J. Allen who treated her child ten times in Jan 1848, three times in Feb 1848 and once in Jun 1848, and "visit & medicine children" in Jul 1848 and treated her [Harriet] in Feb 1848 (pp. 71, 96, noted she paid part of the medical bill in cash in Aug 1848 and paid part of the bill "by washing 9 pieces" in Nov 1848); see John Clarke, q.v.

Green, Henry, Sr., was visited by Dr. John Archer who treated him and Henry Green, Jr. in 1797 (Ledger I, which is missing, was abstracted by Dr. George W. Archer circa 1890; his notes are in the Archives of the Historical Society of Harford County folder "Archer, G. W. Coll. – Ledgers and Day Books"); see Clement Green and Thomas Green, q.v.

Green, Isaac, was treated by Dr. John Archer in Nov 1786 and was prescribed medicine for his wife by Dr. Robert H. Archer on 24 Jan 1801 (Ledger F, p. 127; Rx Book, 1796-1801, p. 28)

Green, James, in Baltimore Town, was treated by Dr. John Archer in Sep 1788 (Ledger F, p. 300)

Green, James, was visited by Dr. John Archer who treated his daughter in May 1779, him in Aug 1779, son James in July 1780, and him [James the father] in Apr and May 1781 and Mar 1786 (Ledger C, p. 50; Ledger F, p. 183)

Green, James, Jr., was treated by Dr. John Archer in May 1781 and Jul 1785 (Ledger D, p. 26, noted "debt forgiven as before")

Green, John, was treated by Dr. John Archer in Apr and May 1781 (Ledger D, p. 23, noted "debt forgiven as before"); see Elizabeth Green, q.v.

Green, John, of John, was visited by Dr. John Archer who treated him and son John at various times in 1798 and 1799 (Ledger I, which is missing, was abstracted by Dr. George W. Archer circa 1890; his notes are in the Archives of the Historical Society of Harford County folder "Archer, G. W. Coll. – Ledgers and Day Books")

Green, Joshua, was inoculated by Dr. John Archer in 1783 [exact date not given] (Ledger D, p.38)

Green, Leonard, was treated by Dr. John Archer in Apr and Jul 1781, Jan and Aug 1782 and Dec 1783 (Ledger D, p. 54) [Leonard Green was a Revolutionary War veteran.]

Green, Michael, was treated by Dr. Robert H. Archer in Baltimore before 1822 [no dates or details were given] (Dr. Archer's "Alphabet to Ledger H" is his booklet [filed in the Archives of the Historical Society of Harford County] that contains his index to Ledger H [which is missing] for his patients in Baltimore City before 1822 and in Harford County after 1822, according to a notation by Dr. George W. Archer.)

Green, Sally, see Henry G. Watters, q.v.

Green, Sarah, see Elizabeth Green, q.v.

Green, Thomas, was visited by Dr. Robert H. Archer who treated a child in March and April 1823 in consultation with Dr. Forwood, and treated his son Henry in July and August 1824 (pp. 61, 62, 115; Ledger F, p. 154)

Green, William (overseer to Thomas Onion), near Onion's Mill [on the Little Gunpowder River at Joppa], was treated by Dr. John Archer in 1798 (Ledger I, which is missing, was abstracted by Dr. George W. Archer circa 1890; his notes are in the Archives of the Historical Society of Harford County folder "Archer, G. W. Coll. – Ledgers and Day Books")

Greenfield, Jacob, see Joseph Everist, q.v.

Greenfield, Louisa, was visited by Dr. Alonzo Preston who treated Sarah [daughter?] in Dec 1824 and Mar 1825 (p. 13)

Greenfield, P. George, was treated by Dr. Robert H. Archer in Baltimore before 1822 [no dates or details were given] (Dr. Archer's "Alphabet to Ledger H" is his booklet [filed in the Archives of the Historical Society of Harford County] that contains his index to Ledger H [which is missing] for his patients in Baltimore City before 1822 and in Harford County after 1822, according to a notation by Dr. George W. Archer.)

Greenland, Richard, was treated by Dr. John Archer in Dec 1778 and Sep 1786 (Ledger C, p. 46, noted that the "debt forgiven by order of testator"; Ledger F, p. 66) [Richard Greenland was a Revolutionary War veteran.]

Greenley, Samuel, on Spesutia Island, was treated by Dr. John Archer in Sep 1786 (Ledger F, p. 82)

Greg, Mrs., see Stephen Hill, q.v.

Gregg, John & Co. (Baltimore) [merchants], had a non-medical account in Dr. John Archer, Jr.'s ledger that mentioned Capt. Elliot, Leven Gale, Thomas Huggins, S. Stump and Capt. White in 1815 and 1816 (p. 49); see Thomas Huggins & Co. and Nathaniel Ramsey, q.v.

Gregg, Mr., see Nathaniel Ramsay, q.v.

Greme, Augustus J., had an account in Dr. Matthew J. Allen's ledger for non-medical matters from Jul 1847 to Sep 1852 and it mentioned him, his wife, Joseph Cole, Daniel McGonigal, Orrick Bagley, Jo. Wilson, William Judd, William Dallam, James Quinlan, Jane A. Greme, James W. Reynolds, E. Reynolds, J. D. Allen, Mr. Gover and Joshua Arthur (p. 66); see Daniel McGonigal and Thomas James, q.v.

Greme, Angus, was treated by Dr. John Archer between 1794 and 1798 [name misspelled Graham] (Ledger I, which is missing, was abstracted by Dr. George W. Archer circa 1890; his notes are in the Archives of the Historical Society of Harford County folder "Archer, G. W. Coll. – Ledgers and Day Books"); see Mrs. Greme, q.v.

Greme, Anna, Miss, was treated by Dr. Matthew J. Allen in Jun 1848 (p. 85)

Greme, Caroline, see Mrs. Greme, q.v.

Greme, Jane A., see Augustus J. Greme, q.v.

Greme, Mary, Mrs., was visited by Dr. Matthew J. Allen who treated her son Ralph in Sep, Oct and Nov 1847 (p. 66, misspelled her name Grene and noted bill "settled by note by Thos. Grene")

Greme, Mr., see James Everist, q.v.

Greme, Mrs., was visited by Dr. Alonzo Preston who treated him at times between 1823 and 1825, Negro John in July 1824, Miss Caroline Greme and Angus Greme in 1825 and 1826; visited by Dr. Robert H. Archer who treated her son Angus and negroes John and Harriet in Apr 1822, and daughter Caroline and son Angus in June 1825 (Dr. Preston, p. 40; Dr. Archer, pp. 64-67, 114, 134, 137; Ledger F, p. 42); see Mr. Smith, q.v.

Greme, Mrs. and Miss, were prescribed medicine by Dr. Robert H. Archer on 22 Jun 1841 (Rx Book, 1825-1851, p. 114)

Greme, Ralph, see Mary Greme, q.v.

Greme, Thomas, was treated by Dr. Matthew J. Allen in May, Jun and Aug 1847 and Sep 1848 (p. 53); see Mary Greme, q.v.

Gresson, Col., of Virginia, was visited by Dr. John Archer who treated him, daughter Maria and an infant in Harford Town in Nov 1787 (Ledger F, pp. 59, 100)

Gresson, Maria, see Col. Gresson, q.v.

Grier, Thomas, was treated by Dr. Matthew J. Allen in the late 1840s [not listed in his ledger] as evidenced by the following statement that was written on a separate page dated 24 Nov 1853 and inserted in the back of Dr. Allen's ledger. The letter, addressed to Major Bond, was signed by I. Day and stated "I have just returned after 3 days ride to look up the Drs. of Dr. Allen and the following is the result." It included several patients and noted "Thos. Grier promises to call & pay you half in a mo. if he can dbl.(?) [illegible three-letter abbreviation] in the spring."]

Griffin, Mr., see Charles Martin, q.v.

Griffith, James, was visited by Dr. Matthew J. Allen who treated his wife (tooth extraction) in Aug 1844 (p. 38) [James Griffith was a War of 1812 veteran.]

Griffith, John, was treated by Dr. John Archer in Jun 1775 and twelve times between 15 Sep and 16 Nov 1779 (Ledger B, p. 61; Ledger C, p. 101, stated "To be paid in wheat at 6 p. per bushel or the value thereof in Continental Dollars" and also noted "debt forgiven by order of testator;" Ledger D, p. 17, noted "debt forgiven as before")

Griffith, Luke [1787-1838], was visited by Dr. Robert H. Archer who treated his wife in Oct 1826 (p. 204) [Luke Griffith was a War of 1812 veteran.]

Griffith, Nathan, was treated by Dr. Robert H. Archer in Baltimore before 1822 [no dates or details were given] (Dr. Archer's "Alphabet to Ledger H" is his booklet [filed in the Archives of the Historical Society of Harford County] that contains his index to Ledger H [which is missing] for his patients in Baltimore City before 1822 and in Harford County after 1822, according to a notation by Dr. George W. Archer.)

Grimes, James, was treated by Dr. Robert H. Archer in Baltimore before 1822 [no dates or details were given] (Dr. Archer's "Alphabet to Ledger H" is his booklet [filed in the Archives of the Historical Society of Harford County] that contains his index to Ledger H [which is missing] for his patients in Baltimore City before 1822 and in Harford County after 1822, according to a notation by Dr. George W. Archer.)

Grimes, John, was treated by Dr. Robert H. Archer in Baltimore before 1822 [no dates or details were given] (Dr. Archer's "Alphabet to Ledger H" is his booklet [filed in the Archives of the Historical Society of Harford County] that contains his index to Ledger H [which is missing] for his patients in Baltimore City before 1822 and in Harford County after 1822, according to a notation by Dr. George W. Archer.)

Grindell, John, "brother to J. L. Gibson," was treated by Dr. John Archer in October 1787 (Ledger F, p. 165, listed him as Jno. Grindel) [account continued in Ledger H, which is missing]

Grossman, Nicholas, at Israel Morris', was visited by Dr. John Archer who treated a child in October 1782 (Ledger D, p. 16, noted "debt forgiven as before")

Grundy, Samuel, see Thomas Hall, q.v.

Gurley, Joseph (Cecil Co.), was visited by Dr. Robert H. Archer who treated his wife in December 1826 (p. 211)

Guyton, Benjamin [1788-1821], appeared on a list of debts dated 26 Dec 1822 and titled "A List of Allen's Claims" that were due and payable to Dr. Richard N. Allen for services rendered [no dates were given] by him to said Guyton (Document filed in Archives of the Historical Society of Harford County folder "R. N. Allen"); see Jane Guyton and John Guyton, q.v.

Guyton, Elenor, see John Guyton, q.v.

Guyton, Elias, see John Guyton, q.v.

Guyton, Elisha, was treated by Dr. Alonzo Preston at various times between 1822 and 1825, but no dates or details were given in the ledger, only entries about various payments (p. 24)

Guyton, Henry, see Jane Guyton, q.v.

Guyton, Isaac, "for Negro Ned in Harford goal" [jail], was treated by Dr. John Archer in Jan 1786 (Ledger F, p. 92) [Isaac Guyton was a Revolutionary War veteran.]

Guyton, James, see John Guyton, q.v.

Guyton, Jane, Mrs. [widow of Benjamin Guyton], was visited by Dr. Alonzo Preston who treated her son Henry in Oct 1825 and mentioned Negro Bob and Jane's woman Hannah in Dr. Robert H. Archer's ledger in Oct 1826; Mrs. Guyton was prescribed medicine for Negro Hannah on 30 Jun 1833 (Dr. Preston, p. 49; Dr. Archer, p. 204, and Rx Book, 1825-1851, p. 109)

Guyton, John (tavern keeper), Bel Air, was treated by Dr. John Archer in 1795 and 1796 and also "by inoculating 4 of yr. children, Benjamin, James, Elenor and Elias" in 1795 (Ledger I, which is missing, was abstracted by Dr. George W. Archer circa 1890; his notes are in the Archives of the Historical Society of Harford County folder "Archer, G. W. Coll. – Ledgers and Day Books")

Hagan, Henry, was treated by Dr. John Archer in Aug 1780 (Ledger D, p. 92, noted "debt forgiven as before")

Hagg, J., see Aquila Paca, q.v.

Hague, Arthur, "at Mr. Bay's Mill moved to the new mills on O," was visited by Dr. John Archer who treated him at various times between Mar and Oct 1774, an infant in Mar 1774 and a child in Apr 1774 (Ledger B, p. 77)

Haily, George (blacksmith), was visited by Dr. John Archer who treated him and his family at various times between 1796 and 1802 (Ledger I, which is missing, was abstracted by Dr. George W. Archer circa 1890; his notes are in the Archives of the Historical Society of Harford County folder "Archer, G. W. Coll. – Ledgers and Day Books")

Haily, John, Jr., was treated by Dr. John Archer in April 1786 (Ledger F, p. 244)

Haily, John, Sr., was treated by Dr. John Archer in July 1786 (Ledger F, p. 361)

Hainy, Patrick, was visited by Dr. John Archer who treated a him and child in Aug 1781, him in Aug 1784, a child in Sep 1784 and him [Patrick] in Feb 1786 (Ledger D, p. 64, noted "account forgiven as before;" Ledger F, p. 127)

Hair, James, was visited by Dr. John Archer who treated him and his wife in Aug 1790 (Ledger F, p. 65)

Hair, Mary, was treated by Dr. John Archer in Jan 1788 (Ledger F, p. 143); see Mary Harr, q.v.

Hair, Robert, was visited by Dr. John Archer who treated him and his wife in Sep 1786 (Ledger F, p. 342) [Robert Hair was a Revolutionary War veteran.]

Hair, Sarah, see Harford County for Pensioners, q.v.

Hale, Charles, was prescribed medicine for his sister [name not given] by Dr. Robert H. Archer on 2 Sep 1802 (Rx Book, 1802-1804, p. 19)

Hale, Stephen, was prescribed medicine by Dr. Robert H. Archer on 4 Feb 1801 (Rx Book, 1796-1801, p. 32)

Haley, Daniel, was visited by Dr. John Archer who inoculated his child in Feb 1782 (Ledger D, p. 65, noted "debt forgiven as before")

Haley, John, was treated by Dr. John Archer in Jun 1778 and Mar 1779 (Ledger C, p. 115, noted "debt forgiven by order of testator")

Haley, Mark, son of John, was treated by Dr. John Archer in Sep 1787 and Dec 1789 (Ledger F, pp. 7, 111) [account continued in Ledger G, which is missing]

Halfpenny, ---- [blank], at Mr. Webb's, was treated by Dr. John Archer in Jul 1775 (Ledger B, p. 47)

Hall, Andrew, was treated by Dr. John Archer in Aug 1773, Oct 1774 and Oct 1780 (Ledger B, p. 30; Ledger D, p. 89, noted "debt forgiven as before")

Hall, Aquila [Jr.] [1750-1815] (attorney, esquire), was visited by Dr. John Archer who treated him in Dec 1781, him and "free George" in Sep 1782, him and children Charlotte, Boby and Nicky in Nov 1787, a child in Dec 1787, and him [Aquila] in Apr 1788 (Ledger D, p. 102 [account continued in Ledger E, which is missing]; Ledger F, pp. 286, 310, 378, 379) [account continued in Ledger G, which is missing]; see John B. Hall, William Hall, Thomas Hall, Edward Hall and John Moore, q.v. [He was styled "Jr." to distinguish himself from his uncle, Col. Aquila Hall.]

Hall, Becky, see William Hall, q.v.

Hall, Benedict, was visited by Dr. Thomas Archer who treated him in Mar 1798, Mar and Apr 1799, Jan, Apr, Jul, Sep and Oct 1801, Feb 1802 ("gonarrea") and Jan 1804, Negro Sam in Sep 1794, Apr 1799 and Sep 1803, a negro at R. Boyce's in Sep 1799, Negro Sam at R. McGaa's in May 1803 and Negro boy Harry in Nov and Dec 1804 (to curing "in lues venerea") (Document in the Archives of the Historical Society of Harford

County folder "Archer, Thomas, Dr., 1768-1821 – Papers" and noted bill was paid in full by Edward Hall at Dairy [Sophia's Dairy] on 5 Feb 1808)

Hall, Benedict Edward [1744-1822], was visited by Dr. John Archer who treated his child in Oct 1781, a negro in Dec 1781, him [Benedict E.] three times in Apr 1785, him and his wife and daughters Caroline, Charlotte and Eliza in 1789; also mentioned, and possibly treated, Jno. Mitchael *(sic)* and Peggy Walker in 1789 (Ledger D, p. 81, listed him as Benedick Edw. Hall and Ledger F, p. 277, listed him as Benedict E. Hall) [account continued in Ledger G, which is missing]; Benedict Hall was visited by Dr. Jacob A. Preston who treated him and his family in Jul 1819, him 12 times between Aug and Dec 1819, negroes in Nov and Dec 1819, him 8 times in Feb 1820, a negro in Mar 1820 and him [Benedict] in Apr and Jul 1820 and 17 times between 7 Oct 1820 and 11 Feb 1821. The bill noted "On this 27th day of January 1822 being since the death of Benedict Hall," Dr. Preston appeared before W. T. Hall, a Justice of the Peace, and swore that the bill was true and just, and the justice confirmed that the said accounts were truly copied from the medical books of Dr. Preston; Major Henry Hall, administrator of Benedict E. Hall, paid his bills at James Park on 23 Jan 1827. It also listed treatment to Negro Troilus in Sep and Dec 1822, Negro Duke in Jun and Jul 1825, Negro Riller in Jan 1826 and Negro Abe in Apr 1826 (Harford County Will Book SR No. 1, p. 256; Documents filed in Historical Society of Harford County Archives folder titled "Preston, Dr. Jacob A.") [Benedict Edward Hall was a Revolutionary War veteran.]

Hall, Betsey, was treated by Dr. John Archer in Oct 1791 (Ledger F, p. 282)

Hall, Betsey, Miss, was treated by Dr. Robert H. Archer in Baltimore before 1822 [no dates or details were given] (Dr. Archer's "Alphabet to Ledger H" is his booklet [filed in the Archives of the Historical Society of Harford County] that contains his index to Ledger H [which is missing] for his patients in Baltimore before 1822 and Harford County after 1822, according to a notation by Dr. George W. Archer.)

Hall, Boby, see Aquila Hall, q.v.

Hall, Capt., see Nathaniel Bond, q.v.

Hall, Caroline, see Benedict Edward Hall, q.v.

Hall, Carvel (negro), near Boner's stone house, was visited by Dr. Robert H. Archer who treated his daughter Mary in Oct 1826 (p. 204)

Hall, Catherine, Mrs., widow of Elihu, was treated by Dr. John Archer in Jan 1791 (Ledger F, p. 199)

Hall, Charlotte, Miss, was treated by Dr. John Archer in Oct 1789 (Ledger F, p. 61, indicated "now married to Col. Ramsay")

Hall, Charlotte, see Aquila Hall and Benedict Edward Hall, q.v.

Hall, Col., see Negro Jacob and Aquila Hall, q.v.

Hall, Delia, see John B. Hall, q.v.

Hall, Dr., was consulted by Dr. John Archer in Feb 1787 (Ledger F, p. 197); see Aquila Paca, q.v.

Hall, Edward [1763-1827] (esquire), son of Aquila, was treated by Dr. John Archer in Feb 1789 (Ledger F, p. 187) and he was visited by Dr. Thomas Archer who treated him in Jul 1809, May and Nov 1810 and Feb 1812, Negro Juniper in Jul and Aug 1808, Negro Rumney [or a negro at Rumney] in Oct 1808 and Feb 1810, Negro Lucy in Jun 1809 and Oct 1810, Negro Hagar in Aug 1809, negro infant in Oct 1801, Negro Nance or Nancy in Mar 1810 and Sep 1811, negro child in Jun 1810, Negro Davy in Sep 1810, Negro Nance's child in Oct 1810, Negro Hannah in Sep 1811 and Negro Sam in Oct 1811 [Thomas Archer's receipt stated "Recd. Dairy 25th Oct 1809 of E. Hall the amount of the above a/c." ["Dairy" did not refer to dairy as a type of payment, but to the Hall family's mansion Sophia's Dairy.] (Document filed in the Archives of the Historical Society of Harford County folder "Medical Papers" [It is interesting to note that the medical bill amounted to £4.4.3 and the amount paid was $11.231/3.]; Document filed in the Archives of the Historical Society folder "Archer, Thomas, Dr., 1768-1821 – Papers"); Edward was also visited by Dr. Joseph Brownley who treated him ("bleeding" and using "febrifuge powders") and Negro man Phillip ("antidysentery pills") in Jul 1817, and he was visited by Dr. Jacob A. Preston who treated his family in Jan, Sep, Nov and Dec 1820, Negro Bidy in Mar 1821, him and Negro Bidy and Negro Charles in Apr 1821, him and Negro Bidy in Jul 1821 and his family in Aug 1821 (Documents filed in the Archives of the Historical Society of Harford County folders "Preston, Jacob A." and "Archer, G. W. Coll. – Medicine #2"); see Benedict Hall and James W. Hall, q.v.

Hall, Edward, "at Cramburry" [Cranberry], was treated by Dr. John Archer in 1799 (Ledger F, p. 83, indicated his executor was Jas. [Jos.?] Hall on 4 Feb 1802)

Hall, Elen or Elenor, see James White Hall, q.v.

Hall, Elihu, Sr. (esquire), was visited by Dr. John Archer who treated him, his wife and child in 1788 (Ledger F, p. 87); see Catherine Hall and Samuel Hall, q.v.

Hall, Eliza, see John B. Hall and Benedict Edward Hall, q.v.

Hall, George W., see Negro Jessee, q.v.

Hall, Elizabeth, was treated by Dr. John Archer in Jan 1787 (Ledger F, p. 287); see William Hall, q.v.

Hall, Harriot, Miss, see James White Hall, q.v.

Hall, Henry (captain), was visited by Dr. William M. Dallam who treated him in Mar and Jul 1817 and Apr 1819, a negro in May and Jun 1819, him [Henry] in Sep 1820, his wife in Dec 1820 and a negro in Jul 1821 (Document filed in the Archives of the Historical Society of Harford County Archives folder "Medical Bills – Dr. William M. Dallam"); see Benedict E. Hall, q.v.

Hall, Hetty, see John B. Hall, q.v.

Hall, I., see John Johnson, q.v.

Hall, Isabella, Mrs. [1774-1827], was visited by Dr. Thomas Archer who treated her in Aug 1804, Jan 1805 "in parturition" [in childbirth] and Mar, Jun and Jul 1805, Negro Manuel in Aug 1804, Negro Maria in Dec 1804, an infant in Feb, Jul and Oct 1805, Negro Ned in Feb 1805 and Negro Jesse in Nov 1805 (Document filed in the Archives of the Historical Society of Harford County folder "Archer, Thomas, Dr., 1768-1821 – Papers")

Hall, James [c1750-1822], was visited by Dr. John Archer who treated a negro boy for a bruised upper jaw in May 1781 (Ledger D, p 24) [account continued in Ledger E, which is missing] [James Hall was a War of 1812 veteran.]; see Edward Hall and John Steel, q.v.

Hall, James White [1754-1808], in Havre de Grace, was visited Dr. Richard Sappington who treated a negro man in Aug 1783 and others not specified between Nov 1783 and Oct 1784 and he was visited by Dr. John Archer who treated him, his wife and daughter Sophia in 1787 and him in 1788; he was visited by Dr. Thomas Archer who treated him in Jun and Aug 1792, Jul and Aug 1794, Aug and Sep 1795, Dec 1797, Jul 1800, Jul, Aug, Sep and Oct 1801, Sep 1805, Nov and Dec 1807 and 13 times between 12 Jan 1808 and 6 Mar 1808, a domestic in Aug 1792, William Stokes in May 1793, an infant in Aug 1792, Jun 1794, Nov 1798 and Feb and Apr 1799, Mrs. Hall in Jan and Aug 1792, Jul and Aug 1794, Feb 1797, Feb, Oct and Nov 1798, Aug 1800, Sep and Dec 1801, Jan 1802, Feb 1804, Aug and Sep 1807, son Mortimer in Jun 1792, Aug 1794, Sep 1795, Mar 1796, May 1800, Jun 1802, Aug 1803 and 40 times between 24 Aug 1806 and 20 Aug 1807, Negro Eli in Aug 1794, Negro Davy in Nov 1794 for "fract. fibul" [broken leg bone], Miss Elenor in Dec 1794, May 1805 and Oct 1807, Miss Julia or Julian in Jun 1792, May 1793, Dec 1794, Nov 1797, Oct 1798, Jun 1800, Jan 1802, Apr 1803 and Aug, Oct and Nov 1807, an unnamed negro in Aug 1792, Jul 1795, Dec 1796, Jul and Aug 1797, Jan, Feb, Apr, Jun and Sep 1798, Jul and Aug 1800, Mar, Apr and Dec 1801, Feb and Aug 1802, Aug 1807, Negro Cupid in Aug 1795, unnamed children in Jun 1792, Nov 1795 and Jul, Oct and Nov 1801, an unnamed child in May 1797, Jan 1798, Apr, Aug and Nov 1799, Apr 1800 and May 1804, daughter Elen in Mar 1796, Jan 1798, May 1800, Jul and Nov 1802, and Nov 1807, daughter Mary in Jun and Nov 1796, Dec 1797, Oct 1798, Aug and Nov 1799, Apr 1800, Mar 1801, Jun 1804, Aug 1806 and Nov 1807, Miss Steven (sic) in Feb 1798, Negro Joe in Feb and Mar 1798 and May 1801, Negro Tom in Aug 1797, unnamed negroes in Jul 1795, Nov 1799 and May 1801, a negro "at Delph" in Aug 1799 and Sep 1801, Negro Jeffery in Mar and Apr 1801, daughter Sophia in Mar 1793 and May 1801, Apr, May and Aug 1802, Negro Jerry in Jun 1801, inoculated "7 of his family" (daughters Sophia, Mary and Elenor and negroes Dina, Robert, Maria and Milcha) in Feb 1802, a negro at J. Ward's(?) in Aug 1802, Negro Hercules "at Delph" in Aug 1793 and Aug 1802, Negro Dina in Apr 1803 and Aug 1807, Negro Harriot in Sep 1805 and Aug 1806, family [no names given] in Aug 1807, Sarah [wife] in Sep 1807 and Negro Milcha in Nov 1807; he was also visited by Dr. William M. Dallam who treated Miss Julian in Jan 1802, his wife in May 1802, a negro in Jul and Dec 1803, Jan, Jun, Sep and Oct 1804, Miss McCubbin in Oct 1804, a negro in Jan 1805, Miss Harriot and a negro in Sep 1805, his [James'] wife and child in Nov 1805, a negro in Dec 1806 and Jan 1807, his [James'] child in Jan and Feb 1807, Mrs. Lewis in Jun 1807, Negro Delph [or negro at Delph] in Mar 1808 and a negro in Aug 1808; the first bill, for the period 1802 to 1805, was paid in full on 25 Jan 1807; the other two bills thereafter stated "Received Harford County 20th August 1810 of Edward Hall, one of the Exrs. of James W. Hall, dec'd., the amount of the above account. Wm. M. Dallam." [One bill was for £4.4.3 and the amount paid was $11.23 and the other was for £4.13.9 and $12.50 was paid.] (Documents filed in the Archives of the Historical Society of Harford County in these folders: (1) "Sappington, Dr. Richard – Accounts, 1783-1830;" (2) "Medical Bills – Dr. William M. Dallam;" and, (3) "Archer, Thomas,

Dr., 1768-1821 – Papers" [Notes in Dr. Thomas Archer's papers stated that James W. Hall paid his 1792-1793 accounts on 15 Jan 1794 and the accuracy of his other accounts were verified by Joseph Brownley, Justice of the Peace, on 14 Nov 1808; they were paid in full by Edward Hall, at Rumney, on 1 Dec 1812]; Dr. John Archer's Ledger F, pp. 217, 328, 362) [account continued in Ledger G, which is missing]; see William Stokes, q.v.

Hall, John, see John B. Hall, Josias Hall, Molly Hall, Thomas Hall and William Hall, q.v.

Hall, John (esquire), was visited by Dr. John Archer who treated a negro "ad obstetricand" [in childbirth] on 12 May 1781, him [John] in Nov 1781, and him, his wife and [daughter] Molly in Mar 1783 and him in Apr 1783 (Ledger D, p. 27) [continued in Ledger E, which is missing]

Hall, John (captain), was visited by Dr. Thomas Archer who treated him in Aug 1793, Sep 1794, Apr, May, Jun and Jul 1795, Sep (for "diarrheam") and Oct 1796, Feb, Mar, Apr, Sep and Oct 1797, Jul 1798, Apr 1799, May 1800, Jan 1801, Aug 1802, Dec 1803, Jan 1804 (for "rheumatols") and Feb 1804 (for "diarr.") in consultation with Dr. Birckhead; also treated Negro Jim in Apr, Jul and Aug 1793, Negro Jacob in Sep 1797 and Jan 1801, "Petre" in Apr 1799, Negro Sal in Apr 1799, Nov 1800 and Jan 1801, and a negro in Feb 1797, Apr 1799, Oct 1800 and Sep 1801 (Document in the Archives of the Historical Society of Harford County folder "Archer, Thomas, Dr., 1768-1821 – Papers" gave the name on the account as "John Hall, dec'd." and also noted a claim was filed in court on 11 Dec 1804 since the bill had not been settled; it was subsequently paid in full by Edward Hall, one of the administrators *de bonis non* of John Hall, at Dairy [Sophia's Dairy] on 5 Feb 1808); Capt. John Hall was also treated by Dr. Thomas H. Birckhead 43 times between 31 Jul 1803 and 11 Feb 1804 [John Hall wrote his will on 12 Feb 1804 and died before 5 Mar 1804 when it was proved.] On 19 Jan 1805 Dr. Birckhead swore to the accuracy of this account before James Wetherall, a Justice of the Peace, who attested on 14 Mar 1805 that it was a true transcript from his book. "Recd. March 21st 1805 of Wm. Hall the contents of the within acct. for the use of Doctr. Thos, Burkhead *(sic)* by me." [No one had signed the note, but in a different handwriting was written "[Matthew Birckhead]" *(sic)*; however, the note looks like it was written by James Wetherall, Justice of the Peace (Document filed in the Archives of the Historical Society of Harford County folder "Birkhead;" Harford County Will Book AJ No. C, p. 206)

Hall, John B. (esquire), was visited by Dr. John Archer who treated him, wife and daughters Eliza, Hetty and Delia and sons John and Aquila in 1789 (Ledger F, pp. 253. 254, noted Josias Hall [brother of John B.] paid the account on 7 Jun 1803 and Aquila Hall, Esq. paid the interest on 21 Oct 1808) [John Beadle Hall was a Revolutionary War veteran.]

Hall, Joseph, at Crambury [Cranberry], was treated by Dr. John Archer in Jul 1787 (Ledger F, p. 199)

Hall, Josias [1752-1832], son of John, was treated by Dr. John Archer in Jun 1788 (Ledger F, p. 157) [account continued in Ledger G, which is missing] [Josias Hall was a Revolutionary War veteran.]; see John B. Hall and Molly Garrettson, q.v.

Hall, Mary, see Sarah Hall and James White Hall, q.v.

Hall, Mary (negro), see Carvel Hall (negro), q.v.

Hall, Molly, Miss, daughter of John, was treated by Dr. John Archer in Mar 1788 (Ledger F, p. 97); see John Hall, q.v.

Hall, Mortimer, see James White Hall, q.v.

Hall, Mrs., see Thomas Hall, q.v.

Hall, Nicky, see Aquila Hall, q.v.

Hall, Patty, was treated by Dr. John Archer in Jan 1787 (Ledger F, p. 168); see Thomas Hall, q.v.

Hall, Polly, see Thomas Hall, q.v.

Hall, Sally, Miss, was treated by Dr. Robert H. Archer in Aug 1827 (p. 244)

Hall, Samuel, son of Elihu, was treated by Dr. John Archer in Jan 1791 (Ledger F, p. 284)

Hall, Sarah, was treated by Dr. John Archer, Jr. in Oct 1815 and Jul 1820 and also mentioned Miss Mary Hall in Jan 1816 (p. 29); see James White Hall, q.v.

Hall, Sophia, Miss, was treated by Dr. John Archer in Feb 1788 (Ledger F, p. 91)

Hall, Sophia, see Thomas Hall, James White Hall and William Hall, q.v.

Hall, Thomas [1752-1804], was visited by Dr. John Archer who treated negroes in Feb, May, Jul and Oct 1780 and Apr, Jul and Sep 1781 (extracted tooth) and May, Jul, Aug (extracted tooth) and Oct 1782 and Jun and Jul (dressed an ear wound) and Aug and Sep (extracted tooth) 1783, and treated him [Thomas] and his daughter Elenor Gordon and his son Aquila Hall in 1788 (Ledger D, p. 43) [account continued in Ledger E, which is missing]; (Ledger F, pp. 270, 271, contained a notation in a different handwriting that Dr. Archer had mistakenly written Elenor's name as Reardon instead of Gordon) [account continued in Ledger G, which is missing]; "Thomas Hall & Mother" also had an account with Dr. Philip Henderson who treated one of them for a dislocated arm in Mar 1781, a "wench in swamps" in May 1781, "Cudger at Mill" and Miss Sophia in Jun 1781, Sam in Jul 1781 (leg dressing), Miss Sophia in Jul 1781, Miss Patty in Aug 1781, Negro boy Neddy and Faney in Aug 1781, "people at home house" and Peter, Faney and John [negroes] in Sep 1781, Miss Sophia and Miss Patty and a "negro in swamps" in Dec 1781, a negro man (by "bleeding") and a negro child in Feb 1782, "Jacob swamps" in Mar 1782, a "negro woman at swamps" in Apr 1782, Miss Patty in Jun 1782, "negro wench at swamp plantation" and John Hall in Jul 1782, Negro boy in Aug 1782, Peter in Sep 1782, William Hall in Oct 1782, Johnny in Nov 1782, Miss Polly and him [Thomas Hall] in Jan 1783; also mentioned Widow Bilings and Robert Smith in Apr 1782 and Samuel Grundy in Jan 1783 in non-medical matters (Document in the Archives of the Historical Society of Harford County folder "Archer, G. W. Coll. – Medicine #2") [Thomas Hall was a Revolutionary War veteran.]; see E. Hall, q.v.

Hall, Thomas G., was treated by Dr. William M. Dallam in Nov and Dec 1806 [The bill was £4.5.9 and the amount paid was $11.43.] "January the 30th 1808, this amount will pass when paid. Abrm. Jarrett, Register of Wills, Harford Co." The bill further stated "Received Harford County 20th August 1810 of Edward Hall, Executor of Thomas Hall, Jr., the amount of the above account in full. Wm. M. Dallam." (Document filed in Historical Society of Harford County Archives folder titled "Medical Bills – Dr. William M. Dallam")

Hall, Thomas W., see Negro Jessee, q.v.

Hall, W., see ---- James, q.v.

Hall, W. Jos., see Patty Garrettson, q.v.

Hall, W. T., see Benedict Hall, q.v.

Hall, William, see Thomas Hall and Capt. John Hall, q.v.

Hall, William, at Swan Town, was visited by Dr. John Archer who treated him, his wife and their sons William and John and daughters Elizabeth and Becky in 1788 (Ledger F, p. 297) [account continued in Ledger G, which is missing]

Hall, William [1756-1818], son of Aquila Hall, was visited by Dr. John Archer who treated him and daughter Sophia in 1791 (Ledger F, p. 223) [account continued in Ledger H, which is missing] [William Hall, of Aquila, was a Revolutionary War veteran.]; see Sophia Presbury, q.v.

Hall, William W. [1797-1819], was visited by Dr. Jacob A. Preston who treated him and his wife in Oct 1818 and him five times between 30 Oct and 7 Nov 1818 in consultation with Dr. Reardon; William died before Jun 1819 and the medical bill submitted by Dr. Preston was acknowledged by Thomas S. Bond, Register of Wills, on 1 Jun 1819, noting "This account will pass when paid." (Document filed in the Archives of the Historical Society of Harford County Archives folder "Preston, Dr. Jacob A.") [His full name was William White Hall.]

Hamer, Michael, near Cooptown, was visited by Dr. John Archer who treated him and his wife in 1790 (Ledger F, p. 30)

Hamilton, James, Jr., was treated by Dr. Robert H. Archer in Sep 1815 (Ledger F, p. 4)

Hamilton, John, at Walter Taylor's, was treated by Dr. John Archer in Sep 1787 (Ledger F, p. 344)

Hamilton, Mrs., near Calvary, was visited on 11 Mar 1827 by Dr. Robert H. Archer who treated her child and then prescribed medicine on 10 Apr 1827 (p. 218; Rx Book, 1825-1851, p. 87, wrote "Harmer" above the name "Hamilton" in ledger)

Hammond, Mrs., was treated by Dr. Robert H. Archer in Baltimore before 1822 [no dates or details were given] (Dr. Archer's "Alphabet to Ledger H" is his booklet [filed in the Archives of the Historical Society of Harford County] that contains his index to Ledger H [which is missing] for his patients in Baltimore before 1822 and Harford County after 1822, according to a notation by Dr. George W. Archer.)

Hammond, William (saddler), was treated by Dr. Matthew J. Allen in Jun 1845 (p. 48)

Hampton, David, was treated by Dr. John Archer in Apr 1787 (Ledger F, p. 267)

Hanby, William (tanner), was treated by Dr. John Archer in 1795 (Ledger I, which is missing, was abstracted by Dr. George W. Archer circa 1890; his notes are in Archives of the Historical Society of Harford County file "Archer, G. W. Coll. – Ledgers and Day Books")

Haney, Patrick (tailor), was visited by Dr. John Archer who treated him in June, July and Aug 1774 and his wife in Nov 1774 and treated him and daughter Susan in 1790 (Ledger B, pp. 29, 343; Ledger F, p. 343) [account continued in Ledger G, which is missing]

Haney, Susan, see Patrick Haney, q.v.

Hanlin, Patrick, was visited by Dr. John Archer who treated him in Jun 1778, Sep 1782 and Apr and Aug 1783, and him and an infant in Jan 1786 (Ledger C, p. 114, spelled his name Hanlin) [account continued in Ledger E, which is missing]; Ledger F, p. 3, spelled his name Handlon) [account continued in Ledger G, which is missing]

Hanlin, Peter, near Mr. Moores, was treated by Dr. John Archer in Aug 1773 (Ledger B, p. 30)

Hanna, Alexander [1752-1829], was visited by Dr. John Archer who treated him in Jul 1775, his wife and a child in Aug 1779, Betsy Golden in Mar 1780 and him in Jul 1781, Mar 1782 and May 1783 (Ledger B, p. 46; Ledger D, p. 7, misspelled his name as Hannah and Betsy's surname as Goolden) [continued in Ledger H, which is missing]; Alexander was also treated by Dr. Alonzo Preston in Jul 1825 and Oct 1828 (p. 45, misspelled his surname Hannah); see John Hanna, q.v.

Hanna, James [1752-1827], was treated by Dr. John Archer in February 1788 (Ledger F, p. 274, misspelled his name as Hannah) [account continued in Ledger H, which is missing] [James Hanna was a Revolutionary War veteran.]; see Samuel Jackson, q.v.

Hanna, James (weaver), was visited by Dr. John Archer who treated him in Jun and Sep 1781, his sister in Nov 1781, him in May (tooth extracted) and Sep 1782 and his brother in Sep 1783 (Ledger D, p. 54) [account continued in Ledger E, which is missing]

Hanna, John, was visited by Dr. John Archer who treated him in 1772 [no dates or details were given], McClure *(sic)* in Sep 1772, John and his mother in Feb and May 1774, a servant man in Mar 1774, John's mother in June 1774, his man in Jun 1776, a child in Jan 1777, a child in Aug 1777, John in Jan 1778 and Jul 1779, a child in Jan 1780, his wife in Feb and Jul 1780, and John in May and Dec 1780 and Jun 1783, and inoculated 7 of his family in 1782 (Ledger B, p. 26, spelled his name Hannah; Ledger C, p. 6, noted "dead & insolvent," but he did not give the date)

Hanna, John, was treated by Dr. John Archer in Oct 1787 (Ledger F, p. 145)

Hanna, John, of Alexander, was visited by Dr. John Archer who treated an infant in 1796 (Ledger I, which is missing, was abstracted by Dr. George W. Archer circa 1890; his notes are in Archives of Historical Society of Harford County file "Archer, G. W. Coll. – Ledgers and Day Books")

Hanna, Mary, was treated by Dr. John Archer in Jun 1793 (Ledger F, p. 130)

Hanna, Mr., was visited by Dr. Robert H. Archer who treated his wife for a "fract. Hum:" [broken arm bone] on 25 Sep 1823 (p. 89)

Hanna, Robert, was visited by Dr. Alonzo Preston who treated his wife in Aug 1825 (p. 52, spelled his surname as Hannah)

Hanna, William [1753-1823], was visited by Dr. John Archer who treated him and his wife in Sep and Oct 1774 and him in Jun 1779, Mar 1780, Dec 1781, Sep 1782 and Mar 1794 (Ledger B, p. 62; Ledger C, p. 35; Ledger F, p. 145)

Hanna, William, Sr. [1789-1878], was treated by Dr. Robert H. Archer in Oct 1823 and was visited by Dr. Alonzo Preston who treated his family [no names given] four times in Feb 1826 and his wife in Feb 1827 (Dr. Archer, pp. 95, 96; Dr. Preston, p. 86, misspelled his surname Hannah; Preston's Ledger F, p. 34) [William Hanna was a War of 1812 veteran]; see James Moores, q.v.

Hanna, William, son of Alexander, was visited by Dr. Robert H. Archer who treated his wife eight times in Oct 1823 (p. 89; Ledger F, p. 78)

Hanson, Benedict, see Mrs. Hanson (widow), q.v.

Hanson, Benjamin, was visited by Dr. John Archer who treated a negro circa 1778 [no date given] and him [Benjamin] in Jul, Aug and Oct 1778 (Ledger C, p. 97, noted "debt forgiven by order of testator"); see John Hanson, q.v.

Hanson, Benjamin, Jr., was visited by Dr. John Archer who treated a negro wench in Feb 1774, a negro in Mar 1774, and him [Benjamin] in Jul 1774 and Jul and Aug 1779 (Ledger B, p. 70; Ledger D, p. 4, noted "debt forgiven as before")

Hanson, Edward, was visited by Dr. John Archer who treated him and his wife in Jun 1775 and him in Sep 1777, Apr and Jul 1780, Jun 1787 and Jul 1788 (Ledger B, p. 59; Ledger C, p. 94, noted that the "debt forgiven by order of testator;" Ledger F, pp. 50, 154) [Edward Hanson was a Revolutionary War veteran.] see Joshua Day, Samuel Jackson and John Day, q.v.

Hanson, Frances (Fanny), see Mrs. Hanson (widow), q.v.

Hanson, Greenberry, see Mrs. Hanson (widow), q.v.

Hanson, Hollis [1750-1789], was visited by Dr. John Archer who treated Joseph Wood in May 1780, him [Hollis] in Aug 1781, a negro in Sep 1781, him [Hollis] in Jul 1782 and Feb and Apr 1783, his wife and a negro in May 1783 and him in Jun 1783 (Ledger D, p. 64) [account continued in Ledger E, which is missing]; Hollis Hanson, "at the Crossroads," was visited by Dr. John Archer who treated him, his wife and an infant in Sep 1787 and him in Sep 1788 (Ledger F, pp. 104, 116) [Hollis Hanson was a Revolutionary War veteran.]; see Mrs. Hanson, q.v.

Hanson, Hollis, of John, in Bush River Neck, was visited by Dr. John Archer who treated him and his wife in May 1789 (Ledger F, p. 29)

Hanson, John, of Benjamin, was visited by Dr. John Archer who treated a child in 1788 and him in Feb 1791 (Ledger F, p. 111)

Hanson, John, see Hollis Hanson, q.v.

Hanson, Mary, was treated by Dr. John Archer in Oct 1779 (Ledger D, p. 34, noted "debt forgiven as before"); see Mrs. Hanson (widow), q.v.

Hanson, Mrs., widow of Hollis, was visited by Dr. John Archer who treated her and children Frances, Greenberry and Benedict at various times between 1795 and 1797 (Ledger I, which is missing, was abstracted by Dr. George W. Archer circa 1890 [who transcribed her children's name as "Fanny, Tony(?) and Benedict" but probate records show them as listed above and his wife was named Mary]; his notes are in the Archives of Historical Society of Harford County folder "Archer, G. W. Coll. – Ledgers and Day Books"); Mrs. Hanson (widow), was treated by Dr. Robert H. Archer in Baltimore before 1822 [no dates or details were given] (Dr. Archer's "Alphabet to Ledger H" is his booklet [filed in the Archives of the Historical Society of Harford County] that contains his index to Ledger H [which is missing] for his patients in Baltimore before 1822 and Harford County after 1822, according to a notation by Dr. George W. Archer.)

Hanswood, James, see William W. Lawrence, q.v.

Haudecouer, Mr., [i. e., C. P. Haudecouer, engineer and map maker], was treated by Dr. John Archer at "sundry times" in 1797 (Ledger I, which is missing, was abstracted by Dr. George W. Archer circa 1890 who listed him as "Monsr. Hodeceur" and noted "Cr. by 1 map of Havre de Grace" [which was printed by Haudecouer in 1799]; Dr. George W. Archer's notes are in the Archives of the Historical Society of Harford County file "Archer, G. W. Coll. - Ledgers and Day Books")

Hardin, Benedict, was visited by Dr. John Archer who treated him and a child in Nov 1790 (Ledger F, p. 71) [account continued in Ledger H, which is missing]

Hardy, Betsy, was visited by Dr. John Archer who treated a negro wench in Apr 1776 and May 1777 (Ledger C, p. 47, noted "debt forgiven by order of testator")

Hardy, Elizabeth, daughter of John, was treated by Dr. John Archer in Jul 1775 (Ledger B, p. 15)

Harford County for Pensioners [name of the account], i. e., those persons treated by Dr. John Archer for whom he billed the county for his services, viz., Mary Reese, Mary Hendricks and Solomon Reese in Apr 1776, John Kelly in Nov 1776, Thomas Reese in Feb 1777, ---- Wogan in Apr and Sep 1777, Sally Elliott "at V. G." [?] and wife of Joseph Jones in Sep 1777, Sarah Hair in Oct 1777, Jane Pace in Jan 1778, Perry ---- [blank] in Feb 1778, Benjamin Pool in Mar 1778, an infant of Joseph Jones and Solomon Reese in Apr 1779 (Ledger C, pp. 38, 111, noted "debt forgiven by order of testator" for Joseph Jones and Solomon Reese aforementioned in 1779)

Hargrove, John (reverend), was treated by Dr. Robert H. Archer in Baltimore before 1822 [no dates or details were given] (Dr. Archer's "Alphabet to Ledger H" is his booklet [filed in the Archives of the Historical Society of Harford County] that contains his index to Ledger H [which is missing] for his patients in Baltimore before 1822 and Harford County after 1822, according to a notation by Dr. George W. Archer.)

Harkins, Joseph (c1785-1850), was visited by Dr. Alonzo Preston who treated his child on 13 Mar 1826 and while the cost of treatment was $2.25 the account was noted as "Denied" (p. 71)

Harkins, Mr. (merchant), was treated by Dr. Robert H. Archer after 1822 [no dates or details were given] (Dr. Archer's "Alphabet to Ledger H" is his booklet [filed in the Archives of the Historical Society of Harford County] that contains his index to Ledger H [which is missing] for his patients in Baltimore City before 1822 and in Harford County after 1822, according to a notation by Dr. George W. Archer.)

Harlan, Jeremiah [1762-1838], was treated by Dr. Robert H. Archer in 1823 (p. 71; Ledger F, p. 22)

Harmer, Mrs., was visited by Dr. Robert H. Archer who treated a child in 1827 (p. 225)

Harmer, see James McNabb, q.v.

Harper, Francis, was treated by Dr. John Archer in Jul 1775 (Ledger B, p. 65) [Francis Harper, Jr. was a Revolutionary War veteran.]

Harr, Kitty, was treated by Dr. John Archer in Mar 1786 and the account was charged to Harford County (Ledger F, p. 160, and then the doctor crossed her name off the ledger)

Harr, Mary, was treated by Dr. John Archer in Mar 1786 and the account was charged to Harford County (Ledger F, p. 160)

Harra, Dr., was consulted by Dr. John Archer in 1788 (Ledger F, p. 298)

Harriott, Andrew, was visited by Dr. John Archer who treated him before 1772 [no details], a child in Aug 1772, him [Andrew] in Dec 1773, Jan 1774 and July 1775, his wife in Nov 1775, him in Dec 1775, his wife in Feb 1777, an infant in Nov 1778, Nelly Pearl in Dec 1782 and him [Andrew] in March 1786 (Ledger B, p. 20; Ledger C, p. 25; Ledger F, p. 149) [Andrew Harriott or Herriott was a Revolutionary War veteran.]

Harris, Arabella, Miss, was treated by Dr. John Archer in Jan 1782 (Ledger D, p. 115, noted "debt forgiven as before")

Harris, Charles (saddler), was treated by Dr. John Archer at times between 1786 and 1794 and was wounded in the head in Nov 1795 (Ledger F, pp. 110, 155; Ledger I, which is missing, was abstracted by Dr. George W. Archer circa 1890; his notes are in the Archives of the Historical Society of Harford County folder "Archer, G. W. Coll. – Ledgers and Day Books")

Harris, Daniel, see Martha Smith, q.v.

Harris, Dr., see Negro ----, q.v.

Harris, Eliza, see Robert Harris, q.v.

Harris, Elizabeth, see Samuel Harris, q.v.

Harris, George, was prescribed medicine by Dr. Robert H. Archer on 6 Mar 1801 (Rx Book, 1796-1801, p. 40); see John D. Harris, q.v.

Harris, Hannah, see John D. Harris, q.v.

Harris, James (blacksmith), was treated by Dr. John Archer in Aug 1773 and Feb 1774 (Ledger B, p. 30, noted "dead and poor," but the date of death was not given)

Harris, James [c1740-1777], was visited by Dr. John Archer who treated him at various times between Aug 1772 and Jun 1775, his brother in Aug 1772, sister Susanna [wife of Matthew McClintock] several times between Oct 1774 and Jun 1775, his sister [unnamed] in Mar 1776 and him from 13 Jan to 17 Jan 1777 and then he died after writing his will (Will Book AJ No. C, p. 273; Ledger B, p. 28; Ledger C, p. 37, noted "debt forgiven by order of testator") [James Harris was a Revolutionary War veteran and signer of the Bush Declaration on March 22, 1775.]

Harris, Jenny, was visited by Dr. John Archer who treated Betsy Fulton in May 1778, Jenny Fulton in Oct 1778, and her [Jenny Harris] in Mar 1779 and Jan and Feb 1780 (Ledger C, p. 35, noted "debt forgiven by order of testator")

Harris, John, of Samuel, was treated by Dr. John Archer in Feb and Aug 1782 (Ledger D, p. 119, spelled his name Harriss and noted "debt forgiven as before")

Harris, John D., was visited by Dr. Alonzo Preston who treated him, George, Hannah and a child at various times in 1825 (p. 18)

Harris, Joseph, was treated by Dr. John Archer in Oct 1802 (Ledger F, p. 317) [Joseph Harris was a Revolutionary War veteran.]

Harris, Mrs. (widow), was treated by Dr. John Archer in May 1789, Nov 1781, Oct 1782 and Jul and Aug 1783 (Ledger D, p. 66) [account continued in Ledger E, which is missing]

Harris, R., Mrs., was prescribed medicine by Dr. Robert H. Archer circa Dec 1804 (Rx Book, 1802-1804, p. 71)

Harris, Richard, see James Gorrell, q.v.

Harris, Robert (captain), was visited by Dr. John Archer who treated him in Nov 1780 and Apr 1783, his wife in May 1781, his daughter Eliza in 1786, him in 1791 and between 1795 and 1801, and his daughter Eliza in 1800 and 1801 (Ledger D, p. 106, noted "debt forgiven as before;" Ledger F, p. 109 [account continued in Ledger H, which is missing, but was abstracted by Dr. George W. Archer circa 1890; his notes are in the Archives of the Historical Society of Harford County file "Archer, G. W. Coll. – Ledgers and Day Books"); [Capt. Robert Harris was a Revolutionary War veteran.] see Capt. Harris, q.v.

Harris, Samuel, was visited by Dr. John Archer who treated him and his daughter Elizabeth in June and July 1781 (Ledger D, p. 34) [account continued in Ledger E, which is missing)

Harris, Samuel, see John Harris, q.v.

Harris, Susanna, see James Harris, q.v.

Harris, Thomas (doctor), had a non-medical account in Dr. John Archer's ledger that mentioned the following: George Vandegrift in Apr 1784, William Smith in Baltimore in July 1786, Edward Prall in July 1786, John Smith in Baltimore in Apr 1790, Robert Amoss (collector) in Apr 1790, and James Bell and Paterson Bell in May 1787; also noted the account and interest were finally settled on 15 Apr 1805 (Ledger C, p. 48)

Harris, Thomas W., see William Lawrence, q.v.

Harrison, Henry L., was treated by Dr. Matthew J. Allen in Calvert County in 1832 (p. 19); see William W. Lawrence and James Kent, q.v.

Harrison, James, see William Lawrence, q.v.

Harrison, Thomas, was visited by Dr. John Archer who treated a negro and a boy [no names were given] in May 1780 (Ledger D, p. 67, noted "debt forgiven as before")

Harrison, William (weaver), was treated by Dr. John Archer in July 1788 (Ledger F, p. 3, indicated he was "dead and poor," but did not give the date of death)

Harrison, William, was treated by Dr. Matthew J. Allen in Calvert County in 1823 (p. 5a)

Harrod, John, was treated by Dr. Robert H. Archer after 1822 [no dates or details were given] (Dr. Archer's "Alphabet to Ledger H" is his booklet [filed in the Archives of the Historical Society of Harford County] that contains his index to Ledger H [which is missing] for his patients in Baltimore City before 1822 and in Harford County after 1822, according to a notation by Dr. George W. Archer.)

Harrod, John, was treated by Dr. Matthew J. Allen in Apr and May 1852 (p. 97)

Harry, John [c1790-1847] (blacksmith), was visited by Dr. John Archer, Jr. who treated him, his wife and an infant in Mar 1815 (p. 3) [John Harry was a War of 1812 veteran.]

Harryman, Mrs., was visited by Dr. Alonzo Preston who treated her at times in 1824 and 1825 and son William in 1825 (p. 44)

Harryman, William, see Mrs. Harryman, q.v.

Hart, Anthony, see Mrs. Hart, q.v.

Hart, Augustus, was treated by Dr. John Archer in Sep 1777 (Ledger C, p. 53, noted "debt forgiven by order of testator")

Hart, Caty, see Mrs. Hart, q.v.

Hart, James, see Aquila Massey, q.v.

Hart, John, was treated by Dr. John Archer in Feb 1782 (Ledger D, p. 54, "debt forgiven as before")

Hart, Joseph, was treated by Dr. John Archer in Aug 1792 and was visited by Dr. James Archer who treated him in Apr 1806 and made nine visits and gave three bleedings and various medicines and advice in Sep and Oct 1806 (Dr. John Archer, Ledger F., p. 264; Dr. James Archer, p. 13) [account continued in Ledger K, which is missing]; see Mrs. Hart, q.v.

Hart, Joseph, was visited by Dr. Robert H. Archer who treated "Lilley" in Oct 1825 and in another account book mentioned Thomas Lilley (p. 163; Ledger F, p. 9)

Hart, Kitty, Miss, was treated by Dr. Robert H. Archer in Aug 1824 (p. 116; listed in Dr. Archer's "Alphabet to Ledger H" [filed in the Archives of the Historical Society of Harford County], but no dates or details were given; the booklet contains his index to Ledger H [which is missing] for his patients in Baltimore City before 1822 and in Harford County after 1822, according to a notation by Dr. George W. Archer.)

Hart, Lilley, see Joseph Hart, q.v.

Hart, Mrs. (widow), was visited by Dr. John Archer who treated her six times in Sep 1772, a child in Feb 1773, Mrs. Hart in Apr and Jun 1773 and Feb and Nov 1774, daughters Caty and Peny in Feb 1777, son Robert in Mar 1778, Mrs. Hart in Feb 1779, sons Joseph and Anthony in Apr 1779, son Joseph nine times from Sep to Nov 1779, Mrs. Hart in Nov 1780, inoculated daughter Anny in Feb 1782 and treated Mrs. Hart in Feb and Apr 1783 and Jul 1795 (Ledger B, p. 38; Ledger C, p. 34; Ledger D, p. 22, transferred to Ledger F, p. 190) [account continued in Ledger I, which is missing]

Hart, Penelope, was treated by Dr. John Archer in Dec 1781, Feb 1784 and Nov 1788 (Ledger D, p. 114, noted "debt forgiven as before;" Ledger F, p. 69) [continued in Ledger G, which is missing]

Hart, Peny, see Mrs. Hart, q.v.

Hart, Robert, see Mrs. Hart, q.v.

Hartgrove, Richard, was visited by Dr. John Archer who treated his wife and child in Aug 1777, his child in 1786, inoculated a daughter, age 16, in 1791 and treated him in 1801 (Ledger C, p. 16; Ledger F, p. 117, mentioned

"Hargrove, Jr." on 25 Oct 1805; also noted that Rheuben Sutton paid the account in 1805); see Ephraim Bayard, q.v.

Harthhorn, John, was visited by Dr. John Archer who treated him in Nov 1779 and a son in Jan 1785 (Ledger D, p. 36, noted "debt forgiven as before")

Hartley, James, at Salt Box, was treated by Dr. John Archer in 1795 (Ledger I, which is missing, was abstracted by Dr. George W. Archer circa 1890; his notes are in the Archives of the Historical Society of Harford County file "Archer, G. W. Coll. – Ledgers and Day Books")

Hartley, Jesse, was treated by Dr. Robert H. Archer in Sep 1822 in consultation with Dr. Coale (p. 21; Ledger F, p. 86)

Hartley, Jonathan, was treated by Dr. Matthew J. Allen in 1848 (p. 88, spelled his name Hartly)

Harvey, Alexander, was visited by Dr. John Archer who treated a child in Jul 1779 (Ledger D, p. 2, noted "debt forgiven as before")

Harvey, Sarah, at Joseph Stokes', was visited by Dr. John Archer who treated her and an infant in Feb 1774 (Ledger B, p. 75)

Harwood, Benjamin, see Rev. Harwood, q.v.

Harwood, John, on J. Moore's place, was treated by Dr. John Archer at various times between 1799 and 1801 (Ledger I, which is missing, was abstracted by Dr. George W. Archer circa 1890; his notes are in the Archives of the Historical Society of Harford County file "Archer, G. W. Coll. – Ledgers and Day Books")

Harwood, Rev., was visited by Dr. John Archer who treated him and son Benjamin at various times between 1795 and 1799 (Ledger I, which is missing, was abstracted by Dr. George W. Archer circa 1890; his notes are in the Archives of the Historical Society of Harford County folder "Archer, G. W. Coll. – Ledgers and Day Books")

Haslem, Mr., was prescribed medicine for his wife by Dr. Robert H. Archer on 31 Aug 1830 (Rx Book, 1825-1851, p. 102)

Haslet, Dr., see William Bond, q.v.

Haslet, Tom (negro), was treated by Dr. Robert H. Archer in Baltimore before 1822 [no dates or details given] (Dr. Archer's "Alphabet to Ledger H" is his booklet [filed in the Archives of the Historical Society of Harford County] that contains his index to Ledger H [which is missing] for his patients in Baltimore before 1822 and Harford County after 1822, according to a notation by Dr. George W. Archer.)

Hassan, John, see John B. Black, q.v.

Hassan, Mary, in a non-medical matter account with Dr. Robert H. Archer in Jul 1822, mentioned her brother Robert Hassan in Aug 1823, Mary Ann Caldwell [actually Calwell] in Nov 1824, and "her mother's" in May 1826 and May 1827 (Ledger F, pp. 55, 162); see James Jackson, q.v.

Hassan, Robert, see Mary Hassan, q.v.

Hasset, William (tailor), was visited by Dr. John Archer who treated him in Sep 1777 and Sep 1780 and him and a child in Sep and Nov 1781 (Ledger C, p. 27; Ledger D, p. 88, noted "debt forgiven as before") [William Hasset or Hassett was a Revolutionary War veteran.]

Hathorn, Samuel, see Thomas Senate, q.v.

Haughey, Barney, was treated by Dr. Robert H. Archer after 1822 [no dates or details were given] (Dr. Archer's "Alphabet to Ledger H" is his booklet [filed in the Archives of the Historical Society of Harford County] that contains his index to Ledger H [which is missing] for his patients in Baltimore City before 1822 and in Harford County after 1822, according to a notation by Dr. George W. Archer.)

Haughey, George, was visited by Dr. Matthew J. Allen who treated him twelve times between 2 Jun and 1 Aug 1845 and treated a child ten times in Aug 1845 (pp. 48, 51, spelled his name Houghy and noted the medical bill totaled $20.12½ and George had paid only 50¢ in Feb 1848) [The following statement was written on a separate page dated 24 Nov 1853 that was inserted in the back of Dr. Allen's ledger. The letter, addressed to Major Bond, was signed by I. Day and stated "I have just returned after 3 days ride to look up the Drs. of Dr. Allen and the following is the result." It mentioned several patients, including this one: "Geo. Hoey (sic) shows a rect. for $7 & says he paid $3 more, in all $17 – will call, make out his act. & prove it & will call on you to pay the bal. in a short time."]

Haughey, Hughy, was treated by Dr. Matthew J. Allen in Jun and Jul 1847 (p. 56) [The following statement was written on a separate page dated 24 Nov 1853 that was inserted in the back of Dr. Allen's ledger. The letter, addressed to Major Bond, was signed by I. Day and stated "I have just returned after 3 days ride to look up the Drs. of Dr. Allen and the following is the result." It mentioned several patients, including this one: "H.

Haughy will call on you to day or so to compromise his jugt." On 20 Mar 1854 "Hughe S. Haughey" [his signature] wrote a note to Ishmael Day: "Sir, I could not attend to that business of Dr. Allen's on the return day on account of sickness in my family. Do nothing in it until I see you. I want you to collect some accounts for me. P.S. I am now at N. W. S. Hays at work and will be in Bell-Air on Saturday next."]

Hawkins, Isaac, appeared on a list of debts dated 26 Dec 1822 and titled "A List of Allen's Claims" that were due and payable to Dr. Richard N. Allen for services rendered [no dates given] by him to Hawkins (Document in Historical Society of Harford County Archives folder "R. N. Allen")

Hawkins, John, was visited by Dr. John Archer who treated a negro child in 1778, him in Aug and Nov 1778, May, Aug and Nov 1780, Aug 1781 and May 1782, son Samuel in Oct 1782 and him [John] in Jun and Jul 1783 (Ledger C, p. 99; Ledger D, p. 106) [account continued in Ledger E, which is missing]

Hawkins, John, was visited by Dr. Matthew J. Allen who treated his wife in Jun, Jul and Aug 1844 (p. 36, noted the bill was paid by cash in full on 19 Nov 1844)

Hawkins, Mrs., "at X Roads," was treated by Dr. Robert H. Archer in 1823 (p. 46; Ledger F, p. 135)

Hawkins, Richard [1753-1806], was treated by Dr. John Archer in Oct 1778 and May 1788 (Ledger C, p. 30; Ledger F, p. 303) [Richard Hawkins was a Revolutionary War veteran.]; see Thomas Hawkins, q.v.

Hawkins, Robert, in Barrens [area in the northwest part of the county near Pennsylvania], was visited by Dr. John Archer who treated him in Dec 1780 and Aug 1781, him and child in Sep 1781 and him in Apr 1782, Oct 1783 and Mar 1786 (Ledger D, p. 108, noted "debt forgiven as before;" Ledger F, p. 152) [Robert Hawkins was a Revolutionary War veteran.]; see Negro Patience, q.v.

Hawkins, Samuel, was treated by Dr. John Archer in Aug 1781 (Ledger D, p. 56, noted "debt forgiven as before") [Samuel Hawkins was a Revolutionary War veteran.]

Hawkins, Samuel, Sr. (negro), was treated by Dr. John Archer, Jr. in July 1816 (p. 32)

Hawkins, Thomas, was visited by Dr. John Archer who treated him several times between May 1773 and Apr 1773, his wife in May 1773, a child in Apr 1774, his wife in Mar 1776, him in Jan 1777 and Mar 1779, his wife in Jun 1781 and him in Mar and Jun 1782 (Ledger B, p. 96; Ledger C, p. 48, noted that the account was paid by Richard Hawkins on 10 Dec 1783)

Hawkins, William, was treated by Dr. John Archer on 1 Jun 1775 (Ledger B, p. 99)

Hawkins, William, near Cox's, was visited by Dr. John Archer who treated his wife in Oct 1777 (Ledger C, p. 51, noted "debt forgiven by order of testator")

Hay, Mrs. (widow), was prescribed medicine by Dr. Robert H. Archer on 29 Dec 1799 (Rx Book, 1796-1801, p. 17)

Hay, Margaret, Mrs., was treated by Dr. Robert H. Archer in Baltimore before 1822 [no dates or details were given] (Dr. Archer's "Alphabet to Ledger H" is his booklet [filed in the Archives of the Historical Society of Harford County] that contains his index to Ledger H [which is missing] for his patients in Baltimore before 1822 and Harford County after 1822, according to a notation by Dr. George W. Archer.)

Hayns, Jacob, see Israel Morris, q.v.

Hays, Archer [1756-1827], was visited by Dr. John Archer who treated him in Jun 1780, his wife in Dec 1780, him in Jan, Jun and Oct 1781, and inoculated his son Thomas in 1782, treated Negro Hagar (tooth extraction) in Aug 1782, him [Archer] in Oct and Nov 1782 and Feb 1783, him, his wife and son John in Jan 1789 and Archer and children named "Darby, Jene[?], Harriet, Patty, Harry, Tommy and John" at various times between 1794 and 1798 [no dates were given and since Archer did not have children named Darby, Jene and Patty they were probably negroes]; Archer was visited by Dr. James Snow who treated a son in Dec 1813, and he was visited by Dr. Robert H. Archer who treated Negro Chloe in Oct 1823 and Jun 1827 ("bleeding & medicines"), Negro Joseph [also called Jo] in Nov 1825, a negro in Jul 1827 and him [Archer] in Jul 1827 "for attendance & medicine for him in last illness" (Dr. John Archer, Ledger D, p. 74 [account continued in Ledger E, which is missing], Dr. John Archer, Ledger F, p. 81; Dr. Robert H. Archer, pp. 86, 167, 235, 237, and his Ledger F, p. 71 [continued in Ledger G, which is missing]; James Snow document filed in Historical Society of Harford County Archives folder "Medical Papers;" Dr. John Archer's Ledger I, which is missing, was abstracted by Dr. George W. Archer circa 1890; his notes are in the Archives of the Historical Society of Harford County folder "Archer, G. W. Coll. – Ledgers and Day Books;" Document filed in Archives of the Historical Society of Harford County folder "Archer, Thomas, Dr., 1768-1821 – Papers," contained an undated note written between Jul 1827 and Mar 1829, signed by Thomas A. Hays, that stated "Dr. Rob. H. Archer was the attending Physician of my late Father's family." [Archer Hays was a Revolutionary War veteran and his mansion and restored springhouse still stand on the Harford Community College campus located between Bel Air and Churchville.]; see John Hays, q.v.

Hays, Charles, see Harry Hays, q.v.

Hays, Emily, see Thomas A. Hays, q.v.

Hays, Frances, see Thomas A. Hays, q.v.

Hays, Hannah, see Thomas A. Hays, q.v.

Hays, Harriet, Miss, was prescribed medicine by Dr. Robert H. Archer on 7 Jun 1832 (Rx Book, 1825-1851, p. 106)

Hays, Harry, was visited by Dr. Robert H. Archer who treated his son Charles five times in June 1828 (pp. 281, 282, 283) [Harry or Henry Hays was a War of 1812 veteran.]; see Archer Hays and John Hays, Sr., q.v.

Hays, James, was treated by Dr. John Archer in Oct 1782 (Ledger D, p. 99, noted "debt forgiven as before")

Hays, John, see Archer Hays, q.v.

Hays, John, near Alexander Rigdon's, in the Barrens [an area in the northwestern part of the county near Pennsylvania], was treated by Dr. John Archer in 1796 (Ledger I, which is missing, was abstracted by Dr. George W. Archer circa 1890; his notes are in the Archives of the Historical Society of Harford County folder "Archer, G. W. Coll. – Ledgers and Day Books")

Hays, John, Jr., was treated by Dr. John Archer at various times between Jul 1779 and Nov 1782 and was inoculated either in 1782 or 1784 when he paid the medical bill by his bond (Ledger D, p. 4)

Hays, John, Sr., was visited by Dr. John Archer who treated his son in Sep and Oct 1774, him [John] in Jan, May and Jun 1775, Negro children in Jun 1775, inoculated his son Archer [no date given], treated him [John] in Jan 1778, his wife in Mar 1778, him in Apr, May, Jun, Nov and Dec 1778, Mar and Nov 1779 and Feb, May and May 1782, son Joseph in Mar 1783, him [John] in Jan 1784, sons Joseph and Harry in Aug 1785, and him [John] in Mar 1790 (Ledger B, p. 69; Ledger C, pp. 99-100; Ledger D, p. 49 [account continued in Ledger E, which is missing]; Ledger F, p. 89) [account continued in Ledger G, which is missing]

Hays, Joseph, was treated by Dr. John Archer in Nov 1796 (Ledger F, p. 92) [account continued in Ledger K, which is missing]; see John Hays, Sr., q.v.

Hays, Mrs., was prescribed medicine for a negro by Dr. Robert H. Archer on 18 Jun 1830 (Rx Book, 1825-1851, p. 101); see Nathaniel W. S. Hays, q.v.

Hays, Nathaniel W. S. [1786-1863], had an account in the ledger as N. and Thomas A. Hays in 1823 and he was visited by Dr. Robert H. Archer who treated him in Dec 1826 and Jan 1827 and a negro in Sep and Oct 1827 in consultation with Dr. Preston; Hays was prescribed medicine for a "man" by Dr. Archer in Aug 1841 (pp. 212, 244, 248, 249; Ledger F, p. 146; Rx Book, 1825-1851, p. 115); Nathaniel was visited by Dr. John T. Archer who treated Wesley [negro?] in Oct 1840, a coloured child in Nov 1840, a coloured boy in Mar 1841 ("dressing foot"), a negro woman in Mar 1841 ("bleeding"), "Ben & extracting tooth for negro man" in Mar 1841, his [Nathaniel's] wife in Mar 1841, coloured girl Hannah in Mar 1841 ("bleeding") and Apr 1841, a coloured girl in Apr 1841 (extracting tooth), coloured children in Nov 1841 (whooping cough), coloured girl Hetty in 1843 [no exact date], Mar 1844, 'in parturentum" [in childbirth] on 25 Jan 1845 and given medication in Feb 1845, coloured boy George in Jan 1845, Negro Sam in Feb 1845 (extracting tooth), and 15 visits to a coloured child at Mrs. Hays in Jul 1845 (Document filed in the Archives of the Historical Society of Harford County folder "Archer, Thomas, Dr., 1768-1821 – Papers") [Nathaniel William Smith Hays was a War of 1812 veteran]; see Abraham Jarrett, Hughy Haughey and John Brown, q.v.

Hays, Parmelia, see Thomas A. Hays, q.v.

Hays, Sally, Miss, was prescribed medicine by Dr. Robert H. Archer on 25 Aug 1828 (Rx Book, 1825-1851, p. 91)

Hays, Thomas, see Archer Hays and Rachel Archer, q.v.

Hays, Thomas A. [1780-1861], was visited by Dr. Robert H. Archer who treated his daughter Sarah (Sally) three times in Jan 1824, once in June 1825, ten times in Aug and Sep 1825 and twice in Apr 1826, and his wife in Jun 1828; he was also visited by Dr. Alonzo Preston who treated his daughter Rachel several times in 1826 and 1827 and once in 1828, his daughters Frances and Parmelia in 1826, his daughter Emily twice in 1827, a Mrs. Jones three times in 1827, Frank Jail [or possibly Frank in jail] in 1827, "a girl at A. Jarrett's" in 1827, a black child [unnamed] and his [Thomas'] daughter Hannah in 1828 and his daughter Sally in May, Jun and Aug 1828 (Dr. Robert H. Archer's ledger, pp. 98, 148-153, 179, 278, 279, 283, 288; Ledger F, p. 94; Dr. Alonzo Preston's ledger, p. 77, noted "This acct. included in settlement of the 8th April 1833 when 2/3 of Mr.

Hays note for $101.03 was paid him by me Wm. B. Bond") [Thomas Archer Hays was a War of 1812 veteran.]; see Archer Hays, Nathaniel W. S. Hays and Abraham Jarrett, q.v.

Hays, William, and his wife, were treated sixteen times by Dr. Robert H. Archer between 27 Sep 1822 and 20 Jun 1823 (pp. 24, 80, 81; Ledger F, pp. 36, 90)

Hays, William S. [1799-1848], was treated by Dr. Robert H. Archer in Jun 1823 (p. 78) [His full name was William Smith Hays.]

Haywood, William, was treated by Dr. Robert H. Archer in Baltimore before 1822 [no dates or details were given] (Dr. Archer's "Alphabet to Ledger H" is his booklet [filed in the Archives of the Historical Society of Harford County] that contains his index to Ledger H [which is missing] for his patients in Baltimore before 1822 and Harford County after 1822, according to a notation by Dr. George W. Archer.)

Heamor, Michael, was visited by Dr. John Archer who treated him and his wife several times between Jan and Sep 1773 and a child in Apr 1773 (Ledger B, p. 27)

Heath, Richard (esquire), was visited by Dr. John Archer who treated him and his wife between 1794 and 1797 (Ledger I, which is missing, was abstracted by Dr. George W. Archer circa 1890; his notes are in the Archives of the Historical Society of Harford County folder "Archer, G. W. Coll. – Ledgers and Day Books") [Dr. George W. Archer added his own note that stated "If this is the Richard Heath who married Miss Hall in 1807 she must have been his second wife."]

Heaton, Jeremiah, in the Barrens [an area in northwest part of the county near Pennsylvania], was treated by Dr. John Archer in 1787 and 1792; Mr. Heaton was prescribed medicine for his wife by Dr. Robert H. Archer on 27 Dec 1802 and 1 Jan, 11 Jan and 24 Feb 1803 (Ledger F, p. 219 listed him as Jeremiah Eaton and p. 345 listed him as Mr. Heaten; Rx Book, 1802-1804, pp. 28, 29, 34); see William Parker, q.v.

Hedrick, Charles (shoemaker), at James Moores', was treated by Dr. John Archer in Nov 1791 (Ledger F, p. 295, spelled his name Hederick)

Hemnor, Michael, was visited by Dr. John Archer who treated a child in Oct 1777 and him in Apr 1780 (Ledger C, p. 76, noted "debt forgiven by order of testator")

Hemphill, John, was treated by Dr. John Archer many times between Dec 1786 and Jan 1788 (Ledger F, pp. 229, 231, 276, 278, 325) [account continued in Ledger G, which is missing]

Henderson, George, was treated by Dr. John Archer in Feb 1791 (Ledger F, p. 280)

Henderson, John [1779-1846], was visited by Dr. Alonzo Preston who treated Negro Orange in 1826 and 1827 (p. 82, noted "This acct. closed by warrant, & acct. in bar produced & proven being exactly same amt. each party agreed to pay half the costs" and signed by W. B. Bond [meaning payment was received by Dr. William B. Bond] [John Henderson was a War of 1812 veteran.]

Henderson, Milkey, see Rebecca Henderson, q.v.

Henderson, Philip (doctor) was consulted by Dr. John Archer in 1782, 1789 and 1792 (Ledger F, pp. 167, 251); see John Paca, Thomas Hall, Francis Holland and Richard Dallam, q.v.

Henderson, Rebecca, was visited by Dr. Alonzo Preston who treated her at various times in 1824 and 1825 and "Milkey" in 1825 (p. 10)

Hendricks, Mary, see Harford County for Pensioners, q.v.

Hendrickson, Mrs. (widow), was visited by Dr. John Archer who inoculated her, Lannah, Rachel, John and Joseph in 1794 or 1795 (Ledger I is missing, but it was abstracted by Dr. George W. Archer circa 1890. His notes are in Archives of the Historical Society of Harford County folder "Archer, G. W. Coll. – Ledgers and Day Books")

Henry, Isaac, above Bald Friar [a landing on the Susquehanna River], was treated by Dr. John Archer in 1788 (Ledger F, p. 290)

Henry, Mary (widow), near Bald Friar [a landing on the Susquehanna River], was treated by Dr. John Archer in 1787 (Ledger F, p. 336, misspelled the location as "Ball Fryar")

Henry, Robert, at Bald Friar Ferry [a landing on the Susquehanna River], was visited by Dr. Robert H. Archer who treated a negro in May 1823 (pp. 71, 72; Ledger F, p. 162)

Henry, Samuel, was treated by Dr. John Archer in Jun and Sep 1781 (Ledger D, p. 40, noted "debt forgiven as before")

Hensil, William, near Darlington, was treated by Dr. Robert H. Archer in Sep 1826 (p. 198)

Herbert, Benjamin, was treated by Dr. John Archer in Sep 1774 (Ledger B, p. 60); see Samuel Gallion, q.v.

Herbert, George, "at X Roads," was treated by Dr. Robert H. Archer in Mar and Apr 1823 and died by 1824; Dr. Archer received $10 from his administrator on 29 Nov 1824 and also cash paid by John Herbert on 6 Dec 1824 (pp. 59, 60, 61, 122; Ledger F, p. 152); see Jane Herbert, q.v.

Herbert, James B. [1794-1830], was visited by Dr. Robert H. Archer who treated an infant and a negro in March 1827 (p. 217) [James Beatty Herbert was a War of 1812 veteran.]

Herbert, Jane, widow of George, was treated by Dr. Robert H. Archer in July and Aug 1823 (p. 85a listed her name "Mrs. Janes Herbert, of George;" Ledger F, p. 50)

Herbert, John (merchant), "at X Roads" [i.e., Lower Cross Roads, once called Herbert's Cross Roads, now called Churchville], was visited by Dr. John Archer who treated his family in 1796 (Ledger I, which is missing, was abstracted by Dr. George W. Archer circa 1890 and it listed his name as Jno. Harburt; Dr. George W. Archer's notes are in Archives of the Historical Society of Harford County folder "Archer, G. W. Coll. – Ledgers and Day Books")

Herbert, John, was treated by Dr. Robert H. Archer in May 1822 (Ledger F, p. 46)

Herbert, John, "at Mrs. Beacham's, Frederick Road" [Baltimore Co.], was treated by Dr. Matthew J. Allen in Aug and Sep 1847 (p. 64)

Herbert, M., Miss, see Mary Ann Smith, q.v.

Herbert, Margaret, Mrs., was treated by Dr. Matthew J. Allen in Jul 1844 and twelve times between 27 Jan and 9 Feb 1845 (p. 37)

Herrington, Mr., was prescribed medicine by Dr. Robert H. Archer on 19 Aug 1803 (Rx Book, 1802-1804, p. 53)

Herron, James, see William B. Bond, q.v.

Herron, James, Jr., was treated by Dr. Matthew J. Allen in Jun 1848 (p. 86, noted the bill was paid "by settlement in full" on 22 Apr 1852); see James Herron, Sr., q.v.

Herron, James, Sr., was visited by Dr. Matthew J. Allen who treated his daughter in Sep, Oct and Nov 1847 and Jul and Sep 1848 (pp. 67, 92, noted that the bill was "settled in full by James Herron, Jr." on 22 Apr 1852)

Hewit, Stephen, was visited by Dr. Matthew J. Allen who treated him and a child in 1848 (p. 95)

Hewitt, Mr. (shoemaker), was noted in Dr. Robert H. Archer's ledger on 8 Aug 1826 as having "paid his a/c in full to this date," but it was probably for a non-medical matter (p. 196)

Hewston, James, son-in-law to James Armstrong, was treated by Dr. John Archer in August 1789 (Ledger F, p. 283) [account continued in Ledger G, which is missing]

Hicks, James, was prescribed medicine for a child by Dr. Robert H. Archer on 2 Feb and 3 Feb 1801 (Rx Book, 1796-1801, p. 31, 32); he was treated by Dr. Robert H. Archer in Baltimore before 1822 [no dates or details were given] (Dr. Archer's "Alphabet to Ledger H" is his booklet [filed in the Archives of the Historical Society of Harford County] that contains his index to Ledger H [which is missing] for his patients in Baltimore before 1822 and Harford County after 1822, according to a notation by Dr. George W. Archer.)

Hill, Alexander, was treated by Dr. John Archer in Jul 1775 (Ledger B, p. 15)

Hill, H., see James Johnson, q.v.

Hill, Herman, was treated by Dr. John Archer in Apr 1788 (Ledger F, p. 333) [Herman or Harmon Hill was a Revolutionary War veteran.]

Hill, Stephen, at Hickory Tavern, was treated by Dr. John Archer in July and Sep 1779 and in Jun 1790; also mentioned Mrs. Greg in 1790 (Ledger B, p. 56, noted "run west," but did not give the date of departure; Ledger F, p. 360) [Stephen Hill was a Revolutionary War veteran.]

Hill, William, was visited by Dr. John Archer who treated him and his wife in 1786 (Ledger F, p. 69)

Hill, William, at William Smith's Bayside, was treated by Dr. John Archer in May 1782 (Ledger D, p. 31, noted "debt forgiven as before")

Hillard, Mrs., see Samuel Wilson, q.v.

Hillen, Solomon, son of Widow Wheeler, was treated by Dr. John Archer in 1787 (Ledger F, p. 301)

Hilles, Major, was prescribed medicine for his wife by Dr. Robert H. Archer in Oct 1804 (Rx Book, 1802-1804, p. 61)

Hilton, Harriet, see Isaac Hilton, q.v.

Hilton, Isaac [c1795-1881] (negro), at Stafford, was visited by Dr. Robert H. Archer who treated his wife Harriet on 15 Oct 1822, 23 Oct 1822 and 24 Oct 1822 and "in partu" [in childbirth] on 3 Nov 1822 (pp. 31, 34; Ledger F, p. 99) [Isaac Hilton and his wife Harriet were both free born.]

Hines, George, was visited by Dr. John Archer, Jr. who treated a child in Jan 1818, his wife in Aug 1818 and him in Oct 1821 (p. 60)

Hinks, Thomas, near John Copeland's, was treated by Dr. John Archer in 1787 (Ledger F, p. 331) [Thomas Hinks was a Revolutionary War veteran.]

Hinkson, Mr., was treated by Dr. Robert H. Archer after 1822 [no dates or details were given] (Dr. Archer's "Alphabet to Ledger H" is his booklet [filed in the Archives of the Historical Society of Harford County] that contains his index to Ledger H [which is missing] for his patients in Baltimore City before 1822 and in Harford County after 1822, according to a notation by Dr. George W. Archer.)

Hipkins, Caleb, was visited by Dr. James Reardon who treated and prescribed medicine for his wife 17 times between 15 Oct and 22 Nov 1826 (Document filed in Historical Society of Harford County Archives folder "Reardon, James Dr.")

Hitchcock, Elizabeth, was visited by Dr. John Archer who treated "Peter Carol:" in Sep 1779 (Ledger D, p. 19, noted "debt forgiven as before")

Hobbs, William, was visited by Dr. John Archer who treated his wife in Mar 1773 (Ledger B, p. 92)

Hobbs, William (weaver), was visited by Dr. John Archer who treated him and a child in 1790 (Ledger F, p. 14)

Hodgkins, L. T., see Jane A. Allen, q.v.

Hodgkins, William C., see William W. Lawrence, q.v.

Hoey, Geo., see George Haughey, q.v.

Hoffman, Peter, on Watson's Island, was treated by Dr. John Archer in 1795 (Ledger I, which is missing, was abstracted by Dr. George W. Archer circa 1890; his notes are in the Archives of the Historical Society of Harford County file "Archer, G. W. Coll. – Ledgers and Day Books")

Hogg, Samuel, was visited by Dr. John Archer, Jr. who treated his son William in March 1816, his [Samuel's] wife in April 1816, "ux mort: nocte" [wife near death or died at night] on 3 Oct 1817, and also treated his son Samuel in April 1819 (p. 48)

Hogg, William, see Samuel Hogg, q.v.

Holland, Eliza, see James Holland, q.v.

Holland, F., see Roger Matthews, q.v.

Holland, Francis [1745-1795] (colonel), was visited by Dr. John Archer who treated him Aug 1780 and Oct 1781, inoculated 13 of his family in Oct 1781, treated his mother in Jan 1782, him in Feb and Jun 1782, a negro in Apr 1782, his mother in Jul 1782 in consultation with Dr. Henderson, him [Francis] in Aug 1782. a negro in Sep1782, him [Francis] in Nov and Dec 1782 and Mar, Apr and May 1783 and Feb 1787, his wife on 21 May 1787 [after childbirth] and him, his wife and son Thomas in Jul 1788 (Ledger C, p. 116; Ledger D, p. 88 [account continued in Ledger E, which is missing]; Ledger F, p. 73, and p. 236 noted in the margin of the ledger in a different handwriting that son Thomas was born on 20 May 1787) [account continued in Ledger G, which is missing] [Francis Holland was a Revolutionary War veteran and a signer of the Bush Declaration on March 22, 1775.]

Holland, Francis [1771-1818] (attorney), was visited by Dr. John Archer who treated him and brother Thomas Holland in Feb 1796 (Ledger I, which is missing, was abstracted by Dr. George W. Archer circa 1890; his notes are in the Archives of the Historical Society of Harford County file "Archer, G. W. Coll. – Ledgers and Day Books") [His full name was Francis Utie Holland.]

Holland, James (boot and shoemaker), was visited by Dr. Matthew J. Allen who treated his son in Jan 1848, a child in Mar 1848, his family [no names given] in Mar 1848, Eliza, Lizzy and Jimmy in Mar and Apr 1848 and Eliza in Jun 1848 (pp. 72, 76, 80)

Holland (Hollond), Jem, see Negro Pompy, q.v.

Holland, Jimmy, see James Holland, q.v.

Holland, John, was treated by Dr. Alonzo Preston in 1827 (p. 88)

Holland, Lizzy, see James Holland, q.v.

Holland, Mr., was visited by Dr. Robert H. Archer who treated him and his wife in Nov 1822 (pp. 34, 36, 37)

Holland, Mrs., see William Holloway, q.v.

Holland, Patrick, was treated by Dr. Robert H. Archer ten times between 1 Oct and 17 Oct 1822 and again in Oct 1823 (p. 95; Ledger F, p. 115)

Holland, Robert W., was visited by Dr. Alonzo Preston who treated his wife "in partu" [in childbirth] on 26 Dec 1824 (p. 5)

Holland, Thomas, see Francis Holland, q.v.

Hollbrook, Samuel, was treated by Dr. Matthew J. Allen on 1 Aug 1847 for a copperhead snake bite and seven more times to 18 Aug 1847, including treatment to "scars and carterising toes" (p. 60)

Holliday, Henry, brother-in-law to George Gale, was treated by Dr. John Archer in 1796 (Ledger I, which is missing, was abstracted by Dr. George W. Archer ca. 1890; his notes are in Archives of the Historical Society of Harford County file "Archer, G. W. Coll. – Ledgers and Day Books")

Holliday, John R., was prescribed medicine by Dr. Robert H. Archer on 26 Jul 1799 (Rx Book, 1796-1801, p. 24, listed him as Jno, R. Halliday); John R, Holliday was treated by Dr. Archer in Baltimore before 1822 [no dates or details were given] (Dr. Archer's "Alphabet to Ledger H" is his booklet [filed in the Archives of the Historical Society of Harford County] that contains his index to Ledger H [which is missing] for his patients in Baltimore City before 1822 and Harford County after 1822, according to a notation by Dr. George W. Archer.)

Hollingsworth, Jacob, see James Hollingsworth, q.v.

Hollingsworth, James, at B. R. Neck [Bush River Neck], was visited by Dr. John Archer who treated him and his son Jacob in 1787 (Ledger F, p. 373)

Hollingsworth, John, was treated by Dr. Matthew J. Allen in Sep 1847 (p. 64)

Hollingsworth, Robert [1784-1863], was visited by Dr. Alonzo Preston who treated his child in Jan 1825 (p. 24)

Hollis, Alonzo, was visited by Dr. Alonzo Preston who treated his wife during the night of 24 Oct 1828 and he returned with Dr. Wilson on 25 Oct, 26 Oct, 27 Oct, 29 Oct and 31 Oct 1828 and also in consultation with Dr. Rearden on 3 Nov 1828; nothing further was recorded regarding treatment (p. 83, noted that the $15.00 medical bill was paid by cash, $10.00 on 15 May 1830 and $5.00 on 3 Sep 1833; the $1.50 interest was still due and it appears it was finally paid later) [Alonzo Hollis was a War of 1812 veteran.]

Hollis, Amos, was visited by Dr. John Archer who treated his son William in 1788 and him [Amos] in Apr 1789 (Ledger F, p. 103, noted that Amos Hollis, Jr. was his executor on 28 Jan 1809) [Amos Hollis was a Revolutionary War veteran.]

Hollis, Clark, see Cyrus Osborn, q.v.

Hollis, Frances, Mrs., was treated by Dr. Matthew J. Allen each day from 30 Jan 1845 (initially at the request of John Barnes) to 8 Feb 1845 (p. 43, noted the bill was paid in full on 24 Feb 1845)

Hollis, Jarret, was visited by Dr. Matthew J. Allen who treated his wife in Aug 1852 (p. 97)

Hollis, Mr., was visited by Dr. Robert H. Archer who treated Miss Osborn in July 1825 (p. 141; Ledger F, p. 137)

Hollis, Richard F., see Negro Jessee, q.v.

Hollis, William, see Amos Hollis and James Gale, q.v.

Hollis, William, Jr., was visited by Dr. John Archer who inoculated six of his family in 1789 and treated him and his wife in Jul 1791 (Ledger F, p. 14) [William Hollis, Jr. was a Revolutionary War veteran.]

Hollis, William, Sr., was treated by Dr. John Archer in Sep 1786 (Ledger F, p. 95, noted the account was paid by William Hollis, Jr. on 7 Aug 1788)

Holloway, William, near Mrs. Holland's, was visited by Dr. John Archer who treated his wife and a child in 1787 and him in 1791 (Ledger F, p. 371) [continued in Ledger H, which is missing]

Holmes, Abram, see James Holmes, q.v.

Holmes, Elizabeth, see James Holmes, q.v.

Holmes, James, "at Crossroads," was visited by Dr. John Archer who treated him in 1794 and also inoculated three of his children, Mary, Elizabeth and Abram (Ledger F, p. 347, spelled his name Holms) [account continued in Ledger I, which is missing]

Holmes, James, was visited by Dr. John Archer who treated him and his sister-in-law in Aug 1772, his wife, daughter and Jen: Bay several times in July 1773, him in Jan and Nov 1778, an infant in Nov 1778, him in Oct 1780 and Jan 1783 when he inoculated 4 children (Ledger B, p. 1, spelled his name Holms, p. 99; Ledger C, p. 99, noted that payment was made "by yr. dividend to the poor of Boston, 14/2") [James Holmes was a Revolutionary War veteran.]

Holmes, James (shoemaker), in Havre de Grace, was visited by Dr. John Archer who treated him and his family in 1796 and James was prescribed medicine by Dr. Robert H. Archer on 29 Dec 1796 (Ledger I, which is missing, was abstracted by Dr. George W. Archer circa 1890; his notes are in the Archives of the Historical Society of Harford County folder "Archer, G. W. Coll. – Ledgers and Day Books;" Dr. Robert H. Archer's Rx Book, 1796-1801, p. 10)

Holmes, Mary, see James Holmes, q.v.

Holmes, Oliver, see Robert H. Archer, q.v.

Honnol, William, was visited by Dr. John Archer who treated him and wife in Sep 1779 (Ledger D, p. 15, had the words "McGuire Security" after his name and noted "debt forgiven as before")

Hood, Frederick &ca *(sic)*, was treated by Dr. Robert H. Archer in Baltimore before 1822 [no dates or details] (Dr. Archer's "Alphabet to Ledger H" is his booklet [filed in the Archives of the Historical Society of Harford County] that contains his index to Ledger H [which is missing] for his patients in Baltimore before 1822 and Harford County after 1822, according to a notation by Dr. George W. Archer.)

Hooper, Abram or Abraham [1756-1820s] (blacksmith), in Abingdon, was treated by Dr. John Archer in July 1787 (Ledger F, p. 365) [Abraham Hooper was a Revolutionary War veteran.]

Hoopman, Christian [1758-1837], Havre de Grace, was treated by Dr. John Archer in Nov 1789 (Ledger F, p. 23) [account continued in Ledger I, which is missing]

Hoopman, Isaac, see Edward Preston, q.v.

Hope, Andrew [1782-c1860], was treated by Dr. Alonzo Preston in Apr 1826 (p. 84) [Andrew Hope was a War of 1812 veteran.]

Hopkins, Charles, was treated by Dr. John Archer in 1793 and was prescribed medicine for his wife by Dr. Robert H. Archer on 31 Jul 1796 (Dr. John Archer, Ledger F, p. 94; Dr. Robert Archer Rx Book, 1796-1801, p. 7, listed him as C. Hopkins) [continued in Ledger H, which is missing]; Charles Hopkins (saddler) and his family [names not given] were treated by Dr. John Archer at times between 1795 and 1802 (Ledger I, which is missing, was abstracted by Dr. George W. Archer circa 1890; his notes are in the Archives of the Historical Society of Harford County file "Archer, G. W. Coll. – Ledgers and Day Books")

Hopkins, David [c1770-1822] (mason), was treated seven times by Dr. Robert H. Archer between 22 Aug 1822 and 17 Oct 1822 and "died insolvent" (pp. 14, 18, 21, 24, 26; Ledger F, p. 69) [David Hopkins, an Englishman, was a poor, unmarried stone mason who built the Archer Hays House in 1808, now known as the Hays-Heighe House on the campus of Harford Community College, and the majestic two-story Smithson-Webster Springhouse, better known as DH Springhouse, on Sandy Hook Road, in 1816; both structures have initialed datestones.]; see Mr. McLaughlin, q.v.

Hopkins, Ephraim [1781-1869], was mentioned in a non-medical matter in Dr. Robert H. Archer's ledger in Mar 1825 (Ledger F, p. 149); see Peggy Morgan, q.v.

Hopkins, Eliza, widow of Joseph, was treated by Dr. John Archer at various times between 1797 and 1799 (Ledger I, which is missing, was abstracted by Dr. George W. Archer circa 1890; his notes are in Archives of the Historical Society of Harford County file "Archer, G. W. Coll. – Ledgers and Day Books"); see Joseph Hopkins and Samuel Hopkins (hatter), q.v.

Hopkins, Gerard, was visited by Dr. John Archer who treated a child in Sep 1779, his wife in Oct 1779, him in Apr 1780, a negro infant in Nov 1780, inoculated son John in Apr 1783, treated infant Marrie(?) in Apr 1784 and him [Gerard], his wife and child in Feb 1791 (Ledger D, p. 12) [account continued in Ledger E, which is missing]; Ledger F, p. 97) [account continued in Ledger H, which is missing]

Hopkins, Hannah, at Mr. Knox, was treated by Dr. Robert H. Archer in Sep 1827 (p. 244)

Hopkins, John, was treated by Dr. John Archer in Feb 1782, Apr and Oct 1783 and Oct 1784 (Ledger D, p. 118) [account continued in Ledger E, which is missing]; see Gerard Hopkins, q.v.

Hopkins, Joseph [1775-1849], was visited by Dr. Robert H. Archer who treated his wife in Apr and May 1824, a child in Apr 1824, a negro "in partu" [in childbirth] in Oct 1825. and his [Joseph's] wife in Oct 1825 and rendered obstetrical services to her on 7 Dec 1825 with follow-up visits on 11, 14 and 17 Dec 1825; also treated his wife several times in May 1827 and him, her and a child in Aug 1827 and rendered obstetrical services to his wife on 17 Sep 1827 with follow-up visits between 20 Sep and 23 Sep 1827, and treated him, his wife and daughter Eliza in May 1828; Joseph was treated by Dr. Matthew J. Allen in Nov 1843 (Dr. Archer's Ledger, pp. 103, 104, 105, 164, 171, 226, 227, 242, 243, 244, 246, 247, 276, 277, 278, and his Ledger F, p. 96; Dr. Allen's Ledger, p. 28); see Negro Duke, William Gardner and Joseph Hopkins, Jr., q.v.

Hopkins, Joseph, Jr., was visited by Dr. John Archer who treated him in Nov 1779 and his wife in Dec 1781, inoculated sons John and Joseph in Jan 1782 and treated a free Negro [name not given] in Aug 1782, him [Joseph] in Aug 1783 and Jul 1784 and his wife in Aug 1784 (Ledger D, p. 35) [account continued in Ledger E, which is missing]

Hopkins, Miss, see William Dallam, q.v.

Hopkins, Mr., was prescribed medicine by Dr. Robert H. Archer circa Dec 1804 (Rx Book, 1802-1804, p. 72)

Hopkins, Mrs., was prescribed medicine by Dr. Robert H. Archer on 22 Dec 1825 (Rx Book, 1825-1851, p. 85)

Hopkins, Prissey, see Samuel Hopkins, q.v.

Hopkins, Rachel, Mrs., see William Hopkins, Sr., q.v.

Hopkins, Richard, brother-in-law to Jo. Gorrell, was treated by Dr. Robert H. Archer in March 1824 (p. 105); see Joseph Gorrell, q.v.

Hopkins, Sally, see Samuel Hopkins, q.v.

Hopkins, Samuel, see William Hopkins, Sr., q.v.

Hopkins, Samuel (hatter), of William, was treated by Dr. John Archer at various times between 1795 and 1801 (Ledger I, which is missing, was abstracted by Dr. George W. Archer circa 1890; his notes are in the Archives of the Historical Society of Harford County file "Archer, G. W. Coll. – Ledgers and Day Books"); Samuel Hopkins (hatter), was also visited by Dr. Robert H. Archer who treated his son William in Aug 1825, in consultation with Dr. Worthington, and treated Samuel and his family, including daughter Eliza, in Sep 1825, Jun 1829, Mar 1830 and Jan 1831; also treated Betsy White in 1825 (pp. 149, 150, 154, 156, 160; Ledger F, p. 112)

Hopkins, Samuel (mason), was visited by Dr. John Archer who treated him in Apr 1780, Aug 1781 and May 1782, a negro in Jul 1782, and inoculated eight children in 1782; treated his [Samuel's] wife in Aug 1782, him in Oct 1782 and Mar 1783, and him and daughters Susanna, Eliza, Prissey and Sally in 1789 (Ledger D, p. 56 [account continued in Ledger E, which is missing]; Ledger F, p. 78) [account continued in Ledger G, which is missing] [Samuel Hopkins was a Revolutionary War veteran.]

Hopkins, Susanna or Susannah, see Samuel Hopkins and William Hopkins, Sr., q.v.

Hopkins, William, see Samuel Hopkins and Daniel Chipman, q.v.

Hopkins, William, Jr., was visited by Dr. John Archer who treated him at various times between January 1776 and July 1783 and William Dun in February 1778 (Ledger C, p. 10)

Hopkins, William, Sr., was visited by Dr. John Archer who treated his daughter Susannah and a negro woman in June 1776, him [William] in Feb 1776, a son in Mar 1776, him in July 1777 and also inoculated two sons; treated him in June 1780, son Samuel in Oct 1781 and Aug 1783, some negroes in Aug 1783, son Samuel in 1788 and him [William] in 1789 (Ledger C, p. 11; Ledger F, pp. 343, 349, and p. 359 noted part of his account was paid in 1790 by Mrs. Rachel Hopkins and the balance was paid by Samuel Hopkins and Joshua Husbands in 1794)

Hopkins, William (saddler), was treated by Dr. John Archer at various times between 1797 and 1801 (Ledger I, which is missing, was abstracted by Dr. George W. Archer circa 1890; his notes are in the Archives of the Historical Society of Harford County folder "Archer, G. W. Coll. – Ledgers and Day Books")

Horford, Samuel (cooper), near T. Jeffrey's, was visited by Dr. Robert H. Archer who treated his wife in May and in June 1828 (pp. 276, 282); see William Hopkins, Sr., q.v.

Horner, see Richard Spence, q.v.

Horner, James (esquire), was listed in Dr. John Archer's ledger circa 1773, but no entries were made in his account; a later ledger account indicated he was visited by Dr. Archer who inoculated 9 of his family in Feb 1777 and treated him in Jan and May 1782, a daughter in Sep 1782, him in Oct 1782, a negro in Feb and Oct 1783, and him [James] in Jun 1779, Feb, Aug and Nov 1780, and Dec 1787 (Ledger B, p. 30; Ledger C, p. 73; Ledger D, p. 117 [account continued in Ledger E, which is missing]; Ledger F, p. 199) [account continued in Ledger G, which is missing]

Horsey, Benjamin (miller), at R. Thomas' Mill, was treated by Dr. John Archer in 1794 (Ledger I, which is missing, was abstracted by Dr. George W. Archer circa 1890; his notes are in the Archives of the Historical Society of Harford County folder "Archer, G. W. Coll. – Ledgers and Day Books")

Horton, Betsy, see Bennett Matthews, q.v.

Horton, Dr., see John Johnson and John Kirk, q.v.

Horton, William, was visited by Dr. John Archer who treated him in Mar 1775 and Sep 1779, a child in Sep 1785 and him in June 1789 (Ledger B, p. 4; Ledger D, p. 24, noted "debt forgiven as before;" Ledger F, p. 166) [continued in Ledger H, which is missing]; see James Ingram, q.v.

Hoskins, Cheyney [1805-1887], was treated by Dr. Robert H. Archer some time after 1822 [no dates or details were given] (Dr. Archer's "Alphabet to Ledger H" is his booklet [filed in the Archives of the Historical Society of Harford County] that contains his index to Ledger H [which is missing] for his patients in Baltimore before 1822 and Harford County after 1822, according to a notation by Dr. George W. Archer.)

Houston, Alexander, was treated by Dr. John Archer in Dec 1786 (Ledger F, p. 156)

Houston, James, see James Hewston, q.v.

Houston, John, see Samuel Willet, q.v.

Houston, Sarah, see Samuel Willet, q.v.

Houzkell(?), ---- (butcher), was treated by Dr. Robert H. Archer in Baltimore before 1822 [no dates or details were given] (Dr. Archer's "Alphabet to Ledger H" is his booklet [filed in the Archives of the Historical Society of Harford County] that contains his index to Ledger H [which is missing] for his patients in Baltimore City before 1822 and in Harford County after 1822, according to a notation by Dr. George W. Archer.)

Howard, Aquila, of Lemuel, brother-in-law to J. Whitaker, was treated by Dr. John Archer circa 1796 [no dates or details were given] (Ledger I, which is missing, was abstracted by Dr. George W. Archer circa 1890; his notes are in the Archives of the Historical Society of Harford County folder "Archer, G. W. Coll. – Ledgers and Day Books")

Howard, Benjamin, Jr., was treated by Dr. John Archer in May and Nov 1781 (Ledger D, p. 33, noted "debt forgiven as before") [Benjamin Howard, Jr. was a Revolutionary War veteran.]

Howard, Benjamin, Sr., was treated by Dr. John Archer in 1781 [no date was given] (Ledger D, p. 33, noted "debt forgiven as before"]; see William Howard, q.v.

Howard, Benjamin (sailor), at John Thompson's, was treated by Dr. John Archer in 1795 (Ledger I, which is missing, was abstracted by Dr. George W. Archer circa 1890 who noted "[Otter Pt.?]" and his notes are in the Archives of the Historical Society of Harford County file "Archer, G. W. Coll. – Ledgers and Day Books")

Howard, Bob (negro), was mentioned in a non-medical matter in Dr. John Archer, Jr.'s ledger and it noted Charles Rutter for "stealing 2 axes" on 5 Mar 1816 and Charles Foard's "manumission of Negro Bob" on 15 Nov 1819 (p. 10)

Howard, F., see F. A. Bond, q.v.

Howard, Fanny, see Thomas Howard, q.v.

Howard, John, was treated by Dr. John Archer in Apr 1788 and the account was charged to Harford County (Ledger F, p. 160) [account continued in Ledger G, which is missing]

Howard, Lemuel, see Aquila Howard, q.v.

Howard, Mary, was treated by Dr. Alonzo Preston at various times between 1825 and 1827 and the $4.50 medical bill was paid in cash in December 1827 (p. 10); see Ann Bond, q.v.

Howard, R., see Thomas Stockdill, q.v.

Howard, Rebecca, see Ann Bond, q.v.

Howard, T. G., see William Bean, q.v.

Howard, Thomas, was visited by Dr. John Archer who treated him and his daughter Fanny in Feb 1788 (Ledger F, p. 60)

Howard, William, was treated by Dr. John Archer in Jun and Aug 1781 (Ledger D, p. 28, noted that his bill for £0.19.0 was transferred to Benjamin Howard's account)

Howe, Mr. (cooper), at Dublin, was visited by Dr. Robert H. Archer who treated his nephew in Feb and Mar 1823 (p. 55 spelled his name How; Ledger F, p. 143, spelled it Howe)

Howe, William, near John Montgomery, was treated by Dr. John Archer in Sep 1777 (Ledger C, p. 4) [William Howe was a Revolutionary War veteran.]

Howell, Samuel, was treated by Dr. John Archer in Dec 1776 and Jan and Feb 1777 (Ledger C, p. 75) [Samuel Howell was a Revolutionary War veteran.]

Howlett, Andrew, was visited by Dr. John Archer who treated him in Jan and Apr 1781, a child in Jun 1783, him in Jul and Nov 1783 and Aug 1794, and his wife and son John in 1794 (Ledger D, p. 117 [account continued in Ledger E, which is missing]; Ledger F, p. 112 [account continued in Ledger I, which is missing] [Andrew Howlet or Howlett was a Revolutionary War veteran.]

Howlett, Catharine, appeared on a list of debts dated 26 Dec 1822 and titled "A List of Allen's Claims" that were due and payable to Dr. Richard N. Allen for services rendered [no dates were given] by him to said Howlett (Document filed in Historical Society of Harford County Archives folder "R. N. Allen"); see Mrs. Howlett, q.v.

Howlett, John, see Andrew Howlett, q.v.

Howlett, Mrs., at Dublin, was treated by Dr. Robert H. Archer seven times between 26 Jan and 12 Feb 1823 (pp. 49-52; Ledger F, p. 138, stated bill was sent to her son on 31 Mar 1824 and noted she was "supposed to have died insolvent"); see Catharine Howlett, q.v.

Howr *(sic)*, Joseph, appeared on a list of debts dated 26 Dec 1822 and titled "A List of Allen's Claims" that were due and payable to Dr. Richard N. Allen for services rendered [no dates were given] by him to said "Howr" (Document filed in Historical Society of Harford County Archives folder "R. N. Allen")

Hoy, James, was prescribed medicine by Dr. Robert H. Archer on 11 Mar 1801 (Rx Book, 1796-1801, p. 42)

Hudson, Benjamin, Bel Air, was treated by Dr. John Archer between 1795 and 1799 (Ledger I, which is missing, was abstracted by Dr. George W. Archer circa 1890; his notes are in the Archives of the Historical Society of Harford County file "Archer, G. W. Coll. - Ledgers and Day Books")

Hudson, Mr., see John Lee Gibson, q.v.

Hufenyzar, Harman, was treated by Dr. Matthew J. Allen in Aug 1844 (p. 38)

Huff, Abram, near Isaac Webster's, was visited by Dr. John Archer who treated his mother in Jul 1777 and him in Aug 1787 (Ledger C, p. 91, noted "debt forgiven by order of testator;" Ledger F, p. 362) [account continued in Ledger G, which is missing]

Huggins, Thomas, was visited by Dr. John Archer, Jr. in 1815 who treated Negro Bob and Negro Daniel, and Sally Evans in Feb 1816 and him in Feb 1816 and Mar 1822; also noted in Dr. Robert H. Archer's ledger that mentioned H. Ferguson in Mar 1821, H. Chamberlaine in Jan 1822 and James Gillespie in Jun 1824; non-medical matters were also noted, including rent due in 1824-1825 and various accounts in 1827-1830 (Dr. John Archer, Jr., pp. 1, 64; Dr. Robert Archer, Ledger F, pp. 29, 133, 152; see Budd White and John Gregg & Co., q.v.

Huggins, Thomas & Co., was a non-medical account in Dr. Robert H. Archer's ledger that mentioned Negro Daniel, James Boyd, Alexander Boyd, D. Simpers, Negro D. Simpers *(sic)*, John Riley, Simon Sears and Capt. Chew in 1815. It was also a non-medical account in Dr. John Archer, Jr.'s ledger that mentioned H. Touchstone and John Gregg & Co. in 1817 and Benjamin Owens, William Taylor, James Simmons, Francis Gillespie, Philip Thomas, and T. McMullen in 1818 (Dr. Robert H. Archer, Ledger F, p. 16; Dr. John Archer, Jr., p. 72)

Hughes & Adlam, see William Evatt, q.v.

Hughes, Abram, was treated by Dr. Robert H. Archer in Baltimore before 1822 [no dates or details were given] (Dr. Archer's "Alphabet to Ledger H" is his booklet [filed in the Archives of the Historical Society of Harford County] that contains his index to Ledger H [which is missing] for his patients in Baltimore before 1822 and Harford County after 1822, according to a notation by Dr. George W. Archer.)

Hughes, James, son-in-law to Mrs. Dines, was treated by Dr. John Archer in Dec 1789 (Ledger F, p. 169, spelled his name Hughs); see Nelly Peril, q.v.

Hughes, John, was visited by Dr. John Archer who inoculated 5 of his family [no names were given] in Feb 1777 (Ledger C, p. 85) [John Hughes was a Revolutionary War veteran.]

Hughes, John Hall [1742-1802], was visited by Dr. John Archer who treated him and his wife in 1787 and his family at various times between 1797 and 1799 (Ledger F, p. 118, spelled his name Jno. Hall Hughs) [account continued in Ledger G, which is missing]; (Ledger I, which is missing, was abstracted by Dr. George W. Archer circa 1890; his notes are in the Archives of the Historical Society of Harford County folder "Archer, G. W. Coll. – Ledgers and Day Books") [John Hall Hughes was a Revolutionary War veteran.]

Hughes, Samuel (esquire), was visited by Dr. John Archer who treated him and his wife in Sep 1787 and him in Apr 1789 (Ledger F, p. 133 spelled his name Hughs, and p. 209 spelled it Hughes); [account continued in Ledger G, which is missing]; Samuel and his family were also treated at various times between 1794 and 1807 – "On 24 Jan 1797 the Dr. excised a tumor from Mr. H.'s head, & dressed it on the 28th & 9 times from that date until 15 Feb. He had a wife, a sister Mrs. Hillard, and a nephew." (Ledger I, which is missing, was abstracted by Dr. George W. Archer circa 1890; his notes are in the Archives of the Historical Society of Harford County folder "Archer, G. W. Coll. – Ledgers and Day Books")

Hughes, William, was visited by Dr. Alonzo Preston who treated his wife in 1826 and 1828 and him in 1828 (pp. 80, 102, noted "This acct. settled by acct. in bar passed the Court $3.00 and by cash $6.00"); see William Coale, q.v.

Hugo, T. B. (captain), was treated by Dr. John Archer in May 1787 (Ledger F, p. 310) [Thomas B. Hugou, of Baltimore County, was a Revolutionary War veteran.]

Humphrey, Mr., see James H. Roberts, q.v.

Hunt, Robert, at Mr. Moores', was visited by Dr. John Archer who treated his wife in Aug 1778 and a child in Jun 1781 and Aug 1782 (Ledger C, p. 121, noted "debt forgiven by order of testator") [Robert Hunt was a Revolutionary War veteran.]

Hunter, Mrs., was treated by Dr. Robert H. Archer in Baltimore before 1822 [no dates or details were given] (Dr. Archer's "Alphabet to Ledger H" is his booklet [filed in the Archives of the Historical Society of Harford County] that contains his index to Ledger H [which is missing] for his patients in Baltimore before 1822 and Harford County after 1822, according to a notation by Dr. George W. Archer.)

Hunter, Peter, at Long Green, was visited by Dr. John Archer who treated his wife in 1776 [exact date was not given] in consultation with Dr. Fitzgerald, a negro in Apr 1781, his [Peter's] wife in Feb 1783, Sep 1785 and Jul 1786 and him and his wife in Oct 1789 (Ledger C, p. 62, noted John Cretin was his security; Ledger D, p. 11; Ledger F, p. 44)

Hurst, Mr., was treated by Dr. Robert H. Archer in Baltimore before 1822 [no dates or details were given] (Dr. Archer's "Alphabet to Ledger H" is his booklet [filed in the Archives of the Historical Society of Harford County] that contains his index to Ledger H [which is missing] for his patients in Baltimore before 1822 and Harford County after 1822, according to a notation by Dr. George W. Archer.)

Hurst, Mrs., in Annapolis, was noted in Dr. Robert H. Archer's ledger with regard to boarding, etc., for Thomas Archer from 1825 to 1827 (Ledger F, p. 122); see Dr. Rafferty, q.v.

Husband, also see Husbands, q.v.

Husband, Joseph, was prescribed medicine by Dr. Robert H. Archer on 3 Feb 1803 (Rx Book, 1802-1804, p. 31)

Husband, Joseph, was treated by Dr. Robert H. Archer in May 1822 and Oct 1823 in consultation with Dr. Worthington and treated his wife in Apr 1825 and Jan 1828 and a child in Aug 1827; also paid for services rendered by the doctor for Henry Smith, quarryman, "left at Rock Run per request" in Aug 1827 (pp. 95, 242; Ledger F, pp. 47, 95, 134, listed as Joseph Husband & Co., May 1822 to Mar 1826) [Joseph Husband was a War of 1812 veteran]; see Joshua Husband, q.v.

Husband, Joseph, Jr., was treated by Dr. Robert H. Archer in Oct 1823 in consultation with Dr. Worthington (Ledger F, p. 75)

Husband, Joseph, Sr., was treated by Dr. Matthew J. Allen in Dec 1843 and Jan 1844 (p. 29)

Husband, Joshua, see Joseph Husbands and Mary Mifflin, q.v.

Husband, William, was prescribed medicine by Dr. Robert H. Archer on 20 Aug 1802 (Rx Book, 1802-1804, p. 15)

Husbands, see Monsr. Dubroceur and also see Husband, q.v.

Husbands, Elizabeth (widow), was visited by Dr. John Archer who treated her in Dec 1781 and inoculated 5 of her family in 1782, treated her in Feb 1782, daughter Rachel in Sep 1782, her [Elizabeth] in Apr 1783, daughter Rachel in May 1783, her [Elizabeth] in Jan and Apr 1784, daughter Rachel in May 1784, her overseer and Negro boy in Sep 1784, her and daughters Eliza, Susan, Polly and Rachel in 1787 and her [Elizabeth] in Feb 1789 (Ledger D, p. 109, identified her as Mrs. Husbands, widow) [account continued in Ledger E, which is missing]; Ledger F, pp. 113, 250) [account continued in Ledger G, which is missing]

Husbands, Joseph, was visited by Dr. John Archer who treated a child in Aug 1781, inoculated his son Joshua in 1782, treated him [Joseph] in May and Sep 1782, a child in Nov 1782, him in Sep and Oct 7813, and him and a child in May 1786 (Ledger D, p. 65 [account continued in Ledger E, which is missing]; Ledger F, p. 4, p. 264 noted that Joseph paid his account on 24 Nov 1800) [account continued in Ledger H, which is missing]; see Joseph Husband, q.v.

Husbands, Joshua [1764-1837], was visited by Dr. John Archer who treated his wife on 29 Nov 1793 (had been in labor) and him and daughter Marian in May 1794 (Ledger F, p. 264) [continued in Ledger I, which is missing]; Joshua Husband was visited by Dr. Robert H. Archer who treated his son Joseph in May 1827 and his [Joshua's] wife in Jul 1827 in consultation with Dr. Worthington (pp. 224, 237, 238 [Joshua Husbands, sometimes spelled Husband, was the founder of Deer Creek Iron Works]; see William Hopkins, Mrs. Mifflin and Joshua Husband, q.v.

Husbands, Marian, see Joshua Husbands, q.v.

Husbands, Mary, was visited by Dr. John Archer who treated her and daughter Mary in 1789 (Ledger F, p. 88)

Husbands, Mrs., see Negro George and Elizabeth Husbands, q.v.

Husbands, Polly, see Elizabeth Husbands, q.v.

Husbands, Rachel, see Elizabeth Husbands, q.v.

Husbands, Susan, see Elizabeth Husbands, q.v.

Hush, John &ca *(sic)*, was treated by Dr. Robert H. Archer in Baltimore before 1822 [no dates or details were given] (Dr. Archer's "Alphabet to Ledger H" is his booklet [filed in the Archives of the Historical Society of Harford County] that contains his index to Ledger H [which is missing] for his patients in Baltimore before 1822 and Harford County after 1822, according to a notation by Dr. George W. Archer.)

Hussy, George, was treated by Dr. Robert H. Archer in Baltimore before 1822 [no dates or details were given] (Dr. Archer's "Alphabet to Ledger H" is his booklet [filed in the Archives of the Historical Society of Harford County] that contains his index to Ledger H [which is missing] for his patients in Baltimore before 1822 and Harford County after 1822, according to a notation by Dr. George W. Archer.)

Hussy, Nathan (wheelwright), was visited by Dr. John Archer who treated him, his wife and a child in 1794 and him and his daughter Peggy at times between 1794 and 1798 (Ledger F, p. 370) [account continued in Ledger I, which is missing, but it was abstracted by Dr. George W. Archer circa 1890; his notes are in the Archives of the Historical Society of Harford County folder "Archer, G. W. Coll. – Ledgers and Day Books")

Hussy, Peggy, see Nathan Hussy, q.v.

Huston, Alexander, was treated by Dr. John Archer in Jun, Aug and Sep 1781 (Ledger D, p. 36, noted the bill was paid in full by cradling wheat in Jul 1786)

Huston, John, near Joppa, was treated by Dr. John Archer in Jun 1782 (Ledger D, p. 96, noted "debt forgiven as before") [John Huston was a Revolutionary War veteran.]

Hutcheson, William, was treated by Dr. John Archer in May 1780 (Ledger D, p. 70, noted "debt forgiven as before")

Hutchins, John, see William W. Lawrence, q.v.

Hutton, Mr., see Joshua Strickland, q.v.

Iley, Jacob, was visited by Dr. Matthew J. Allen who treated a child in Aug 1848 (p. 91)

Indian Mary, see Samuel Webster, Jr., q.v.

Ingram, James, near William Horton's, was visited by Dr. John Archer who treated him and his wife in Mar 1774, him in May 1774 and inoculated sons Richard and James in 1791 (Ledger B, p. 6; Ledger F, p. 335)

Ingram, John (doctor), was visited by Dr. John Archer who treated his mother in June 1778 and him in Jul 1780 and Apr 1784 (Ledger C, p. 15, noted "debt forgiven by order of testator;" Ledger D, p. 82, identified him simply as John Ingram)

Ingram, Mrs. (widow), was visited by Dr. John Archer who treated her in Sep 1778, a servant in Jul 1781 and her in Feb 1783 and Aug 1787 (Ledger C, p. 123, noted "debt forgiven by order of testator; Ledger F, p. 9)

Ingram, Richard, see James Ingram, q.v.

Ireland, Gilbert, was treated by Dr. Matthew J. Allen in 1823 in Calvert County (p. 13a)

Ireland, John, was visited by Dr. John Archer who treated him and his wife in Jan 1789 and the account also mentioned Caleb Dorsey (Ledger F, p. 95) [account continued in Ledger G, which is missing]; Mr. Ireland was prescribed medicine for his child by Dr. Robert H. Archer on 18 Feb 1801 (Rx Book, 1796-1801, p. 34); Rev. John Ireland was treated by Dr. Robert H. Archer in Baltimore before 1822 [no dates or details were given] (Dr. Archer's "Alphabet to Ledger H" is his booklet [filed in the Archives of the Historical Society of Harford County] that contains his index to Ledger H [which is missing] for his patients in Baltimore City before 1822 and Harford County after 1822, according to a notation by Dr. George W. Archer.); see Monsr. Tixier, q.v.

Irons, John, was treated by Dr. John Archer in Jul and Aug 1780 (Ledger D, p. 83, noted "debt forgiven as before") [John Irons was a Revolutionary War veteran.]

Irons, Polly, was inoculated by Dr. John Archer in Feb 1782 (Ledger D, p. 96, noted "debt forgiven as before")

Irons, Widow, was treated by Dr. John Archer in Sep 1782 (Ledger D, p. 83, noted "debt forgiven as before")

Irwin, James, Sr., was visited by Dr. John Archer who treated him and sons Joseph, Solomon and Thomas at various times between 1797 and 1799 (Ledger I, which is missing, was abstracted by Dr. George W. Archer circa 1890; his notes are in the Archives of the Historical Society of Harford County folder "Archer, G. W. Coll. – Ledgers and Day Books"); see Samuel Willet, q.v.

Irwin, Joseph, see James Irwin, q.v.

Irwin, Mrs., near Little Falls Quaker Meeting, was treated by Dr. John Archer in June 1787 (Ledger F, p. 326)

Irwin, Solomon, see James Irwin, q.v.

Irwin, Thomas, see James Irwin, q.v.

Irwin, William, see Samuel Willet, q.v.

Irwine, Andrew, was treated by Dr. John Archer in Oct 1772 (Ledger B, p. 19, noted that 15 sh. cash was received from Hugh Beatty)

Irwine, James (weaver), near Ashmead's, was treated by Dr. John Archer in Jun and Sep 1778 (Ledger C, p. 106)

Jackson & Fox, had an account in the ledger of Dr. John Archer, Jr. that mentioned S. Jackson and Polly Barrat in Apr 1815, Mrs. Jackson between Jan 1816 and May 1818, P. Fox in Dec 1816, Mary Ann Donn in Jan 1817, son Philip Jackson in Feb 1818 and son John Jackson in Sep 1818 (p. 4); see Fox & Jackson, q.v.

Jackson, Betsy, see Peggy Jackson, q.v.

Jackson, Edward, was visited by Dr. John Archer, Jr. who treated him and children in Sep 1815 and his wife at various times between 9 Sep 1818 and 25 Aug 1821 (p. 2)

Jackson, Edward, of James, was treated by Dr. Robert H. Archer in Sep 1821 (Ledger F, p. 10)

Jackson, George (negro), was treated by Dr. John Archer, Jr. in Aug 1817 and mentioned Ben York [also a negro] (p. 65)

Jackson, Hugh, was visited by Dr. John Archer, Jr. who treated him and a child in Jul 1816 and mentioned Samuel Kerr and C. Little in Mar 1819 (p. 57)

Jackson, James, see Skipwith Coale and Edward Jackson, q.v.

Jackson, James, distiller at Mr. Webb's, was treated by Dr. John Archer in Dec 1778 (Ledger C, p. 126, noted part of bill was paid in cash on 15 Dec 1779 and the balance was forgiven)

Jackson, James, near Octoraro [in Cecil Co.], was treated by Dr. John Archer, Jr. in Apr 1817 and also noted "paid to Mary Hassan" on 18 Feb 1821 (p. 78)

Jackson, John, stepson to John Caine, was visited by Dr. John Archer who treated him and his family at various times between 1796 and 1803 (Ledger I, which is missing, was abstracted by Dr. George W. Archer circa 1890; his notes are in the Archives of the Historical Society of Harford County folder "Archer, G. W. Coll. – Ledgers and Day Books")

Jackson, John, was visited by Dr. John Archer, Jr. who treated him in Mar 1816, his wife at times between 1 Mar 1816 and 8 Aug 1819, son Ned ("dressing wound") on 11 Jun 1816, daughter Nancy in Aug 1817, son John in Sep 1819 and son William in Oct 1821 (p. 8)

Jackson, Mr., see John Massey, q.v.

Jackson, Mrs., see Jackson & Fox, q.v.

Jackson, Nancy, see John Jackson, q.v.

Jackson, Ned, see John Jackson, q.v.

Jackson, Peggy, was visited by Dr. John Archer, Jr. who treated her in May 1817, daughter Betsy in Jul 1818 and also mentioned P. Fox in May 1816 (p. 50); see Jackson & Fox, q.v.

Jackson, Philip, see Jackson & Fox, q.v.

Jackson, Robert, was visited by Dr. John Archer, Jr. who treated him, his wife and children in June 1816 (p. 53)

Jackson, S., see Jackson & Fox, q.v.

Jackson, Samuel, at Dismal [a swamp at the mouth of Swan Creek], son-in-law to Edward Hanson, was treated by Dr. John Archer in 1791 (Ledger F, p. 347)

Jackson, Samuel, near James Hanna's, was treated by Dr. John Archer in 1786 (Ledger F, p. 343)

Jackson, William, see John Jackson, q.v.

Jail(?), Frank, see Thomas A. Hays, q.v.

James ---- [blank] (cabinet maker), was treated by Dr. Robert H. Archer in Baltimore before 1822 [no dates or details were given] (Dr. Archer's "Alphabet to Ledger H" is his booklet [filed in the Archives of the Historical Society of Harford County] that contains his index to Ledger H [which is missing] for his patients in Baltimore before 1822 and Harford County after 1822, according to a notation by Dr. George W. Archer.)

James, ---- [blank], near W. Hall, was treated by Dr. Robert H. Archer in Baltimore before 1822 [no dates or details were given] (Dr. Archer's "Alphabet to Ledger H" is his booklet [filed in the Archives of the Historical Society of Harford County] that contains his index to Ledger H [which is missing] for his patients in Baltimore before 1822 and Harford County after 1822, according to a notation by Dr. George W. Archer.)

James, George, see Jacob James, q.v.

James, Jacob, was visited by Dr. Robert H. Archer who treated him and his wife in July 1822 (p. 8; Ledger F, p. 51)

James, Jacob, was visited by Dr. Matthew J. Allen who treated his sons George, William and Jarvis in Sep 1844 (p. 39) [The following statement was written on a separate page dated 24 Nov 1853 that was inserted in the back of Dr. Allen's ledger. The letter, addressed to Major Bond, was signed by I. Day and stated "I have just returned after 3 days ride to look up the Drs. of Dr. Allen and the following is the result." It mentioned several patients, including: "Jacob James agrees to pay $10 on his act. to you & to be in full as soon as he can make the money."]

James, Jarvis, see Jacob James, q.v.

James, John, was listed in Dr. John Archer's ledger circa 1773, but no dates or entries were made in his account (Ledger B, p. 36); John James "in the Barrens" [an area in the northwestern part of Harford County near Pennsylvania] was treated by Dr. John Archer in April 1776 (Ledger C, p. 46, noted "debt forgiven by order of testator"); see ---- Paxton, q.v.

James, John, was treated by Dr. Matthew J. Allen in Apr 1848 (p. 79); see Livssey James, q.v.

James, Livssey (sic), was visited by Dr. Matthew J. Allen who treated a child in May and Jul 1845 and daughter Mary (tooth extraction) and son John (tooth extraction) in Jun 1845 (p. 47)

James, Mary, see Livssey James, q.v.

James, Richard, near Slate Ridge, was treated by Dr. John Archer in May and Jul 1774 and 1777 [exact date not given] (Ledger B, p. 17); see Sedgwick James, q.v.

James, Samuel, appeared twice on a list of debts dated 26 Dec 1822 and titled "A List of Allen's Claims" that were due and payable to Dr. Richard N. Allen for services rendered [no dates were given] by him to said James (Document filed in Historical Society of Harford County Archives folder "R. N. Allen"); Samuel was also visited by Dr. Alonzo Preston who treated Sarah James on 7 Jul 1827 (p. 91)

James, Sarah, see Samuel James, q.v.

James, Sedgwick, near William Ashmore's, was treated by Dr. John Archer in Oct 1777 and in Feb, Aug and Sep 1778 (Ledger C, p. 55, noted "to his father's account from Ledger B, fol. 17") [thus, his father was Richard James, q.v.] [Sedgwick James was a Revolutionary War veteran.]

James, Sedgwick, Jr., appeared on a list of debts dated 26 Dec 1822 and titled "A List of Allen's Claims" that were due and payable to Dr. Richard N. Allen for services rendered [no dates were given] by him to said James (Document filed in Historical Society of Harford County Archives folder "R. N. Allen") [Sedgwick James was a War of 1812 veteran.]

James, Thomas, on Jos. Lee's place, was treated by Dr. John Archer in Feb 1790 (Ledger F, p. 257) [Thomas James, Jr. was a Revolutionary War veteran.]

James, Thomas, was visited by Dr. Matthew J. Allen who treated him in Jun and Aug 1847 (p. 54, noted that the $4 medical bill was paid by A. J. Greme)

James, William, see Jacob James, q.v.

Jameson, Adam (pump maker), was treated by Dr. Robert H. Archer in Aug 1823 and also mentioned his brother [no name given] and M. Frazier in June 1827 (p. 237; Ledger F, p. 48)

Jameson, Alexander, was treated by Dr. John Archer in Sep 1782, Apr 1785 and Jul 1799 (Ledger D, p. 87, noted "debt forgiven as before;" Ledger F, p. 113)

Jameson, John (farmer), was treated by Dr. John Archer in Aug and Sep 1772, and in Feb and July 1773, his daughter in July 1773 and him and a child in Apr and May 1775 (Ledger B, pp. 35, 50) [John Jamison (farmer) was a Revolutionary War veteran.]

Jameson, John (tavern keeper), was visited by Dr. John Archer who treated him nine times between Jan 1774 and June 1775, his brother and his [John's] wife in Mar 1774, his daughter in July 1774, his mother in Nov 1774, a child in May 1775, him [John] in Jan 1776 and Jan 1777, his brother in Mar 1778, his [John's] wife in May 1778, his mother in Oct 1778, his brother in Feb 1779 and him [John] in Sep 1779 and Aug 1780 (Ledger B, p. 95; Ledger C, p. 26) [John Jamison (innkeeper) was a Revolutionary War veteran.]

Jameson, Joseph, was prescribed medicine by Dr. Robert H. Archer on 27 Feb 1801 and 18 Apr 1803 and for his child on 22 Oct 1802 and on 18 Jun and 18 Aug 1803 (Rx Book, 1796-1801, p. 38; Rx Book, 1802-1804, pp. 23, 40, 44, 53)

Jameson, Mrs., was visited by Dr. John Archer who treated her in Feb and Aug 1781 and inoculated 4 of her family in 1782 (Ledger D, p. 122, noted "debt forgiven as before")

Janney, Joseph, see Thomas Wilson, q.v.

Jarrett, A., see Thomas A. Hays, q.v.

Jarrett, Abraham [1785-1832], was visited by Dr. Alonzo Preston who treated a child in 1826, Archer and Mary Jarrett and a black girl in 1827 and his wife and Archer Jarrett in 1828 (p. 85, noted "This acct. settled by order on Jarrett in favour of T. A. & N. W. S. Hays [and] in favour of Mr. Gover – both by Dr. P. in his life time. W.B.B.") [referring to Dr. William B. Bond]; Abraham Jarrett, Jr., was visited by Dr. Robert H. Archer who treated his wife in Sep 1826 and Aug 1828 and a negro in Oct 1827 (pp. 202, 249, 288) [Abraham Jarrett was a War of 1812 veteran.]; see Garrett Garrettson and John Forwood, of Jacob, q.v.

Jarrett, Archer, see Abraham Jarrett, q.v.

Jarrett, Bennett, see Jesse Bussey, q.v.

Jarrett, Mary, see Abraham Jarrett, q.v.

Jarvis, James, was treated by Dr. John Archer in Dec 1780 (Ledger D, p. 109, noted "debt forgiven as before") [James Jarvis was a Revolutionary War veteran.]

Jarvis, James, was prescribed medicine by Dr. Robert H. Archer on 5 Sep 1796 (Rx Book, 1796-1801, p. 9)

Jarvis, Joseph, see John Moorn, q.v.

Jay, Eliza, see Stephen Jay, q.v.

Jay, Samuel [1768-1818], was treated by Dr. Robert H. Archer in Baltimore before 1822 [no dates or details were given] (Dr. Archer's "Alphabet to Ledger H" is his booklet [filed in the Archives of the Historical Society of Harford County] that contains his index to Ledger H [which is missing] for his patients in Baltimore before 1822 and Harford County after 1822, according to a notation by Dr. George W. Archer.)

Jay, Samuel, was treated by Dr. Robert H. Archer in Nov 1826 (p. 210) [Samuel Jay was a War of 1812 veteran.]

Jay, Samuel, son of Thomas, was treated by Dr. Robert H. Archer in Jul and Nov 1823 (pp. 92, 93; Ledger F., p. 28)

Jay, Stephen, was visited by Dr. John Archer who treated him in Jun and Sep 1781, his wife, son and daughter in Aug 1784, him in Sep 1784, him and son Thomas in Nov 1787 and him, wife and daughter Eliza in June 1790 (Ledger D, p. 35 spelled his name Jay and p. 76 misspelled his name as Jaye) [account continued in Ledger E, which is missing]; Ledger F, p. 54 [account continued in Ledger G, which is missing]

Jay, Steven, see Thomas Jay, q.v.

Jay, Thomas, was visited by Dr. John Archer who treated him and son Steven at times between 1798 and 1805 (Ledger I, which is missing, was abstracted by Dr. George W. Archer circa 1890; his notes are in the Archives of the Historical Society of Harford County folder "Archer, G. W. Coll. – Ledgers and Day Books"); see Samuel Jay and Stephen Jay, q.v.

Jay, Thomas, was visited by Dr. Robert H. Archer who treated his wife and child in Oct 1822 (p. 30; Ledger F, p. 10); see Martha Wilson, q.v.

Jay, Thomas, of Thomas, was visited by Dr. Robert H. Archer who treated him in July 1823 and a child in Nov 1823 at C. Wilson's (p. 84 listed him as Mr. Jay, of Thomas, and on p. 92 the doctor wrote the name Samuel over Thomas in the ledger)

Jeffrey, Alexander, was treated by Dr. John Archer in Jun 1779, Mar 1781, Jun 1783 and Feb 1790 (Ledger C, p. 49, and Ledger F, p. 251, both spelled his name Jeffry) [Alexander Jeffrey was a Revolutionary War veteran.]

Jeffrey, Hugh, was visited by Dr. John Archer who treated him in Feb and Mar 1773, a "man" in 1773, him [Hugh] in Mar and Apr 1774 in consultation with Dr. Andrews and in June and Oct 1779, his wife "ad obstetricand" [in childbirth] on 3 Jul 1780, and treated him in Feb, Apr, May, Sep and Oct 1781 and five times in Jul 1782 (Ledger B, p. 33, spelled his name Jeffry; Ledger D, p. 31, spelled his name Jeffery) [account continued in Ledger E, which is missing]

Jeffrey, James, see William Jeffrey, q.v.

Jeffrey, Jim, see William W. Lawrence, q.v.

Jeffrey, John, was visited by Dr. Alonzo Preston who treated his family [no names were given] in Dec 1826 (p. 87)

Jeffrey, Martha, was visited by Dr. John Archer who treated her and son Robert in June 1773 (Ledger B, p. 34, spelled her name Jeffry)

Jeffrey, Mrs. (widow), was visited by Dr. John Archer who treated her in Sep 1782, Nov 1784 and Oct 1785 and her and a child in Sep 1788 (Ledger D, p. 105, noted "debt forgiven as before" and spelled her name Jeffry; Ledger F, p. 101, spelled her name Jeffery)

Jeffrey, Robert, was visited by Dr. John Archer who treated him and his wife in Dec 1772, him in Nov 1773 and Sep 1774, his wife in Sep 1779, him and his wife in Oct 1779 and him in Feb and Jun 1780, Mar 1781 and Apr 1782 (Ledger B, p. 32, spelled his name Jeffry; Ledger D, p. 13, spelled it Jeffry and noted "debt forgiven by order as before"); see William W. Lawrence, Samuel Jeffrey and Martha Jeffrey, q.v.

Jeffrey, Robert, Jr., was treated by Dr. John Archer in Mar 1781 (tooth extraction) and Aug 1785 (Ledger D, p. 124, spelled his name Jeffry) [account continued in Ledger G, which is missing]

Jeffrey, Samuel, was visited by Dr. John Archer who treated him in Oct 1772 and Mar 1774 and his brother Robert in July 1772 (Ledger B, p. 31, spelled his name Jeffry)

Jeffrey, Thomas [1753-1832], was treated by Dr. John Archer at various times from 1772 to 1779, in Jul 1780, Aug 1782, May 1784, Apr and Aug 1785, a negro child in Jul 1785 and him [Thomas] in 1788 and 1790 (Ledger B, p. 34; Ledger C, p. 66, spelled his name Jeffry; Ledger D, p. 80, spelled his name Jeffery [account continued in Ledger E, which is missing]; Ledger F, pp. 226, 242, spelled his name Jeffry and Jeffrey) [account continued in Ledger G, which is missing]

Jeffrey, Thomas, was visited by Dr. Robert H. Archer who treated a negro in Sep 1824, Thomas at various times between Aug 1824 and Oct 1825 and in Dec 1827 (prescribed medicine on 20 Dec 1827) and son Thomas in Apr 1828 and Negro Grace in Apr and May 1828 (pp. 121, 166, 257, 258, 272, 273, 274, 275; Ledger F, p. 105; Rx Book, 1825-1851, p. 91, spelled his name Jeffery) [account continued in Ledger G, which is missing]; see Samuel Horford, q.v.

Jeffrey, William, was visited by Dr. Matthew J. Allen who treated him in Mar, Jun and Oct 1848 and James Jeffry (sic) in Mar 1848 (p. 77 spelled his name Jeffrie; p. 97 spelled his name Jeffry and noted that the account was paid in Jul 1852)

Jeffries, Samuel, was treated by Dr. Robert H. Archer in Sep 1815 (Ledger F, p. 10)

Jenkins, Francis, was treated by Dr. John Archer in Jun 1778, Aug 1781 and Jun and Jul 1782 (Ledger C, p. 113) [account continued in Ledger E, which is missing] [Francis Jenkins was a Revolutionary War veteran.]

Jenkins, Thomas, was treated by Dr. John Archer in Feb 1775 and also mentioned William Kelly (Ledger B, p. 37)

Jenkins, Thomas (free negro), was murdered in 1834: "State of Maryland, Harford County, sct: An Inquisition taken at Point Concord in the County and State aforesaid on the 24th day of April in the year Eighteen hundred & thirty four before me Warren L. Nicoll one of the Justices of the Peace in & for the County aforesaid upon the view of the body of Thomas Jenkins, a free black man, then and there lying dead upon the Oaths of … good and lawful men of the County aforesaid who being sworn upon the Holy Evangely of Almighty God and charged to enquire when, where, how and after what manner the said Thomas Jenkins came to his death do say upon their oaths that the said Thomas Jenkins came to his death by a blow inflicted on his head with an oak club by John Clark, a free black man, on Saturday the 19th day of April instant at the County aforesaid. In Witness whereof as well the aforesaid Warren L. Nicoll Justice as aforesaid as the Jurors aforesaid have to this Inquisition put their hands and seals on the day and year aforesaid and at the place aforesaid. Inquisition on the body of Thomas Jenkins. Received and Recorded May 2nd Eighteen hundred and thirty four in Liber H. D. No. 17, folio 116, one of the Land Record Books of Harford County." ("Slavery Inquisitions" file in the Archives Department of the Historical Society of Harford County)

Jervis, see Jarvis, q.v.

Jervis, James, son of John, was visited by Dr. John Archer who treated him and his wife in Sep 1786 (Ledger F, p. 35)

Jervis, John, was visited by Dr. John Archer who treated him four times between 6 Jul 1773 and 26 Feb 1775, his wife in Mar 1775, him in Jul 1779, Feb 1780 and Mar 1780, son Johan [John] in Jan 1782, him in Jun and Oct 1782, Minta Jervis in Apr 1783 and him in Feb 1787 (Ledger B, p. 99; Ledger D, p. 1, noted "debt forgiven by order of the testator in his last will and testament;" Ledger F); see James Jervis, q.v.

Jervis, Joshua, was listed in Dr. John Archer's ledger circa 1773, but no entries were made in his account (Ledger B, p. 39)

Jervis, Minta, see John Jervis, q.v.

Jessop, Mrs., was prescribed medicine by Dr. Robert H. Archer on 15 Mar 1803 and then noted "to be sent to Mrs. Wells" (Rx Book, 1802-1804, p. 39)

Jewell, George [c1750-1820] (blacksmith), was visited by Dr. John Archer who treated him and children Jemima, Mary, George, John, Sally and Joseph at times between 1794 and 1799 [no dates were given] (Ledger I, which is missing, was abstracted by Dr. George W. Archer circa 1890; his notes are in the Archives of the Historical Society of Harford County folder "Archer, G. W. Coll. – Ledgers and Day Books; spelled his name Jewel); George Jewell was prescribed medicine for his wife by Dr. Robert H. Archer on 7 Oct 1802 and his child on 18 Oct 1802 (Rx Book, 1802-1804, pp. 6, 22); George Jewel &ca (sic) was treated by Dr. Archer in Baltimore [no dates were given; he returned to Harford County where he died on 2 Jul 1820] (Dr. Archer's "Alphabet to Ledger H" is his booklet [filed in Archives of the Historical Society of Harford

County] that contains his index to Ledger H [which is missing] for his patients in Baltimore City before 1822 and Harford County after 1822, according to a notation by Dr. George W. Archer.)

Jewett, Thaddeus, was treated by Dr. David Dick in Sep and Nov 1778 and Feb, Mar and Jun 1779; Dr. Dick swore to the accuracy of this account before magistrate A. Whitaker on 29 Nov 1780. (Historical Society of Harford County, Court Records Department, Document File 4.18.15)

Jewitt, Ann, Mrs., was treated by Dr. John Archer in Apr 1787 (Ledger F, p. 250)

Jibb, John, was visited by Dr. John Archer who treated him at various times between Aug 1772 and Mar 1774 and treated an infant and a girl in Aug 1772, a child in Mar 1773, a man in May 1773 and May 1774, him and family [names not given] in June 1773, a child in Sep and Dec 1774, him in Jan and Dec 1777, his wife in Jun 1777 and him in Jul, Sep and Dec 1778, Patty in Oct 1779, daughter in Aug 1780 and May 1781, him in Aug and Sep 1781 and Mar 1782, daughter in Jun 1782, him in Jul 1790 and him and his family at various times between 1797 and 1803 (Ledger B, p. 37; Ledger C, p. 82, noted that part of the bill was paid "by your proportion of the money you paid for the poor of Boston £1.4.9" on 10 Jun 1777; Ledger D, p. 29 [account continued in Ledger E, which is missing]; Ledger F, p. 144 [account continued in Ledger H, which is missing]; Ledger I, which is also missing, was abstracted by Dr. George W. Archer circa 1890; his notes are in the Archives of the Historical Society of Harford County folder "Archer, G. W. Coll. – Ledgers and Day Books") [John Jibb was a Revolutionary War veteran.]

Johns, ----, see Daniel McGlaughlin, q.v.

Johns, Anney, see Skipwith Johns, q.v.

Johns, Caroline, see Aquila Massey, q.v.

Johns, Cassey, see Skipwith Johns, q.v.

Johns, Drucilla, see Henry H. Johns, q.v.

Johns, Ephraim, see Henry H. Johns, q.v.

Johns, Henry, was visited by Dr. John Archer who treated him in Jul and Aug 1781 and Jun 1783 and him and a child in 1790 (Ledger D p. 38; Ledger F, p. 335) [account continued in Ledger G, which is missing]; see Richard Johns, q.v.

Johns, Henry H. [1794-1861], was visited by Dr. Alonzo Preston who treated him at times in 1825 and 1826, his wife many times and a child and Mary several times in 1826, Mrs. Johns "in partu" [in childbirth] on 20 Jul 1826, Ephraim, John, Mary and Drucilla in 1827 and his wife and Mary in 1828 (pp. 37, 38, 87, noting "This acct. settled by note for the balance above [$37.11] struck Dec 19, 1832" and signed by Wm. B. Bond) [referring to Dr. William B. Bond] [Henry Hosier Johns was War of 1812 veteran.]

Johns, John, see Henry H. Johns, q.v.

Johns, Mary, see Henry H. Johns, q.v.

Johns, Molly, see Skipwith Johns, q.v.

Johns, Nat., see Negro Will, q.v.

Johns, Nathan, was treated by Dr. Robert H. Archer in Baltimore before 1822 [no dates or details were given] (Dr. Archer's "Alphabet to Ledger H" is his booklet [filed in the Archives of the Historical Society of Harford County] that contains his index to Ledger H [which is missing] for his patients in Baltimore before 1822 and Harford County after 1822, according to a notation by Dr. George W. Archer.)

Johns, Nathaniel, was visited by Dr. John Archer who treated his wife and child in Jan 1777, his daughter in Nov 1779, him in Mar 1781, his wife and a child in 1786 and him and a child in 1790 (Ledger C, p. 79, noted "debt forgiven by order of testator;" Ledger D, p. 35, noted "debt forgiven as before;" Ledger F, p. 119)

Johns, Richard, was visited by Dr. John Archer who treated him in Dec 1776 and Jan 1777 and his daughter and Miss Chew in Oct 1779 (Ledger C, p. 76, noted "deliver to Henry Johns, exec." and also "debt forgiven by order of testator")

Johns, Sally, see Skipwith Johns, q.v.

Johns, Skipwith, was visited by Dr. John Archer who treated his wife and daughters Cassey, Anney, Molly and Sally in Mar and Apr 1788 and him in Jul 1788 (Ledger F, p. 223, 233, 263, 265) [account continued in Ledger G, which is missing]

Johns, Stephen, was treated by Dr. Robert H. Archer in Baltimore before 1822 [no dates or details were given] (Dr. Archer's "Alphabet to Ledger H" is his booklet [filed in the Archives of the Historical Society of Harford County] that contains his index to Ledger H [which is missing] for his patients in Baltimore before 1822 and Harford County after 1822, according to a notation by Dr. George W. Archer.)

Johns, William (clerk's office), was treated by Dr. Robert H. Archer in June 1828 in consultation with Dr. Preston (p. 280)

Johnson, ----[blank] (watchman), was treated by Dr. Robert H. Archer in Baltimore before 1822 [no dates or details were given] (Dr. Archer's "Alphabet to Ledger H" is his booklet [filed in the Archives of the Historical Society of Harford County] that contains his index to Ledger H [which is missing] for his patients in Baltimore before 1822 and Harford County after 1822, according to a notation by Dr. George W. Archer.)

Johnson, ---- [blank], son-in-law &ca *(sic)*, was treated by Dr. Robert H. Archer in Baltimore before 1822 [no dates or details were given] (Dr. Archer's "Alphabet to Ledger H" is his booklet [filed in the Archives of the Historical Society of Harford County] that contains his index to Ledger H [which is missing] for his patients in Baltimore before 1822 and Harford County after 1822, according to a notation by Dr. George W. Archer.)

Johnson, Ann, "widow of John, now Rigdon," was visited by Dr. John Archer who inoculated 3 of her family in 1777 and treated her son and a negro in Feb 1780 and her in Jun 1780 (Ledger C, p. 65, noted "debt forgiven by order of testator;" Ledger D, p. 50, noted "debt forgiven as before")

Johnson, Barnett, appeared on a list of debts dated 26 Dec 1822 and titled "A List of Allen's Claims" that were due and payable to Dr. Richard N. Allen for services rendered [no dates were given] by him to said Johnson (Document filed in Historical Society of Harford County Archives folder "R. N. Allen"); see Thomas Johnson, q.v.

Johnson, Barney, see Thomas Johnson, q.v.

Johnson, C. [Caleb] (reverend), "Yanker," was visited by Dr. John Archer who treated him and his wife at various times between 1796 and 1803 (Ledger I, which is missing, was abstracted by Dr. George W. Archer circa 1890; his notes are in the Archives of the Historical Society of Harford County folder "Archer, G. W. Coll. – Ledgers and Day Books")

Johnson, Caroline, see Charles D. W. Johnson, q.v.

Johnson, Charles, near Trap [i. e. Trappe, an area south of Dublin, west of Darlington, near Trappe Church], was visited by Dr. Robert H. Archer who treated a child in May 1823 (p. 72)

Johnson, Charles D. W., was visited by Dr. Alonzo Preston who treated him at various times between 1824 and 1827, and his wife, an unnamed child and son James in 1824 and 1825, and his wife "in partu" [in childbirth] on 18 Jun 1825; also treated her in Feb 1827 and Aug 1828, daughter Caroline in 1827 and 1828 and vaccinated their children in Jun 1827 (pp. 21, 39)

Johnson, Dr., see James Smith and Carvill H. Prigg, q.v.

Johnson, Elisha, near Trap [i. e., Trappe, an area south of Dublin, west of Darlington, near Trappe Church], was visited by Dr. Robert H. Archer who treated a child in May 1823 (Ledger F, p. 26)

Johnson, Elizabeth, was prescribed medicine by Dr. Robert H. Archer on 13 Sep 1841 (Rx Book, 1825-1851, p. 116)

Johnson, Elizabeth, Mrs., appeared on a list of debts dated 26 Dec 1822 and titled "A List of Allen's Claims" that were due and payable to Dr. Richard N. Allen for services rendered [no dates were given] by him to said Elizabeth (Document filed in Archives of the Historical Society of Harford County folder "R. N. Allen")

Johnson, James, see Charles D. W. Johnson, q.v.

Johnson, James, over Deer Creek, was treated by Dr. John Archer in Sep and Nov 1775 (Ledger B, p. 60); "Jas. Johnson" was visited by Dr. John Archer who treated him and children Joseph and Susan at times between 1794 and 1800 [no dates were given] (Ledger I, which is missing, was abstracted by Dr. George W. Archer circa 1890; his notes are in the Archives of the Historical Society of Harford County folder "Archer, G. W. Coll. – Ledgers and Day Books")

Johnson James, was treated by Dr. Robert H. Archer in Baltimore before 1822 [no dates or details were given] (Dr. Archer's "Alphabet to Ledger H" is his booklet [filed in the Archives of the Historical Society of Harford County] that contains his index to Ledger H [which is missing] for his patients in Baltimore before 1822 and Harford County after 1822, according to a notation by Dr. George W. Archer; "James Johnson, H. Hill" was also indexed on a different page.)

Johnson, John, was visited by Dr. John Archer who treated him and his wife several times in Aug 1774 (Ledger B, p. 25) [John Johnson was a Revolutionary War veteran.]

Johnson, John, near Delph, was visited by Dr. John Archer who treated him and his wife in 1787 (Ledger F, p. 372) [John Johnson was a Revolutionary War veteran.]

Johnson, John [1783-1865], was visited by Dr. Robert H. Archer who treated his wife and "Jud:" in Mar 1823 in consultation with Dr Preston (pp. 56, 58; Ledger F, p. 145); he was also treated by Dr. Thomas H. Birckhead prior to 10 Mar 1828 on which date James Reardon acknowledged that he had "Received of John Johnson thirty five dollars the amount of his account in full with Dr. Thos. H. Birckhead." John was also visited by Dr. William L. Horton who treated him in 1829 [no details were given in the medical bill, just an amount due for the year] and also for "bleeding & reducing fractured clavicle (I. Hall)" in Jul 1830 and "opening abscess (boy)" in Aug 1830 (Documents filed in the Archives of the Historical Society of Harford County folder "Medical Papers") [John Johnson was a War of 1812 veteran.]; see John Slee, q.v.

Johnson, John, Mrs. (widow), was treated by Dr. John Archer in Dec 1774 and May 1779 (Ledger B, p. 5); see Ann Johnson and Mrs. Johnson (widow), q.v.

Johnson, Joseph, see James Johnson, q.v.

Johnson, Joseph &ca *(sic)*, was treated by Dr. Robert H. Archer in Baltimore before 1822 [no dates or details were given] (Dr. Archer's "Alphabet to Ledger H" is his booklet [filed in the Archives of the Historical Society of Harford County] that contains his index to Ledger H [which is missing] for his patients in Baltimore City before 1822 and in Harford County after 1822, according to a notation by Dr. George W. Archer.)

Johnson, London (negro), was treated by Dr. Robert H. Archer after 1822 [no dates or details given] (Dr. Archer's "Alphabet to Ledger H" is his booklet [filed in the Archives of the Historical Society of Harford County] that contains his index to Ledger H [which is missing] for his patients in Baltimore before 1822 and in Harford County after 1822, according to a notation by Dr. George W. Archer.)

Johnson, Matthew, was treated by Dr. Matthew J. Allen in Jan, May, Jun and Jul 1847 (pp. 56, 57, noted the medical bill was partly paid by cash on 6 Sep 1847 and settled in full "by draft on J. W. and L. Reynolds" on 13 Jan 1848)

Johnson, Moses, see Thomas and Moses Johnson, q.v.

Johnson, Mrs. (widow), mother of Thomas, was treated by Dr. John Archer in Aug 1774 (Ledger B, p. 45); see Mrs. John Johnson (widow), q.v.

Johnson, Mrs., widow of William, was treated by Dr. John Archer in Mar 1789 (Ledger F, p. 62)

Johnson, Susan, see James Johnson, q.v.

Johnson, Thomas, was visited by Dr. John Archer who treated him in Jul 1781 and son Barney in Nov 1781 (Ledger D, p. 47, noted "debt forgiven as before" and also noted part paid "By cash for his and Barnet Johnson's account" on 12 Sep 1783) [Thomas Johnson was a Revolutionary War veteran.]; see Mrs. Johnson, q.v.

Johnson, Thomas (esquire), was visited by Dr. John Archer who treated him and son William at times in 1794 and 1796 [no dates were given] (Ledger I, which is missing, was abstracted by Dr. George W. Archer circa 1890; his notes are in the Archives of the Historical Society of Harford County folder "Archer, G. W. Coll. – Ledgers and Day Books")

Johnson, Thomas and Moses, appeared together on a list of debts dated 26 Dec 1822 and titled "A List of Allen's Claims" that were due and payable to Dr. Richard N. Allen for services rendered [no dates were given] by him to the said Thomas and Moses Johnson (Document in the Archives of the Historical Society of Harford County folder "R. N. Allen")

Johnson, Widow, see John Lyon, Mrs. Johnson and Mrs. John Johnson, q.v.

Johnson, William, see Thomas Johnson and Mrs. Johnson, q.v.

Johnson, William, was treated by Dr. John Archer at various times in 1798 and 1799 (Ledger F, p. 298) [continued in Ledger I, which is missing, but abstracted by Dr. George W. Archer circa 1890; his notes are in the Archives of the Historical Society of Harford County folder "Archer, G. W. Coll. – Ledgers and Day Books")] [William Johnson was a Revolutionary War veteran.]

Johnson, William, was treated by Dr. Matthew J. Allen in 1833 in Calvert County (p. 26) [William Johnson was a War of 1812 veteran.]

Johnson, William, son of Thomas, was treated by Dr. John Archer in Feb 1793 (Ledger F, p. 290)

Johnston, Bernet, son of Thomas, was visited by Dr. John Archer who treated him and a child in 1788 (Ledger F, p. 125)

Johnston, Robert, son of Thomas, was visited by Dr. John Archer who treated his wife in Oct 1777 (Ledger C, p. 97)

Johnston, Thomas, see Bernet Johnston and Robert Johnston, q.v.

Johnston, Thomas, Sr., was visited by Dr. John Archer who treated a child in 1788 and him in Sep 1791 (Ledger F, p. 88) [account continued in Ledger H, which is missing] [Thomas Johnston was a Revolutionary War veteran.]

Joice, Thomas, was listed in Dr. John Archer's ledger circa 1773, but no entries were made in his account (Ledger B, p. 38)

Jolly, Edward, was treated by Dr. John Archer in May 1789 (Ledger F, p. 362)

Jolly, Elizabeth, was treated by Dr. John Archer in April 1793 (Ledger F, p. 346)

Jolly, John, was treated by Dr. John Archer in June 1779 (Ledger C, p. 66, noted "debt forgiven by order of testator") [John Jolly was a Revolutionary War veteran.]; see Charles Beaver, q.v.

Jolly, John, was prescribed medicine for his child by Dr. Robert H. Archer on 17 Feb, 13 Sep and 14 Sep 1803 (Rx Book, 1802-1804, pp. 33, 55, spelled his name Jolley)

Jolly, Widow, was visited by Dr. John Archer who treated her in Jul 1781 and Aug 1782, her daughter in Sep 1782, a negro in Dec 1782 and her son William in Sep 1783 (Ledger D, p 50) [account continued in Ledger E, which is missing]

Jolley, William, dec'd., appeared on a list of debts dated 26 Dec 1822 and titled "A List of Allen's Claims" that were due and payable to Dr. Richard N. Allen for services rendered [no dates were given] by him to the said Tolley (Document filed in Historical Society of Harford County Archives folder "R. N. Allen"); see Widow Jolly, q.v.

Jones, Amos [1754-1827], "near W. Hall" [referring to White Hall, but he actually lived on Bond's Forest near White House in Fallston], was visited by Dr. John Archer who treated him and children Nancy, Sally and Daniel at times between 1798 and 1800 (Ledger I, which is missing, was abstracted by Dr. George W. Archer circa 1890; his notes are in Archives of the Historical Society of Harford County file "Archer, G. W. Coll. – Ledgers and Day Books") [Amos Jones was a Revolutionary War veteran.]

Jones, Aquila, was visited by Dr. John Archer who treated his wife in Mar 1773 (Ledger B, p. 91) [Aquila Jones, Jr. and Aquila Jones, Sr. were both Revolutionary War veterans.]

Jones, Asbury, was prescribed medicine for a lady by Dr. Robert H. Archer on 2 May 1803 (Rx Book, 1802-1804, p. 41, actually stated "To a lady sick at Asbury Jones's b. Row")

Jones, Benjamin, at Bynum Run, was treated by Dr. John Archer between 1794 and 1807 (Ledger I, which is missing, was abstracted by Dr. George W. Archer circa 1890; his notes are in Archives of Historical Society of Harford County file "Archer, G. W. Coll. – Ledgers and Day Books")

Jones, Benjamin G., was visited by Dr. Alonzo Preston who treated a black boy in 1826 (p. 69)

Jones, Betty, see Stephen Jones, q.v.

Jones, Capt., Havre de Grace, was visited by Dr. John Archer who treated him and his family in 1797 (Ledger I, which is missing, was abstracted by Dr. George W. Archer circa 1890; his notes are in the Archives of the Historical Society of Harford County folder "Archer, G. W. Coll. – Ledgers and Day Books")

Jones, Carvil, see William Jones, Sr., q.v.

Jones, Daniel [1784-1848], was treated by Dr. Matthew J. Allen twenty-two times between 24 May and 2 Jul 1847 for hemorrhoids, and a tooth extraction in Jun 1857 (p. 52); see Amos Jones, q.v.

Jones, Eliza, see Gilbert Jones and William Jones, Sr., q.v.

Jones, Gilbert, was visited by Dr. John Archer who treated him and his daughter Eliza in Jan 1791 (Ledger F, p. 263) [Gilbert Jones was a Revolutionary War veteran.]

Jones, Griffith, was treated by Dr. John Archer in 1786 (Ledger F, p. 187); see Widow Thorn, q.v.

Jones, Isaac, at Bush Town, was treated by Dr. John Archer in June 1787 (Ledger F, p. 314) [Isaac Jones and Isaac Jones, of William, were Revolutionary War veterans.]; he appeared on a list of debts dated 26 Dec 1822 and titled "A List of Allen's Claims" that were due and payable to Dr. Richard N. Allen for services rendered [no dates given] to said Jones (Document filed in Historical Society of Harford County Archives folder "R. N. Allen"); see William Jones, q.v.

Jones, James [1793-1860], was treated by Dr. Robert H. Archer in Mar and Sep 1828 and was prescribed medicine on 8 Sep 1828 (pp. 266, 295; Rx Book, 1825-1851, p. 92) [James Jones was a War of 1812 veteran.]; see Aquila Paca, q.v.

Jones, James, son of Reuben, was treated by Dr. Robert H. Archer in Apr 1823 and Sep 1828 (Ledger F, p. 2)

Jones, Jane, servant to Isaac Blake, was treated by Dr. John Archer in Apr 1787 (Ledger F, p. 317, noted "now married to Philip Quinlan," but did not give the date of marriage)

Jones, Jinny, was treated by Dr. John Archer in Jan 1794 (Ledger F, p. 104, noted "now married to Isaac Blake," but did not give the date of marriage)

Jones, John, at Harford Town, was treated by Dr. John Archer in Oct 1778 (Ledger C, p. 124, noted "debt forgiven by order of testator")

Jones, John, at Ring Factory [on Winters Run, west of Bel Air], was visited by Dr. Matthew J. Allen who treated a child ten times between 10 Sep 1848 and 3 Oct 1848 (p. 93)

Jones, Jos., Mrs., see Harford County for Pensioners, q.v.

Jones, Joseph (Quaker preacher), was treated by Dr. John Archer in Dec 1777 (Ledger C, p. 80, noted "debt forgiven by order of testator")

Jones, Joseph, was visited by Dr. John Archer who treated an infant in Feb 1779 and then charged his services to Harford County (Ledger C, p. 111) [Joseph Jones was a Revolutionary War veteran.]

Jones, Joseph, was visited by Dr. Robert H. Archer who treated his wife "in partu" [in childbirth] on 22 Jun 1827 and him and his child in Apr 1828 (pp. 235, 272, 273)

Jones, Joshua, was visited by Dr. John Archer who treated his wife in labor on 29 Jan 1773 and her again on 7 Feb 1773 and again in Nov 1773, and him in Oct 1774 and June 1778 (Ledger B, p. 23; Ledger C, p. 115, noted "debt forgiven by order of testator"); see Reubin Jones, q.v.

Jones, Maggy, see William Jones, Sr., q.v.

Jones, Mary (widow), was treated by Dr. Robert H. Archer in Baltimore before 1822 [no dates or details were given] (Dr. Archer's "Alphabet to Ledger H" is his booklet [filed in the Archives of the Historical Society of Harford County] that contains his index to Ledger H [which is missing] for his patients in Baltimore before 1822 and Harford County after 1822, according to a notation by Dr. George W. Archer.)

Jones, Mr., son-in-law to Mrs. Nevill, was visited by Dr. Robert H. Archer who treated his wife on 8 Sep 1822 in consultation with Dr. Worthington (p. 17)

Jones, Mr., was prescribed medicine by Dr. Robert H. Archer on 8 May 1851 (Rx Book, 1825-1851, p. 121)

Jones, Mr., Cedarfield, was treated by Dr. Robert H. Archer after 1822 [no dates or details were given] (Dr. Archer's "Alphabet to Ledger H" is his booklet [filed in the Archives of the Historical Society of Harford County] that contains his index to Ledger H [now missing] for his patients in Baltimore before 1822 and Harford County after 1822, according to a notation by Dr. George W. Archer.)

Jones, Mrs., in Baltimore, was prescribed medicine by Dr. Robert H. Archer on 21 Apr 1803 (Rx Book, 1802-1804, p. 40)

Jones, Mrs., in Bel Air, was prescribed medicine by Dr. Robert H. Archer on 19 Mar 1834 (Rx Book, 1825-1851, p. 110); see Thomas A. Hays, q.v.

Jones, Nancy, see Amos Jones, q.v.

Jones, Priscilla, at Slate Ridge, was treated by Dr. John Archer in 1790 (Ledger F, p. 104)

Jones, Reuben (post fence maker), was visited by Dr. Robert H. Archer who treated a child in Jul 1823 (p. 83; Ledger F, p. 74, "insolvent"); see James Jones and Simon Brown, q.v.

Jones, Reubin, was visited by Dr. John Archer who treated him in Jan 1781 (laxative pill) and May 1783 ("hamorrhoid") and treated him and his wife in 1790 (Ledger D, p. 113, listed him as Rubin Jones and noted "transferred from your father's acct., B. 23" [i. e., Ledger B, p. 23] which was in Joshua Jones' name [Reubin's account was continued in Ledger E, which is missing] [Reuben Jones was a Revolutionary War veteran.]; Ledger F, p. 329) see Joshua Jones, q.v.

Jones, Sally, see Amos Jones, q.v.

Jones, Samuel, was visited by Dr. Robert H. Archer who treated his wife in Sep 1822 (p. 19; Ledger F, p. 75)

Jones, Stephen, see Daniel Buckley, q.v.

Jones, Stephen, was visited by Dr. Alonzo Preston who treated Betty "in partu" [in childbirth] on 1 Dec 1825 (p. 33)

Jones, Thomas, at John Ruff's in Bush River Neck, was treated by Dr. John Archer in Jun 1788 (Ledger F, p. 37) [Two men named Thomas Jones were Revolutionary War veterans.]

Jones, William, was visited by Dr. John Archer who inoculated 10 of his family in Feb 1776, treated him in Aug 1777, Oct 1779, Feb 1780, May 1781, Jun 1783, Jul and Sep 1784, son Isaac in Feb 1785 and him [William] in May 1785 (Ledger C, p. 27; Ledger D, p. 45, noted "debt forgiven as before") [Two men named William Jones were Revolutionary War veterans.]

Jones, William, near William Hollins, was treated by Dr. John Archer in Jan 1786 (Ledger F, p. 86)

Jones, William, Sr., at B. Run [probably Bynum Run], was visited by Dr. John Archer who treated him, his wife, sons William and Carvil and daughters Eliza and Maggy in 1788, his daughter Eliza, son William and a grandson [name not given] in 1791 and him [William] in May 1798 (Ledger F, pp. 252, 316, 322, 338) [account continued in Ledger K, which is missing]

Jordan, John, see William Jordan, q.v.

Jordan, Mary, Miss, was visited by Dr. Matthew J. Allen who treated Miss Sarah in May 1848 and her [Mary] in Jun 1848, mentioned the balance from S. Jordan's account from p. 52, and treated Mary in Aug 1848 and Mary and sister Sarah in Sep 1848 (p. 82, noted the bill was reduced and the doctor was paid "by 5 bushels of oats in full" on 26 Oct 1848); see William Jordan, q.v.

Jordan, Samuel, see William Jordan, q.v.

Jordan, Sarah, Miss, see Mary Jordan, q.v.

Jordan, Simon, was treated by Dr. John Archer in Jul 1781 (Ledger D, p. 53, noted "debt forgiven as before") [Simon Jordin or Jordon was a Revolutionary War veteran.]

Jordan, Sophia, Miss, was treated by Dr. Matthew J. Allen nineteen times between 23 May 1847 and 7 Aug 1847 (p. 52, noted "see fol. 82," which mentioned her in the account of Mary Jordan)

Jordan, William, was visited by Dr. Alonzo Preston who treated him at times between 1822 and 1825 [no details were given] and his wife, son John and Mary and Samuel in 1825 (p. 32)

Jordan, William, was visited by Dr. Matthew J. Allen who treated him seven times in Apr 1848 and once in May 1848 and rendered obstetrical services to his wife on 1 Jun 1848 and gave her medicine on 8 Jun 1848 (p. 81)

Jourdan (Jordon), Mr. (sub-sheriff), was treated by Dr. Robert H. Archer in Aug and Sep 1824 in consultation with Dr. Preston (pp. 119, 120, and p. 65 noted "Ran off")

Judd, Daniel, was treated by Dr. John Archer in May and Jun 1775 (Ledger B, p. 27)

Judd, Daniel, Jr., was treated by Dr. John Archer in Jul 1788 (Ledger F, p. 158)

Judd, Edward, was visited by Dr. Alonzo Preston who treated his wife on 12 Jun 1827 (p. 8, noting he was paid $2 and the balance of $3 was carried over from another ledger and later marked "Denied") [Edward Judd was a War of 1812 veteran.]

Judd, John [1798-1870], was noted in a non-medical matter in Dr. Robert H. Archer's ledger when the doctor "paid him for shoemaker" *(sic)* in Jun 1827 (p. 232); see John F. Wheeler, q.v.

Judd, Joshua, on D. Lee's place, was treated by Dr. John Archer in Jul 1791 (Ledger F, p. 349)

Judd, Matthew, was visited by Dr. John Archer who treated him and his family at various times between 1796 and 1804 (Ledger I, which is missing, was abstracted by Dr. George W. Archer circa 1890; his notes are in Archives of the Historical Society of Harford County folder "Archer, G. W. Coll. – Ledgers and Day Books"); also mentioned in a non-medical matter in Dr. Robert H. Archer's ledger when Matthew was "paid by building chimney & pointing underpinning house where Ewing lives" in Apr 1823 (Ledger F, p. 156)

Judd, William, near Daniel Dunnavan, was visited by Dr. John Archer who treated him and his wife in 1787 and him in 1791 (Ledger F, pp. 32, 126)

Judd, William, was treated by Dr. Matthew J. Allen eleven times in Apr and May 1848, twice in Jun 1848 and once in Jul 1848 (pp. 79, 85, noted "paid to A. Greme"); see Augustus J. Greme, q.v.

Judd, William, Jr., was treated by Dr. John Archer in Jun 1791 (Ledger F, p. 139)

Justice, Joseph, was treated by Dr. Robert H. Archer in Baltimore before 1822 [no dates or details were given] (Dr. Archer's "Alphabet to Ledger H" is his booklet [filed in the Archives of the Historical Society of Harford County] that contains his index to Ledger H [which is missing] for his patients in Baltimore before 1822 and Harford County after 1822, according to a notation by Dr. George W. Archer.)

Karr, William, son-in-law to William Dyer, near the Little Falls Quaker Meeting House, was treated by Dr. John Archer in 1795 and 1796 (Ledger I, which is missing, was abstracted by Dr. George W. Archer circa 1890; his notes are in the Archives of the Historical Society of Harford County folder "Archer, G. W. Coll. – Ledgers and Day Books")

Karr, William &ca *(sic)*, was treated by Dr. Robert H. Archer in Baltimore before 1822 [no dates or details were given] (Dr. Archer's "Alphabet to Ledger H" is his booklet [filed in the Archives of the Historical Society of Harford County] that contains his index to Ledger H [which is missing] for his patients in Baltimore before 1822 and Harford County after 1822, according to a notation by Dr. George W. Archer.)

Kean, John, appeared on a list of debts dated 26 Dec 1822 and titled "A List of Allen's Claims" that were due and payable to Dr. Richard N. Allen for services rendered [no dates were given] by him to the said Kean (Document filed in Historical Society of Harford County Archives folder "R. N. Allen"); John Kean (former sheriff) was also visited by Dr. Robert H. Archer who treated a child in July 1825 in consultation with Dr. Forwood (p. 141; Ledger F, p. 110)

Kearns, Thomas, see Matthew Bonar, q.v.

Keech, Mr., see John Magness and Negro Nero, q.v.

Keeports, George P. [in Baltimore], was prescribed medicine for his wife by Dr. Robert H. Archer on 24 Feb and 1 Jun 1803 (Rx Book, 1802-1804, pp. 34, 43)

Keirle, John W., was treated by Dr. Robert H. Archer in Sep 1815 (Ledger F, p. 11, partially torn)

Kell, Thomas [1772-1846] (esquire), was treated by Dr. Robert H. Archer in Baltimore before 1822 [no dates or details were given] (Dr. Archer's "Alphabet to Ledger H" is his booklet [filed in the Archives of the Historical Society of Harford County] that contains his index to Ledger H [which is missing] for his patients in Baltimore before 1822 and Harford County after 1822, according to a notation by Dr. George W. Archer.) [Thomas Kell was a War of 1812 veteran.]

Kellen, ---- [blank] (tailor), was treated by Dr. Robert H. Archer in Baltimore before 1822 [no dates or details were given] (Dr. Archer's "Alphabet to Ledger H" is his booklet [filed in the Archives of the Historical Society of Harford County] that contains his index to Ledger H [which is missing] for his patients in Baltimore before 1822 and Harford County after 1822, according to a notation by Dr. George W. Archer.)

Kelly, ---- [blank] (merchant), was treated by Dr. Robert H. Archer in Baltimore before 1822 [no dates or details were given] (Dr. Archer's "Alphabet to Ledger H" is his booklet [filed in the Archives of the Historical Society of Harford County] that contains his index to Ledger H [which is missing] for his patients in Baltimore before 1822 and Harford County after 1822, according to a notation by Dr. George W. Archer.)

Kelly, ---- [blank] (potter), was treated by Dr. Robert H. Archer in Baltimore before 1822 [no dates or details were given] (Dr. Archer's "Alphabet to Ledger H" is his booklet [filed in the Archives of the Historical Society of Harford County] that contains his index to Ledger H [which is missing] for his patients in Baltimore before 1822 and Harford County after 1822, according to a notation by Dr. George W. Archer.)

Kelly, Alexander, was visited by Dr. John Archer who treated him and his wife and child in 1792 (Ledger F, p. 72)

Kelly, Andrew, was treated by Dr. John Archer in Feb 1781 (Ledger D, p. 124) [account continued in Ledger G, which is missing]

Kelly, James (tailor), over Deer Creek, was treated by Dr. John Archer in Aug 1782 (Ledger D, p. 69, noted the doctor was paid in trade by Kelly "making a nankeen coat for Tommy")

Kelly, John, see Harford County for Pensioners, q.v.

Kelly, John, was prescribed medicine by Dr. Robert H. Archer on 29 Mar 1803 (Rx Book, 1802-1804, p. 38)

Kelly, John (weaver), was treated by Dr. John Archer in Jan 1781 (Ledger D, p. 118, noted "debt forgiven as before")

Kelly, Lawrence, was treated by Dr. Robert H. Archer in Baltimore before 1822 [no dates or details were given] (Dr. Archer's "Alphabet to Ledger H" is his booklet [filed in the Archives of the Historical Society of Harford County] that contains his index to Ledger H [which is missing] for his patients in Baltimore before 1822 and Harford County after 1822, according to a notation by Dr. George W. Archer.)

Kelly, Martha, see Thomas Kelly, q.v.

Kelly, Patty, see Thomas Kelly, q.v.

Kelly, Robert, was visited by Dr. John Archer who treated him in Mar 1781, his wife in Jun, Jul and Aug 1783 and him, his wife and a child in Sep 1783 (Ledger D, p. 128) [account continued in Ledger E, which is missing] [Robert Kelly was a Revolutionary War veteran.]

Kelly, Thomas, at A. Redding's, was treated by Dr. Matthew J. Allen in Feb 1845 (p. 44)

Kelly, Thomas, was visited by Dr. Alonzo Preston who treated him at times between 1824 and 1828, his wife in 1825, Patty and daughter Martha [same person?] in 1827 and youngest child [not named] in 1828 (p. 47, spelled his name Kelley)

Kelly, Valentine, was treated by Dr. John Archer in 1786 (Ledger F, p. 321)

Kelly, William (tailor), was treated by Dr. John Archer in July 1773 (Ledger B, p. 56)

Kelly, William, was visited by Dr. Alonzo Preston who treated him, his sister and a boy in 1828 (p. 21, spelled his name Kelley); see Thomas Jenkins, q.v.

Kelso, John, was prescribed medicine for his child by Dr. Robert H. Archer on 25 Aug 1802 (Rx Book, 1802-1804, p. 16) and he was treated by Dr. Archer in Baltimore before 1822 [no dates or details were given] (Dr. Archer's "Alphabet to Ledger H" is his booklet [filed in the Archives of the Historical Society of Harford

County] that contains his index to Ledger H [which is missing] for his patients in Baltimore before 1822 and Harford County after 1822, according to a notation by Dr. George W. Archer.)

Kelso, Mrs., High Street [Baltimore], was prescribed medicine by Dr. Robert H. Archer on 16 May 1798 (Rx Book, 1796-1801, p. 11)

Kenard, Joseph, near the Quaker Meeting House in Pennsylvania, was treated by Dr. John Archer in Aug 1788 (Ledger F, p. 182)

Kenley, ---- [blank], of Richard, son-in-law of Mr. T. McCann, was visited by Dr. Robert H. Archer who treated his wife in Sep 1823 and son in May 1824 (pp. 91, 105; Ledger F, p. 30)

Kenley, Daniel (schoolmaster), was visited by Dr. John Archer who treated him in Sep 1779 and May, Jul, Aug, Sep and Oct 1780, Jun and Jul 1781 and Apr 1782, a child in Apr and May 1783, his wife in May 1784, Miss Polly Kenley in May 1786, his wife in Mar 1788 and him in Jan and May 1791 (Ledger D, p. 20, noted "debt forgiven as before") [account continued in Ledger E, which is missing]; Ledger F, p. 20 spelled his name Kenley and p. 272 spelled it Kenly. It was noted in a different handwriting that his wife died in 1788, but the date of death was not given); see Mr. Willson and Polly Kenley, q.v.

Kenley, Polly, daughter of Daniel, was treated by Dr. John Archer in 1798 (Ledger I, which is missing, was abstracted by Dr. George W. Archer circa 1890; his notes are in the Archives of the Historical Society of Harford County file "Archer, G. W. Coll. – Ledgers and Day Books"); see Daniel Kenley, q.v.

Kenley, Richard [1761-1825], was visited by Dr. John Archer who treated him and his wife and child in 1788; was prescribed medicine for his wife by Dr. Robert H. Archer on 1 Jun 1796 (Ledger F, p. 61 and Rx Book, 1796-1801, p. 6, spelled his name Kenly); Richard appeared on a list of debts dated 26 Dec 1822 and titled "A List of Allen's Claims" that were due and payable to Dr. Richard N. Allen for services rendered [no dates were given] by him to said Kenley (Document filed in Historical Society of Harford County Archives folder "R. N. Allen" spelled his name Kenly); Richard was also visited by Dr. Robert H. Archer who treated his wife in Oct 1822 (p. 32; Ledger F, p. 113) [Richard Kenley was a Revolutionary War veteran.]; see ---- Kenley, q.v.

Kennedy, Ann, see James Kennedy, q.v.

Kennedy, Elihu B., see James Kennedy, q.v.

Kennedy, Hannah, widow of Robert, near Alexander Rigdon's, was treated by Dr. John Archer at various times between 1796 and 1800 (Ledger I, which is missing, was abstracted by Dr. George W. Archer circa 1890; his notes are in the Archives of the Historical Society of Harford County folder "Archer, G. W. Coll. – Ledgers and Day Books")

Kennedy, James, was visited by Dr. John Archer who treated him many times between Feb and Aug 1773, a child in Jan 1774, a "man" in Jan 1775, him [James] on 11 Feb 1778 ("cutting out a ganglion in his knee"), his sister in Jul 1778, and him in Sep 1779, Jul 1780 and Jul 1781 (Ledger B, p. 46; Ledger C, p. 102) [account continued in Ledger E, which is missing]

Kennedy, James, was treated by Dr. John Archer between 1794 and 1798 and inoculated his wife and five children, Ann, Thomas, William, Lavinia and Elihu B. Kennedy; also had a daughter Jenny (Ledger I, which is missing, was abstracted by Dr. George W. Archer circa 1890; his notes are in the Archives of the Historical Society of Harford County folder "Archer, G. W. Coll. – Ledgers and Day Books")

Kennedy, Jane, was treated by Dr. Matthew J. Allen in Mar and Apr 1848 (p. 78, spelled her name Kenneday and noted that part of the bill was paid in cash in Jul 1852 and the balance was paid "by making 3 shirts" in Dec 1852)

Kennedy, Jenny, see James Kennedy, q.v.

Kennedy, Lavinia, see James Kennedy, q.v.

Kennedy, Nathaniel (weaver), was treated by Dr. John Archer in Apr 1789 (Ledger F, p. 88) [account continued in Ledger G, which is missing]; see Philip Quinlan, q.v.

Kennedy, Robert, see Hannah Kennedy, q.v.

Kennedy, Thomas, was treated by Dr. Alonzo Preston in 1825 (p. 20); see James Kennedy, q.v.

Kennedy, William, was prescribed medicine by Dr. Robert H. Archer in Mar 1801 (Rx Book, 1796-1801, pp. 45, 48); he was treated by Dr. Archer in Baltimore before 1822 [no dates or details] (Dr. Archer's "Alphabet to Ledger H" is his booklet [filed in the Archives of the Historical Society of Harford County] that contains his index to Ledger H [which is missing] for his patients in Baltimore City before 1822 and Harford County after 1822, according to a notation by Dr. George W. Archer.); see James Kennedy, q.v.

Kent & Company, was mentioned by Dr. Matthew J. Allen in 1823 in Calvert County (p. 3a)

Kerr, Samuel, see Hugh Jackson, q.v.

Kent, Daniel, Esq., was treated by Dr. Matthew J. Allen in 1823 in Calvert County (p. 14a)

Kent, James, was treated by Dr. Matthew J. Allen in 1832 in Calvert County and mentioned William Williams and H. L. Harrison (p. 24)

Kent, Mrs., was treated by Dr. Matthew J. Allen in 1823 in Calvert County (p. 12b)

Kent, Robert, was treated by Dr. Robert H. Archer in Baltimore before 1822 [no dates or details were given] (Dr. Archer's "Alphabet to Ledger H" is his booklet [filed in the Archives of the Historical Society of Harford County] that contains his index to Ledger H [which is missing] for his patients in Baltimore before 1822 and Harford County after 1822, according to a notation by Dr. George W. Archer.)

Kerr, ---- [blank], at Knox's, was visited by Dr. Robert H. Archer who treated his wife in Oct and Nov 1827 (pp. 252, 253)

Kerr, Alexander, was visited by Dr. Robert H. Archer who treated his wife in Nov 1827 (p. 254)

Kerr, Robert, at Union X Roads, was visited by Dr. Robert H. Archer who treated Peggy Tate in Sep 1822 (pp. 21, 22; Ledger F, p. 84, misspelled his name Carr and noted "intemperate and good for nothing") [Robert Kerr was a War of 1812 veteran, so apparently he was good for something!]

Kerr, William, was treated by Dr. Robert H. Archer in Nov 1827 and Feb 1828 (pp. 253, 254, 263)

Kertice, ---- [blank], was visited by Dr. Alonzo Preston who treated him and his wife in 1825, 1826 and 1828 (p. 56)

Kidd, George, was visited by Dr. John Archer, Jr. who treated his wife on 7 Sep 1816 and rendered obstetrical services [in childbirth] on 16 Sep 1816; treated Mrs. Smith (aunt) in Mar 1818, a child in Feb 1818 and a child in Apr 1819; George was also treated by Dr. Robert H. Archer seven times in Nov and Dec 1822 "trans fluis" ["across the water," meaning across the Susquehanna River in Cecil Co.] (Dr. John Archer, Jr., p. 26; Dr. Robert Archer, pp. 39-43, Ledger F, p. 124); see Mrs. James Kidd and Lloyd Bailey, q.v.

Kidd, James, Mrs. (widow), was visited by Dr. Robert H. Archer who treated a child in Oct 1821 and also mentioned George Kidd (Ledger F, p. 16)

Kile, William, was treated by Dr. John Archer in Dec 1780 (Ledger D, p. 111, noted "debt forgiven as before")

Killan, ----, see Robert Nesbitt, q.v.

Kimberry, John, near Josias William Dallam's, was treated by Dr. John Archer in Jun 1787 (Ledger F, p. 242)

Kimble, Giles, was treated by Dr. John Archer in Dec 1790 (Ledger F, p. 102) [Giles Kimble was a Revolutionary War veteran.]

Kimble, James [c1740-c1778], was treated by Dr. John Archer in May 1778 (Ledger C, p. 112, noted "debt forgiven by order of testator") [James Kimble was a Revolutionary War veteran.]

King, Francis, was treated by Dr. John Archer in Feb 1776 and in 1777 [exact date not given] (Ledger C, p. 35)

King, Mary (widow), was treated by Dr. John Archer in Aug and Dec 1779 and Jun 1781 (Ledger D, p. 6, noted her bill was paid by Benjamin Silver on 16 Jul 1791)

King, Mr., was prescribed medicine by Dr. Robert H. Archer on 15 Sep and 17 Oct 1804 (Rx Book, 1802-1804, pp. 58, 59)

King, Thomas, near James McCandless, was visited by Dr. John Archer who treated a child in 1786 and him [Thomas] in 1790 (Ledger F, p. 106)

Kirk, John, was visited by Dr. Robert H. Archer who treated his wife in Aug 1828 in consultation with Dr. Horton (p. 290); see James McGaw and Samuel Prichard, q.v.

Kirk, William, at Davis' Mill, was visited by Dr. Matthew J. Allen who treated his son by extracting a fishing hook from his nose on 25 Jul 1845 (p. 37, noted the $1 bill was paid in full in Jul 1845)

Kirkpatrick, Edward, was treated by Dr. John Archer, Jr. in Aug 1816 (p. 3)

Kirkpatrick, H., see Andrew Whitesides, q.v.

Kirkpatrick, Hugh, was visited by Dr. John Archer who treated a child in Aug 1772, a man in Jul 1775, and him [Hugh] in Feb 1777, Jun 1777 and Jul 1782 (Ledger C, p. 80; Ledger B, p. 44) [Hugh Kirkpatrick was a Revolutionary War veteran.]; see Robert Young, q.v.

Kirkpatrick, James, was visited by Dr. John Archer who treated his wife in 1775 (Ledger B, p. 77)

Kitely, Rachel, was treated by Dr. John Archer in May 1786 (Ledger F, p. 251)

Kitely, William, was visited by Dr. John Archer who treated a child in Oct 1780 and him in Nov and Dec 1782 (Ledger D, p. 100, noted the £8.18 bill was paid "by cash received of Charles Waters by the *(sic)* James Wetherel" on 4 Feb 1789)

Knight, Hannah, was visited by Dr. John Archer who treated her and sons James and Thomas in 1794 [no dates were given] (Ledger I, which is missing, was abstracted by Dr. George W. Archer circa 1890; his notes are in the Archives of the Historical Society of Harford County folder "Archer, G. W. Coll. – Ledgers and Day Books")

Knight, Thomas, at Upper Ferry, was treated by Dr. John Archer from 1794 to 1798 (Ledger I, which is missing, was abstracted by Dr. George W. Archer circa 1890; his notes are in Archives of the Historical Society of Harford County folder "Archer, G. W. Coll. – Ledgers and Day Books")

Knox, Evan [c1790-1833], was treated by Dr. Robert H. Archer in Sep 1826, Mar 1827 and Apr 1829 (pp. 199, 220, and p. 306, listed his name as Eving) [Evan Knox was a War of 1812 veteran.]

Knox, Mr., was treated by Dr. Robert H. Archer eight times in Apr and May 1826 and once in Aug 1826 (pp. 181, 182, 185, 187, 188, 196); see Hannah Hopkins and---- Kerr, q.v.

Knox, William, see James Ward (tailor), q.v.

Kroesen, Betsey, see Richard Kroesen, q.v.

Kroesen, Catherine, see Richard Kroesen, q.v.

Kroesen, Garret, see John Kroesen, q.v.

Kroesen, John, was visited by Dr. John Archer who treated him in June 1775, a man in Mar 1776, him [John] and a man in Apr 1776, him in Jan 1777 and him and son Garret in Sep 1790 (Ledger B, p. 43; Ledger C, p. 49; Ledger F, p. 66) [account continued in Ledger H, which is missing] [John Kroesen or Croesen was a Revolutionary War veteran.]

Kroesen, Michael, son of John, was visited by Dr. John Archer who treated him and his wife in 1789 and him in 1790 (Ledger F, p. 66 spelled his Kroesen, and p. 118 spelled his name Krosen) [account continued in Ledger H, which is missing]

Kroesen, Nicholas, was treated by Dr. John Archer in Jan and Feb 1774, June and July 1775, May, Aug, Sep, Oct and Dec 1778, Feb, Mar and Apr 1779 and Oct 1786 (Ledger B, p. 6; Ledger C, p. 76, and the account was continued in Ledger D, p. 103, where his name was spelled Crosin; Ledger F, p. 258); see Nicholas Crosin, q.v.

Kroesen, Richard, was visited by Dr. John Archer who treated him five times between Jan 1773 and Jun 1775, daughter Betsey in Jan 1773, his wife in Oct 1773, daughter Catherine in Jan 1774, him [Richard] in Aug 1776, Joseph Stiles' child in Dec 1776 and Jan 1777, and him [Richard] in Aug 1778 (Ledger B, p. 47; Ledger C, p. 18) [Richard Kroesen or Croesen was a Revolutionary War veteran.]; see Richard Crossin, q.v.

Krooks, Henry, see Henry Crooks, q.v.

Krooks, William, see Henry Crooks, q.v.

L. M. Academy, Trustees of, were mentioned in the ledger of Dr. Matthew J. Allen in 1832 in Calvert County (p. 19)

Lacy, Thomas, near Upper X Roads, was visited by Dr. John Archer who treated him in Apr 1782 and his wife in Aug 1783 (Ledger D, p. 120) [account continued in Ledger E, which is missing] [Thomas Lacy was a Revolutionary War veteran.]

Lamborn, Daniel [paper mill owner near Bel Air], was visited by Dr. Alonzo Preston who treated him at various times between 1824 and 1825, a son in 1825 and a girl named Maria in 1827 (p. 8)

Laming, Eleanor, was treated by Dr. Robert H. Archer in Baltimore before 1822 [no dates or details were given] (Dr. Archer's "Alphabet to Ledger H" is his booklet [filed in the Archives of the Historical Society of Harford County] that contains his index to Ledger H [which is missing] for his patients in Baltimore before 1822 and Harford County after 1822, according to a notation by Dr. George W. Archer.); "Mrs. Laming" was prescribed medicine by Dr. Robert H. Archer on 14 Feb 1803 (Rx Book, 1802-1804, p. 32)

Lamphear, Asael, was treated by Dr. Matthew J. Allen seven times in Oct 1848 (p. 94, spelled his name Asel Lampher)

Lamphear, Daniel, "Abraham's overseer," was treated by Dr. John Archer in 1794 and 1795 (Ledger I, which is missing, was abstracted by Dr. George W. Archer circa 1890, spelled his name Danl. Lamphers; George's notes are in the Archives of the Historical Society of Harford County folder "Archer, G. W. Coll. – Ledgers and Day Books")

Lamphear, John, at Ring Factory [on Winters Run, west of Bel Air], was visited" from the road" by Dr. Matthew J. Allen who treated a child in Sep 1847 (p. 67)

Lamphear, William, was visited by Dr. Matthew J. Allen who treated his wife in Jun, Jul and Oct 1848 (p. 87)

Lancaster, Christianna, alias McKenny, at Mr. Dorsey's, was treated by Dr. John Archer in Sep 1787 (Ledger F, p. 15)

Lancaster, Nathaniel, was treated by Dr. Alonzo Preston on 3 Feb 1826 (p. 67) [Nathan Lancaster was a War of 1812 veteran]

Lancaster, Thomas [1785-c1806], at Mr. Gash's, was treated by Dr. John Archer eight times from 26 Nov 1774 to 12 Jan 1775 (Ledger B, p. 96) [Thomas Gash was a Revolutionary War veteran.]

Lansdale, Dr., was consulted by Dr. John Archer in 1786 (Ledger F, p. 123)

Lardner, Robert, was visited by Dr. John Archer who treated him in Sep 1772 and his wife in May and Sep 1773 (Ledger B, p. 24)

Laughlin, Peter, was treated by Dr. John Archer in Jun 1778, Feb 1779 and Jul 1780 (Ledger C, p. 94) [Peter Laughlin was a Revolutionary War veteran.]

Laughrey, George, was treated by Dr. Robert H. Archer in Aug 1823 and was mentioned as the brother of John Laughray in John's account with Dr. Archer in Nov 1823 (pp. 86, 93, spelled his name Laughray); see John Laughrey, q.v.

Laughrey, John, was treated by Dr. Robert H. Archer in Jul 1822 and mentioned his brother George, his sisters and mother, and treated him in Sep 1823 (pp. 8, listed him as Mr. Laughry and pp. 93, 94, spelled his name Laughray; Ledger F, p. 54, spelled it Laughrey); see George Laughrey, q.v.

Laughrey, Mrs., see Mr. ----, q.v.

Lawrence, Henry (nailer) [nailmaker], at Mr. Gale's [in Cecil Co.], was visited by Dr. John Archer who treated him and his family in 1795 and 1796 (Ledger I, which is missing, was abstracted by Dr. George W. Archer circa 1890; his notes are in the Archives of the Historical Society of Harford County folder "Archer, G. W. Coll. – Ledgers and Day Books")

Lawrence, James (shoemaker), on Isaac Webster's place, was visited by Dr. John Archer who treated him and his wife in 1788 (Ledger F, p. 121)

Lawrence, John, was visited by Dr. John Archer who treated his son in Dec 1775 ("by setting of his thigh"), him [John] in Sep 1782 and him and a child in 1786 (Ledger C, p. 16; Ledger F, p. 76) [John Laurence or Lawrence was a Revolutionary War veteran.]

Lawrence, William (colonel), was visited by Dr. Matthew J. Allen in Calvert County who treated him, a child and negroes Charles, John and Betty in 1832; the account also mentioned James Harrison, William G. Spicknall, Thomas W. Harris and Isaac Nindes (pp. 21-22)

Lawrence, William W., was treated by Dr. Matthew J. Allen in 1832 in Calvert County and the account also mentioned William C. Hodgkins, H. L. Harrison, Jim Jeffry, Robert Jeffry, John Hutchins, Dr. Dorsey, James Hanswood and James Thompkins (p. 21)

Lawson, Richard, was prescribed medicine by Dr. Robert H. Archer on 1 Jan 1803 (Rx Book, 1802-1804, p. 29) and he was treated by Dr. Archer in Baltimore before 1822 [no dates or details were given] (Dr. Archer's "Alphabet to Ledger H" is his booklet [filed in the Archives of the Historical Society of Harford County] that contains his index to Ledger H [which is missing] for his patients in Baltimore before 1822 and Harford County after 1822, according to a notation by Dr. George W. Archer.)

Leach, John, was treated by Dr. Matthew J. Allen in 1823 in Calvert County (p. 4b)

Leage, Mrs., sister of Mr. Massey, was treated by Dr. Robert H. Archer in Oct 1823 and Nov 1823 in consultation with Dr. Worthington (p. 87 spelled her name Leake, p. 88 spelled it Leage, p. 89 spelled it Leag and Leage, pp. 90 and 92 spelled it Leage; Ledger F, p. 77, spelled it Leage)

Leathim, William, was treated by Dr. John Archer in Jan 1790 (Ledger F, p. 214)

LeBarron, Dr., see Samuel McMullen, q.v.

Lee, Anne, see Parker Hall Lee, q.v.

Lee, Archer, see Josiah (Josias) Lee, q.v.

Lee, Betsey, Miss, was treated by Dr. Robert H. Archer in March 1824; account noted John Lochary in March 1823 and Negro man Duke in July 1823 (pp. 67, 99, 100; Ledger F, p. 160)

Lee, Billy, see Parker Hall Lee, q.v.

Lee, C. H., see Negro Adam, q.v.

Lee, Charles, was visited by Dr. John Archer who treated him and daughter Nancy at various times between 1796 and 1798 (Ledger I, which is missing, was abstracted by Dr. George W. Archer circa 1890; his notes are in Archives of the Historical Society of Harford County folder "Archer, G. W. Coll. – Ledgers and Day Books")

Lee, Corbin, was treated by Dr. John Archer in 1789 (Ledger F, p. 282) [account continued in Ledger G, which is missing]; see James Lee, Jr., q.v.

Lee, David [1740-1816], was visited by Dr. John Archer who treated his son Ralph in 1788 and him in 1797 (Ledger F, p. 368); see John Mason, Joshua Judd, Joseph Dubree and William Lee, q.v.

Lee, David (negro), was treated by Dr. Robert H. Archer in May 1823 (Ledger F, p. 33)

Lee, Dr., see Benjamin Osborn, q.v.

Lee, Edward, near Robert Morgan's, was treated by Dr. John Archer in 1798 (Ledger I, which is missing, was abstracted by Dr. George W. Archer circa 1890; his notes are in the Archives of the Historical Society of Harford County folder "Archer, G. W. Coll. – Ledgers and Day Books")

Lee, Eliza, Mrs., was treated by Dr. John Archer in Aug 1788 (Ledger F, p. 105, and then crossed her name off the ledger)

Lee, Elizabeth, Mrs. (widow), was visited by Dr. John Archer who treated her in May 1781 and "Aur:"[?] in Jun 1782, her [Elizabeth] in Sep and Oct 1782 and Sep 1782, a grandson in Jun 1785, her in Sep 1785, son Jacob in Oct 1785 and her and a child named Vanclief in Aug 1790 (Ledger D, pp. 21, 79, noted "debt forgiven as before;" Ledger F, p. 93) [account continued in Ledger G, which is missing]

Lee, Fras.(?) H., was prescribed medicine "for Elizabeth" by Dr. Robert H. Archer on 27 Aug 1850 (Rx Book, 1825-1851, p. 120)

Lee, George, see Letitia Lee, q.v.

Lee, Hannah, Mrs., was visited by Dr. Matthew J. Allen who treated her son and Reverdy and Miss Sally in Feb and Mar 1848, Miss Sally in Apr 1848 a child in May and Jun 1848, a negro boy in Jun 1848 and Negro woman Emma in Sep 1848 (pp. 75, 84)

Lee, Henry D., of Parker, was treated by Dr. Robert H. Archer after 1822 [no dates or details were given] (Dr. Archer's "Alphabet to Ledger H" is his booklet [filed in the Archives of the Historical Society of Harford County] that contains his index to Ledger H [which is missing] for his patients in Baltimore before 1822 and Harford County after 1822, according to a notation by Dr. George W. Archer.)

Lee, Jacob, see Samuel Lee, Elizabeth Lee and Milcah Lee, q.v.

Lee, James (doctor), see Milcah Lee, q.v.

Lee, James (shoemaker), was visited by Dr. John Archer who treated him in Sep 1777, his wife in Sep 1779 and Mar 1780 and inoculated their two children in 1782 (Ledger C, p. 52; Ledger D, p. 92, noted "debt forgiven as before")

Lee, James, was treated by Dr. John Archer in Sep 1790 (Ledger F, p. 8)

Lee, James, was visited by Dr. Robert H. Archer who treated him (for a hydrocele) in Jun 1824, a negro in Apr 1826 and him [James] several times between 28 Dec 1830 and 6 Jan 1831, and also mentioned Parker Lee in Apr 1831 (p. 108, Ledger F, p. 97) [James Lee was a War of 1812 veteran and James Lee, of Samuel, was a Revolutionary War veteran.]

Lee, James, Jr., was visited by Dr. John Archer who treated him at various times between Dec 1772 and Apr 1775, Negro Jo in Dec 1772, a man in Aug 1773, his [James'] wife in Feb, Apr and May 1774 and Jan and Apr 1775, his son Corbin in Jul 1774, Negro Nell in Feb 1775, him [James] in Jan 1776, inoculated his wife and 6 children in Mar 1776 and treated him in Jan 1777, a negro in Feb 1778, a negro wench in Jan 1779, his wife in Jul and Aug 1779, a child in May 1780, him in May 1781, and Samuel and Phil in Sep 1782 (Ledger B, p. 42; Ledger C, p. 33)

Lee, James, Sr., was visited by Dr. John Archer who inoculated twelve of his family circa 1777 [date illegible] (Ledger C, p. 40)

Lee, James, of Josias, was treated by Dr. John Archer between 1796 and 1799 (Ledger I, which is missing, was abstracted by Dr. George W. Archer circa 1890; his notes are in the Archives of the Historical Society of Harford County file "Archer, G. W. Coll. – Ledgers and Day Books")

Lee, James C., was treated by Dr. Robert H. Archer after 1822 [no dates or details were given] (Dr. Archer's "Alphabet to Ledger H" is his booklet [filed in the Archives of the Historical Society of Harford County] that contains his index to Ledger H [which is missing] for his patients in Baltimore City before 1822 and in Harford County after 1822, according to a notation by Dr. George W. Archer.)

Lee, John (tailor), was treated by Dr. John Archer in Jul 1788 (Ledger F, p. 149, listed his name as "Jno. Lee, taylor") [John Lee was a Revolutionary War veteran.]

Lee, John [in Baltimore], was prescribed medicine for his child by Dr. Robert H. Archer on 23 Apr 1803 (Rx Book, 1802-1804, p. 41)

Lee, Joseph, see Josiah Lee, q.v.

Lee, Josiah (Josias), was visited by Dr. John Archer who treated him in Nov 1774, a child in Mar 1776, inoculated three negroes in Mar 1776, treated a negro in Feb 1777, his [Josiah's] wife in Feb 1778, son Samuel in Mar 1778, a negro in Sep 1778, a child in Oct 1778, a negro in Aug 1780, him [Josiah] and a negro in Sep 1780, him [name spelled Josias] in Sep, Oct and Nov 1780, his wife and a negro (tooth extraction) in Jan 1781, him [name spelled Josias] in Apr 1781 his wife on 10 Sep 1781 (obstetrical services), and inoculated "ten of yr. Family African" in 1782; also treated his wife three times in May 1782 and on 7 Jun 1782 (obstetrical services) and visited her again on 16 Jun 1782, him [name spelled Josias] in Jul 1782, son James in Aug 1782, him [name spelled Josiah], his wife and child in 1786, him [name spelled Josiah], wife, son Joseph, a child [name illegible], an infant in 1786, 1787 and 1788 and him [name spelled Josias] and sons Archer and Samuel from 1794 to 1797 [no dates were given] (Ledger B, p. 35; Ledger C, p. 42; Ledger D, p. 89 [account continued in Ledger E, which is missing]; Ledger F, pp. 75. 122, 139) [continued in Ledger G, which is missing]; Ledger I, which is missing, was abstracted by Dr. George W. Archer circa 1890; his notes are in the Archives of the Historical Society of Harford County folder "Archer, G. W. Coll. – Ledgers and Day Books") [Josiah Lee was a Revolutionary War veteran.]; see Elisha Daws, q.v.

Lee, Josias, see Samuel W. Lee and Josiah Lee, q.v.

Lee, Letitia, was visited by Dr. John Archer who treated her and son George in 1789 (Ledger F, p. 1) [account continued in Ledger G, which is missing]

Lee, M., Mr., was prescribed medicine by Dr. Robert H. Archer on 8 May 1851 (Rx Book, 1825-1851, p. 121)

Lee, Mary, Mrs., of Parker, was treated by Dr. Robert H. Archer after 1822 [no dates or details were given] (Dr. Archer's "Alphabet to Ledger H" is his booklet [filed in the Archives of the Historical Society of Harford County] that contains his index to Ledger H [which is missing] for his patients in Baltimore before 1822 and Harford County after 1822, according to a notation by Dr. George W. Archer.)

Lee, Milcah, widow of Dr. James Lee, was visited by Dr. John Archer who treated her and son Jacob in 1788 and her and a child in 1789 (Ledger F, pp. 141, 153); [account continued in Ledger G, which is missing]

Lee, Nancy, see Charles Lee, q.v.

Lee, Pamelia, see William D. Lee, q.v.

Lee, Parker, see James Lee, Mrs. Mary Lee, Henry D. Lee and Richard Dallam, q.v.

Lee, Parker Hall [1759-1829], was visited by Dr. John Archer who treated his wife in Jul 1781 and Jan 1782, an infant in Mar 1782, a negro in Jan 1783, his [Parker's] wife in Feb 1783, him in Apr and May 1783, him and son William in 1787, him and his wife and his son William, daughter Anne Lee and Nancy Matthews in 1788 and also treated him [Parker] in 1789 and 1790 and sons Sam and Billy in 1789 (Ledger D, p. 48) [account continued in Ledger E, which is missing] and Ledger F, pp. 19, 108, 356) [account continued in Ledger G, which is missing); Parker was also treated by Dr. Robert H. Archer in Jul 1822 (mentioned negroes Forrester, Stephen and Jacob in May 1822) and in Aug and in Oct 1825, Negro Jacob in Aug 1823 and him [Parker] and Negro Matilda in Aug 1828, Parker was prescribed medicine on 8 Jul 1825, 21 Sep 1825, 22 Nov 1825, 12 Jan 1826 and 3 Jun 1829 (Dr. John Archer, Jr., pp. 11, 88, 151, 152, 161, 291, 293; Dr. Robert H. Archer's Rx Book, 1825-1851, pp. 81, 84, 85, 86, 94; Ledger F, p. 44; Dr. Robert H. Archer's "Alphabet to Ledger H" is his booklet [filed in the Archives of the Historical Society of Harford County] that contains his index to Ledger H [which is missing] for his patients in Baltimore before 1822 and Harford County after 1822, according to a notation by Dr. George W. Archer.) [Parker Hall Lee, a Revolutionary War veteran, died 6 Jun 1829, just 3 days after being treated.]

Lee, Presbury, see Samuel Lee, q.v.

Lee, R. D., see Big Bill, q.v.

Lee, Rachael, was listed in Dr. John Archer's ledger circa 1773, but no entries were made in her account (Ledger B, p. 41)

Lee, Ralph, see David Lee, q.v.

Lee, Reverdy, see Hannah Lee, q.v.

Lee, Richard, was visited by Dr. Robert H. Archer who treated him in Aug 1823, Negro Maria in Sep 1825, a negro "in partu" [in childbirth] during the night of 16 Apr 1826, and his [Richard's] wife in Aug and Sep 1827 (pp. 88, 159, 181, 247; Ledger F, p. 47)

Lee, Sally, see Hannah Lee, q.v.

Lee, Sam or Samuel, see Parker Hall Lee, Josiah (Josias) Lee and John Fleharty, q.v.

Lee, Samuel, was visited by Dr. John Archer who treated him at various times between 1772 and June 1775 and Jos. Stone's wife in Dec 1772, a child several times in Aug and Sep 1772, son Samuel in Sep 1772 and June 1775, an infant in Aug 1774 and June 1775, inoculated a daughter in 1775, and treated a negro wench in Oct 1777, him [Samuel] in Feb 1778, Negro Bob in Apr 1778, a negro in Jul 1778, son Jacob in Dec 1778, his [Samuel's] wife in Jan 1780, him twelve times between Jan 1780 and Feb 1780, and again in Jul, Sep, Oct and Dec 1780 and Jan and Mar 1781; also rendered service "for mill right" and James in May 1781,him [Samuel] in Jun, Sep and Oct 1781, a child in Oct and Nov 1781, him in Mar 1782 and a negro in Apr 1782 (Ledger B, p. 40; Ledger C, pp. 3-4; Ledger D, p. 73) [account continued in Ledger E, which is missing]

Lee, Samuel, was visited by Dr. John Archer who treated him and sons Presbury and Jacob in Dec 1791 and was prescribed medicine for a child by Dr. Robert H. Archer on 26 Nov 1802 (Ledger F, p. 173; Rx Book, 1802-1804, p. 26)

Lee, Samuel M., was treated by Dr. Robert H. Archer after 1822 [no dates or details were given] (Dr. Archer's "Alphabet to Ledger H" is his booklet [filed in the Archives of the Historical Society of Harford County] that contains his index to Ledger H [which is missing] for his patients in Baltimore City before 1822 and in Harford County after 1822, according to a notation by Dr. George W. Archer.)

Lee, Samuel W., was prescribed medicine for his child on 9 Mar 1803 by Dr. Robert H. Archer (Rx Book, 1802-1804, p. 35) and he was treated by Dr. Robert H. Archer in Baltimore before 1822 [no dates or details were given] (Dr. Archer's "Alphabet to Ledger H" is his booklet [filed in the Archives of the Historical Society of Harford County] that contains his index to Ledger H [which is missing] for his patients in Baltimore before 1822 and Harford County after 1822, according to a notation by Dr. George W. Archer.)

Lee, Samuel W., son of Josias, was visited by Dr. John Archer who treated him and daughter Mary in 1796 and 1797 (Ledger I, which is missing, was abstracted by Dr. George W. Archer circa 1890; his notes are in the Archives of the Historical Society of Harford County folder "Archer, G. W. Coll. – Ledgers and Day Books")

Lee, T: (sic), see Micajah Mitchell, q.v.

Lee, Vanclief, see Elizabeth Lee, q.v.

Lee, William, near D. Lee's Mill, Little Falls [i. e., David Lee's Jerusalem Mills on Little Gunpowder River], was visited by Dr. John Archer who treated him and his wife in 1786 (Ledger F, p. 337)

Lee, William, father-in-law to Joseph Reese, was treated by Dr. John Archer in 1796 (Ledger I, which is missing, was abstracted by Dr. George W. Archer circa 1890; his notes are in the Archives of the Historical Society of Harford County folder "Archer, G. W. Coll. – Ledgers and Day Books"); see Parker Hall Lee, q.v.

Lee, William D. [1785-1828], was visited by Dr. Robert H. Archer who treated daughter Pamelia and Negro Mark in July 1826, Negro Grace in Oct 1827 and him five times in Aug 1828 [William died on 23 Aug 1828] (pp. 192, 193, 252, 292, 293) [William Dallam Lee was a War of 1812 veteran.]; see Priscilla Bryarly, q.v.

LeFlet, Peter, "X Roads," was visited by Dr. John Archer who treated him and his family at various times between 1796 and 1799 (Ledger I, which is missing, was abstracted by Dr. George W. Archer circa 1890; his notes are in the Archives of the Historical Society of Harford County folder "Archer, G. W. Coll. – Ledgers and Day Books")

Legget, John, was prescribed medicine by Dr. Robert H. Archer on 6 Jun 1803 (Rx Book, 1802-1804, p. 44)

Lemmon, Jacob, was treated by Dr. John Archer for "cutting a thumb and finger off" in 1773 [exact date was not given] and also treated an infant in Jun 1775 (Ledger B, p. 37)

Lemon, Mrs., mother-in-law to William McCandless, Slate Ridge, was treated by Dr. John Archer in 1798 (Ledger I, which is missing, was abstracted by Dr. George W. Archer circa 1890; his notes are in Archives of the Historical Society of Harford County file "Archer, G. W. Coll. - Ledgers and Day Books")

Lendrum, Robert, was treated by Dr. John Archer in May, Nov 1773 and Jan 1774 (Ledger B, p. 93)

Lendrum, Robert Burney, was visited by Dr. John Archer who treated his daughter in Sep and Oct 1779, him and a child in Apr 1780 and him and his wife in Feb 1782 (Ledger C, p. 13, noted "debt forgiven by order of testator")

Lester, ----, son-in-law to Mrs. Curswell [or Criswell] at the Susquehanna, was treated by Dr. John Archer in 1795 (Ledger I, which is missing, was abstracted by Dr. George W. Archer circa 1890; his notes are in Archives of the Historical Society of Harford County file "Archer, G. W. Coll. - Ledgers and Day Books")

Lester, William, see William Luster, q.v.

Letter, Thomas, was treated by Dr. Robert H. Archer in Baltimore before 1822 [no dates or details were given] (Dr. Archer's "Alphabet to Ledger H" is his booklet [filed in the Archives of the Historical Society of

Harford County] that contains his index to Ledger H [which is missing] for his patients in Baltimore before 1822 and Harford County after 1822, according to a notation by Dr. George W. Archer.)

Levering, C., see Reuben H. Davis, q.v.

Levy, John (hatter), in Havre de Grace, was visited by Dr. John Archer, Jr. who treated him and his wife in Feb 1829 (p. 17)

Lewis, Charles, was treated by Dr. Robert H. Archer in Baltimore before 1822 [no dates or details were given] (Dr. Archer's "Alphabet to Ledger H" is his booklet [filed in the Archives of the Historical Society of Harford County] that contains his index to Ledger H [which is missing] for his patients in Baltimore before 1822 and Harford County after 1822, according to a notation by Dr. George W. Archer.)

Lewis, Eli, see Mrs. Lewis, q.v.

Lewis, Eliza, Miss, was treated by Dr. Birckhead in 1807 and the receipt stated: "1807, Dr. Wm. Hall to Dr. Birckhead, To medicine & attendance administered to Miss Eliza in Oct & Nov ... Ds. 20 … Recd. payt. in full. Wm. Birckhead." On the reverse side of the tri-folded paper was written "Mr. John Lewis" as if it had been addressed to him and "Miss Eliza" was his daughter (Document filed in the Archives of the Historical Society of Harford County folder "Birkhead")

Lewis, George, near Samuel Forwood's, was treated by Dr. John Archer in 1787 (Ledger F, p. 113)

Lewis, John, see Eliza Lewis, q.v.

Lewis, John, was treated by Dr. John Archer in May 1779 and May, Sep and Oct 1780 (Ledger C, p. 108, noted "debt forgiven by order of testator") [John Lewis was a Revolutionary War veteran.]

Lewis, John (shoemaker), was visited by Dr. John Archer who treated him and his wife in Aug 1788 (Ledger F, p. 14)

Lewis, John W., was treated by Dr. John Archer in Jul 1786 (Ledger F, p. 362) [Jonathan W. Lewis was a Revolutionary War veteran.]

Lewis, Joseph [1753-1791], was treated by Dr. John Archer in Jul 1788 (Ledger F, p. 13) [Joseph Lewis was a Revolutionary War veteran.]

Lewis, Mr., was prescribed medicine for his child by Dr. Robert H. Archer on 23 Feb 1801 (Rx Book, 1796-1801, p. 35)

Lewis, Mrs. (widow), in Baltimore, was visited by Dr. John Archer who treated her and son Eli at various times between 1796 and 1799; Mrs. Lewis was also treated by Dr. Robert H. Archer in Baltimore before 1822 [no dates or details given] (Ledger I, which is missing, was abstracted by Dr. George W. Archer circa 1890; his notes are in the Archives of the Historical Society of Harford County folder "Archer, G. W. Coll. – Ledgers and Day Books;" Dr. Archer's "Alphabet to Ledger H" is his booklet [filed in the Archives of the Historical Society of Harford County] that contains his index to Ledger H [which is missing] for his patients in Baltimore City before 1822 and in Harford County after 1822, according to a notation by Dr. George W. Archer.)

Lilley, Eliza, see Thomas Lilley, q.v.

Lilley, Fanny, see Thomas Lilley, q.v.

Lilley, Henry, see Thomas Lilley, q.v.

Lilley, James, see Thomas Lilley, q.v.

Lilley, John, was visited by Dr. Matthew J. Allen who treated his child in Apr 1844 (p. 34 noted the bill was paid "by cash in full through S. Maccatee" in Jun 1844); see Sylvester Macatee, q.v.

Lilley, Mr., was prescribed medicine by Dr. Robert H. Archer on 13 Oct 1825 and 18 Jul 1834 (Rx Book, 1825-1851, p. 84 spelled his name Lilley and p. 112 spelled it Lilly); see Joseph Hart, q.v.

Lilley, Thomas, was visited by Dr. Matthew J. Allen who treated his expectant wife on 19 Feb 1844 and "from Feb 27th to March 1st, wife with twins" and treated her through 11 Mar 1844; treated him [Thomas] in Aug, Sep, Nov and Dec 1844 (eye wash), his wife and mother [possibly his wife's mother] in Jan 1845, a child in Feb, Mar and Apr 1845, his wife and child in Jun 1845 (noted part of the bill was paid "by order on Mrs. Smith"), his wife in Jul 1845 (eye wash), his wife and child in Jul 1847, him in Aug 1847 ("leaching"), rendered obstetrical services to his wife on 24 and 25 Dec 1847, treated his son in Feb and Mar 1847, James in Mar 1848, Eliza and infant in Mar 1848 and Eliza and Fanny or Henry [illegible] and an infant in Apr 1848 (pp. 31, 42, 58, spelled his name Lilley, and p. 78 spelled it Lilly); see Joseph Hart, q.v.

Linam, James, was visited by Dr. John Archer who treated him in Feb 1776 ("opening his finger") and inoculated a child at Dutch Jacob's [most likely referring to John Jacob Albert, Dutchman shoemaker, q.v.] (Ledger C, p. 32, noted "debt forgiven by order of testator") [James Linam was a Revolutionary War veteran.]

118

Lindsay (Linsay), Mr., was prescribed medicine by Dr. Robert H. Archer on 27 Feb 1801 and 17 May 1803 (Rx Book, 1796-1801, p. 38; Rx Book, 1802-1804, p. 43)

Lindsey (Linsey), Andrew, was visited by Dr. John Archer who treated him in May 1779, Mar 1780, Apr 1782, Feb 1783 and Feb 1785 and a child in Aug 1785 (Ledger C, p. 9, noted "debt forgiven by order of testator," Ledger D, p. 49, noted "debt forgiven as before") [Andrew Lindsey was a Revolutionary War veteran.]

Lindsey, John [1759-1814], at Widow Barrow's in Long Green, was treated by Dr. John Archer in 1787 (Ledger F, p. 158)

Lindsey, William, was visited by Dr. James Archer who treated him four times between July 1805 and Jan 1806 (p. 14)

Lingum, Mr. (well digger), was visited by Dr. Robert H. Archer who treated his wife in July 1828 in consultation with Dr. Allen (p. 287)

Lisby, Widow, was treated by Dr. John Archer in 1776 [no date was given] (Ledger C, p. 62, account was titled "Widow Lisby or Tudor Chalk")

Lisly, George, was visited by Dr. John Archer who treated him and his wife in 1783 and mentioned that R. Thomas was his security (Ledger F, p. 320)

Litle, Ephraim, was visited by Dr. Alonzo Preston who treated him at times between 1825 and 1828, "uxor Jn. Parker" [wife of John Parker] in 1825, a black boy named Frank in 1826, Mrs. Litle "in partu" [in childbirth] on 2 May 1827, Virginia Litle in 1827 and 1828, and Helen Mar and Mrs. Litle in 1828 (p. 60, noting "Settled by acct. in bar")

Litle, Virginia, see Ephraim Litle, q.v.

Little, Adam, see Christopher Little, q.v.

Little, Christopher, was visited by Dr. John Archer, Jr. him and his daughter Mary in Nov 1815 and his wife in Oct 1817; also mentioned William Simco in Dec 1815 and Adam Little in Apr 1816 (p. 36); see Hugh Jackson, q.v.

Little, James, at Matthew McClintock's, was treated by Dr. John Archer in March 1786 (Ledger F, p. 54)

Little, John, appeared on a list of debts dated 26 Dec 1822 and titled "A List of Allen's Claims" that were due and payable to Dr. Richard N. Allen for services rendered [no dates] by him to said Little (Document filed in Historical Society of Harford County Archives folder "R. N. Allen") [John Little was a War of 1812 veteran.]

Little, Mary, see Christopher Little, q.v.

Little, Mr., in Bellaire [Bel Air], was visited by Dr. Robert H. Archer who treated him and wife in 1823 (Ledger F, p. 43)

Litton, John, was treated by Dr. John Archer in Mar 1782 and Oct 1783 (Ledger D, p. 112, noted "debt forgiven as before")

Litton, Samuel, was treated by Dr. John Archer in Jun 1781 (Ledger D, p. 111, noted "debt forgiven as before")

Livingston, John, near the Slate Ridge Meeting House, was treated by Dr. John Archer in Jan 1791 (Ledger F, p. 298)

Livsey(?), James, was visited by Dr. Matthew J. Allen who treated a child in May and Jul 1845 and daughter Mary (tooth extraction) and son John (tooth extraction) in Jun 1845 (p. 47)

Livsey, John, see James Livsey, q.v.

Livsey, Mary, see James Livsey, q.v.

Lochary, George, was treated by Dr. Robert H. Archer in March and April 1826 and June 1827 and was prescribed medicine on 27 Mar 1826 and 8 Oct 1832; George paid off a $30 medical bill in 1827 "by building basement story of barn and ice house and carriage house" [at *Maiden's Bower*, the home of Dr. Robert H. Archer] (p. 167; Rx Book, 1825-1851, pp. 87, 107; Ledger F, pp. 120, 125); see John Lochary, q.v.

Lochary, John [1798-1850], was visited by Dr. Robert H. Archer who treated him in Jul 1824 and his brother George's knee wound on 23 Jun 1825; also mentioned George Smith, John Archer, M. [Matthew] Cain, William Stephenson and H. [Henry] Ruff in non-medical matters in 1825; treated John's wife in May 1826 and "in partu" [in childbirth] on 31 Mar 1827 and visited her again on 5 Apr and 8 May 1827 (was prescribed medicine on 18 May 1827), treated a child in June 1828, his wife in Nov 1828 and his wife and child in Apr 1829; was prescribed medicine for his niece on 13 July 1833 (pp. 114, 136, 184, 220, 224, 284, 300, 306; Rx Book, 1825-1851, pp. 90, 109; Ledger F, p. 111); see Betsey Lee, q.v.

Lochary, Michael, was treated by Dr. Robert H. Archer twice in Aug 1826 (pp. 195, 196)

Lochary, Mrs. (widow) was treated by Dr. Robert H. Archer in Oct 1826 and was prescribed medicine on 2 Dec and 6 Dec 1831 (Ledger, p. 206; Rx Book, 1825-1851, pp. 103-104)

Lochary, Thomas, was mentioned in the ledger of Dr. Robert H. Archer in a non-medical matter in 1826 and was prescribed medicine by Dr. Archer on 20 May 1830 (Ledger F, p. 160; Rx Book, 1825-1851, p. 100); see John McKenney, q.v.

Loflin, Daniel, see Mrs. Loflin, q.v.

Loflin, Mr. (constable), was visited by Dr. Robert H. Archer who treated a child in July 1823 (p. 84)

Loflin, Mrs., wife of Daniel Loflin, was prescribed medicine by Dr. Robert H. Archer on 2 Aug 1841 (Rx Book, 1825-1851, p. 116)

Logan, Samuel, was treated by Dr. Robert H. Archer in Baltimore before 1822 [no dates or details were missing] (Dr. Archer's "Alphabet to Ledger H" is his booklet [filed in the Archives of the Historical Society of Harford County] that contains his index to Ledger H [which is missing] for his patients in Baltimore before 1822 and Harford County after 1822, according to a notation by Dr. George W. Archer.)

Logue, C., Miss, was prescribed medicine by Dr. Robert H. Archer on 17 Oct 1799 (Rx Book, 1796-1801, p. 25)

Logue, Johanna, see William Webb, q.v.

Logue, Mary, was treated by Dr. John Archer in May 1781 and July 1783; Mary Logue (widow) was treated by Dr. Archer in Oct 1788 (Ledger D, p. 31, noted "debt forgiven as before;" Ledger F, p. 111) [account continued in Ledger G, which is missing]

Logue, William, was visited by Dr. John Archer who treated him at various times between Feb 1773 and Aug 1774, his wife in Apr 1773, a daughter in May 1773, a child in Oct 1773, son William in Mar 1774, him in Sep 1777, his wife in Mar and Aug 1778, and him in Jul and Aug 1779 (Ledger B, p. 71; Ledger C, p. 45, mentioned "7 years interest" in Nov 1780) [William Logue was a Revolutionary War veteran.]

Loney, Capt., see John Forwood, q.v.

Loney, Moses, was visited by Dr. John Archer who treated him and his son in Apr 1791 (Ledger F, p. 119, indicated William Loney was Moses Loney's executor on 5 Jul 1804) [Moses Loney was a Revolutionary War veteran.]

Loney, Mrs. (widow), was treated by Dr. John Archer in May 1787 (Ledger F, p. 204)

Loney, William, was visited by Dr. John Archer who treated him and wife in Mar and Aug 1788 (Ledger F, pp. 91, 98) [account continued in Ledger G, which is missing] [William Loney was a Revolutionary War veteran.]; see Moses Loney, q.v.

Long, Daniel, of John, at John Cox's, was treated by Dr. John Archer in 1794 [no dates were given] (Ledger I, which is missing, was abstracted by Dr. George W. Archer circa 1890; his notes are in the Archives of the Historical Society of Harford County folder "Archer, G. W. Coll. – Ledgers and Day Books")

Long, John (Crier of the Court), was treated by Dr. John Archer in Sep 1781 (Ledger D, p. 77, noted the medical bill was paid in full in 1788 "by the iniquitous insolvent act") [John Long was a Revolutionary War veteran.]; see Daniel Long, q.v.

Long, Mr., at Ignatius Wheeler, Esq., was treated by Dr. John Archer in June 1788 (Ledger F, p. 275)

Love, Bennett [1776-1852], appeared on a list of debts dated 26 Dec 1822 and titled "A List of Allen's Claims" that were due and payable to Dr. Richard N. Allen for services rendered [no dates were given] by him to the said Love (Document filed in Historical Society of Harford County Archives folder "R. N. Allen"); Bennett was visited by Dr. Alonzo Preston who treated his wife in Feb 1825 and the account also mentioned a black man named Corbin (p. 26) [Bennett Love was a War of 1812 veteran.]

Love, James, had an account in the ledger of Dr. Matthew J. Allen in a non-medical matter in Apr 1848 (p. 81, had only one entry that noted "April 26th 1848, To balance on feed paid" 23 cents) [James Love was a War of 1812 veteran.]

Love, John [c1730-1793] (esquire), was treated by Dr. John Archer in Aug 1774 and at various times between Sep 1778 and Mar 1780 (Ledger B, p. 97; Ledger C, p. 2) [John Love was a Revolutionary War veteran.]

Love, Margaret, Mrs., was visited by Dr. John Archer who treated her and her children Molly and Bennett at times between 1794 and 1807 [no dates were given] (Ledger I, which is missing, was abstracted by Dr. George W. Archer circa 1890; his notes are in the Archives of the Historical Society of Harford County folder "Archer, G. W. Coll. – Ledgers and Day Books")

Love, Margaret, was visited by Dr. Alonzo Preston who treated her at various times between 1823 and 1826 and Hannah and Peter in 1825 (p. 16, noted the $19.00 medical bill was paid in cash on 1 Aug 1829 and the receipt was signed by Wm. B. Bond) [referring to Dr. William B. Bond]

120

Love, William, appeared on a list of debts dated 26 Dec 1822 and titled "A List of Allen's Claims" that were due and payable to Dr. Richard N. Allen for services rendered [no dates given] to said Love (Document filed in Historical Society of Harford County Archives folder "R. N. Allen")

Low, Deborah, was treated by Dr. John Archer in February 1789 (Ledger F, p. 60)

Lowe, Margaret, Mrs., was treated by Dr. Robert H. Archer in Baltimore before 1822 [no dates or details were given] (Dr. Archer's "Alphabet to Ledger H" is his booklet [filed in the Archives of the Historical Society of Harford County] that contains his index to Ledger H [which is missing] for his patients in Baltimore before 1822 and Harford County after 1822, according to a notation by Dr. George W. Archer.)

Lowman, Mrs., was treated by Dr. Robert H. Archer in Baltimore before 1822 [no dates or details were given] (Dr. Archer's "Alphabet to Ledger H" is his booklet [filed in the Archives of the Historical Society of Harford County] that contains his index to Ledger H [which is missing] for his patients in Baltimore before 1822 and Harford County after 1822, according to a notation by Dr. George W. Archer.)

Lowrey, Dennis, see Robert Sanders (Saunders), q.v.

Lowry, Robert, see George Benjamin, q.v.

Luckey, John, see William Luckey, q.v.

Luckey, William, was visited by Dr. John Archer who treated him and his wife in Aug 1778, him in Jul and Dec 1779, a child in Apr 1780, him and sister in Aug 1780, him in Dec 1780 and Feb 1781, a child in Mar 1781, an infant in Oct 1781, him in Nov 1781, Mar, Apr and Aug 1782 and May and Jun 1783, and him, his wife and sons William and John in 1790 (Ledger C, p. 120; Ledger D, p. 116 [account continued in Ledger E, which is missing]; Ledger F, p. 63) [account continued in Ledgers E and H, which are missing]

Luckie, William, see Francis Spriard(?) and Robert Culver, q.v.

Lukins, Benjamin, appeared on a list of debts dated 26 Dec 1822 and titled "A List of Allen's Claims" that were due and payable to Dr. Richard N. Allen for services rendered [no dates] to said Lukins (Document in Historical Society of Harford County Archives folder "R. N. Allen")

Lukins, Eli, appeared on a list of debts dated 26 Dec 1822 and titled "A List of Allen's Claims" that were due and payable to Dr. Richard N. Allen for services rendered [no dates] by him to said Lukins (Document filed in Historical Society of Harford County Archives folder "R. N. Allen")

Luster (Lester), William, was murdered in 1807: "State of Maryland, Harford County, to wit: An inquisition taken at the house of the late William Luster in the County & State aforesaid on the 12 day of May 1807 before me Jno. Jolley one of the Justices of the Peace of the said State for the County aforesaid (now acting as Coroner) upon the view of the body of William Luster then and there lying dead, upon the oaths of ... good and lawful men of Harford County aforesaid, who being sworn on the Holy Avengely *(sic)* of Almighty God, & charged to inquire, when, where, how, and after what manner the said Wm. Luster, came to his death do say upon their oaths, that on this said 12 day of May in the year of our Lord 1807 about the hour of 3 o'clock in the afternoon, that a certain Edward Dorsey, of Greenbury discharged the contents of a large fowling piece, loaded with powder & shott at the door of the said Wm. Luster at the space of a few feet distance into the right breast of the said Wm. Luster about one inch above the nipple, making an orifice about the size of the circumference of a cent, of which the said William Luster died a few minutes after. In witness whereof as well the aforesaid Coroner, as the jurors aforesaid, have to this inquisition putt *(sic)* their hands & seals, on the day & year aforesaid, and at the place aforesaid. Jno. Jolley, Coroner. Inquisition on the body of William Lester *(sic)*. Received & Recorded the 28th day of July Eighteen hundred and seven in Liber HD No. T, folio 269, one of the Land Record Books of Harford County." (Document filed in the Lester folder in the Archives Department of the Historical Society of Harford County)

Lynch, James, was treated by Dr. John Archer in Aug 1780 and Nov 1782 (Ledger D, p. 90)

Lynch, James, was treated by Dr. Robert H. Archer in Sep 1821 (Ledger F, p. 5, page partially torn)

Lynch, John, was visited by Dr. John Archer who treated his son in Feb 1772, his wife in Feb and Mar 1774, and him at various times between 1772 and 1775 [no dates or details were given] and in Jan and Feb 1777, and also mentioned Mrs. Mary Sims (Ledger B, p. 39; Ledger C, p. 77)

Lynch, John, was prescribed medicine for his wife by Dr. Robert H. Archer on 18 Sep 1802 (Rx Book, 1802-1804, p. 5)

Lyon, John, at Widow Johnson's, was treated by Dr. John Archer in March and June 1779 (Ledger C, p. 122) [John Lyon was a Revolutionary War veteran.]

Lytle, see George Chancey and also see Lyttle, q.v.

Lytle, George, was treated by Dr. John Archer in June 1790 (Ledger F, p. 51) [account continued in Ledger G, which is missing] [George Lytle was a Revolutionary War veteran.]

Lytle, James, was visited by Dr. Matthew J. Allen who rendered obstetrical services to his wife on 20 Jun 1845 (p. 50, noted that part of the bill was paid "by order on Wm. G. Burk" on 20 Jul 1848, part was paid in cash in Oct 1850 and the balance was paid in cash in Feb 1851)

Lytle, Thomas [1788-1853], was visited by Dr. Matthew J. Allen who treated a child in 1847 (p. 55)

Lyttle, Francis, was treated by Dr. Robert H. Archer in May 1825 (Ledger F, p. 87)

Lyttle, John, was visited by Dr. James Archer who treated his wife thirteen times from Apr to Sep 1806 for hysteria (p. 15)

Lyttle, Mr., at Bellaire [Bel Air], was visited by Dr. Robert H. Archer who treated his wife in June 1823 (p. 78)

Lyttle, William, appeared on a list of debts dated 26 Dec 1822 and titled "A List of Allen's Claims" that were due and payable to Dr. Richard N. Allen for services rendered [no dates] by him to said Lyttle (Document filed in Historical Society of Harford County Archives folder "R. N. Allen") [William Lytle was a Revolutionary War veteran.]

Macatee, also see McAtee, q.v.

Macatee, George, living near Ignatius Wheeler, was visited by Dr. John Archer who treated a negro in Dec 1781 and him [George] in Jan and Feb 1784 (Ledger D, p. 107, noted "debt forgiven as before") [account continued in Ledger E, which is missing]

Macatee, Henry, see Sylvester Macatee, q.v.

Macatee, Sylvester [1803-1880], was visited by Dr. Matthew J. Allen who treated him in Dec 1843 and Jan 1844, his wife and son in Jan 1844, his son in Feb and Apr 1844, son Henry in May 1844 (noted $5 paid "cash through John Lilley" in Jun 1844) and treated his wife in Aug 1844 and him in Oct and Nov 1844 and Jan to Mar 1845 (pp. 28, 29, 45); see Robert Cantlin (Cantling), q.v.

Mackall, James, was visited by Dr. Matthew J. Allen who treated him and his son Richard in 1823 in Calvert County; also mentioned Capt. Graham (p. 9a)

Mackall, Richard, see James Mackall, q.v.

Mackenheimer, Peter [c1756-1801], was treated by Dr. Robert H. Archer in Baltimore before 1801 [no dates or details were given] (Dr. Archer's "Alphabet to Ledger H" is his booklet [filed in the Archives of the Historical Society of Harford County] that contains his index to Ledger H [which is missing] for his patients in Baltimore before 1822 and Harford County after 1822, according to a notation by Dr. George W. Archer.) [Peter Mackenheimer was a Revolutionary War veteran.]

Mackey, George, was treated by Dr. John Archer in Jun 1773 and Aug and Sep 1780 (Ledger B, p. 95; Ledger D, p. 93, noted "debt forgiven as before")

Mackey, Molley, was treated by Dr. Alonzo Preston in 1825 (p. 13) [name was indexed as Macke, but written in the ledger as Mackey]

Macubbin, Ellen, Miss, was treated by Dr. Robert H. Archer in Sep 1821 (Ledger F, p. 2)

Madden, Joseph, was visited by Dr. Matthew J. Allen who treated his wife four times in May 1844 (p. 36, noted that most of the bill was paid "by order on H. Whittimore" on 28 Oct 1848)

Madden, Philip, was treated by Dr. John Archer in Jan 1789 (Ledger F, p. 365) [Philip Madden was a Revolutionary War veteran.]

Magaw, Mrs., see Mrs. Finney, q.v.

Magness, ---- [blank], was treated by Dr. Matthew J. Allen in Oct 1848 (p. 94)

Magness, Amanda, see Samuel Magness, q.v.

Magness, Harriet, see Thomas Magness, q.v.

Magness, John's Negro Joshua was treated by Dr. Matthew J. Allen "at Keech's" in Jul 1848 (p. 88)

Magness, John McComas, Jr., was visited by Dr. [Thomas H.] Birckhead who treated a friend with "sundry medicines" in Sep 1799, him [John] in Apr, Aug and Nov 1810 and Oct 1811 and Robert in Feb 1813 (Document filed in Archives of the Historical Society of Harford County folder "Reardon, James R.")

Magness, Milly, see Samuel Magness, q.v.

Magness, Moses (lieutenant), was visited by Dr. John Archer who treated him and his family at various times between 1797 and 1801 (Ledger I, which is missing, was abstracted by Dr. George W. Archer circa 1890; his notes are in the Archives of the Historical Society of Harford County folder "Archer, G. W. Coll. – Ledgers and Day Books")

Magness, Robert, see John McComas Magness, Jr., q.v.

Magness, Samuel, was visited by Dr. Alonzo Preston who treated him at various times between 1822 and 1825 [no dates or details were given], Amanda in Aug 1825 and Milly in Jul 1828 (p. 45) [Samuel Magness was a War of 1812 veteran.]

Magness, Thomas, was visited by Dr. Alonzo Preston who treated his family [no names were given] in Mar 1822 and Harriet in Sep 1827 (p. 54) [Thomas Magness was a War of 1812 veteran.]

Magraw, see Rose Bond, q.v.

Magraw, James (reverend), was visited by Dr. Robert H. Archer who treated his daughter Jane in Oct 1826 in consultation with Dr. J. Archer, Dr. Allen and Dr. Broughton (p. 206)

Magraw, Jane, see James Magraw, q.v.

Magraw, Mr., at West Nottingham [in Cecil Co.] was treated by Dr. John Archer, Jr. in Sep 1821 (Ledger F, p. 27); see Mary Reynolds, q.v.

Maiden's Bower, a land tract owned by Dr. Robert H. Archer, was mentioned in his medical ledger with regards to various non-medical matters handled between 1786 and 1796 (Ledger F, p. 120)

Malady, Bridget, near Ashmead's Mill, was treated by Dr. John Archer in 1786 (Ledger F, p. 256)

Mar, Helen, see Ephraim Litle, q.v.

March, P., was prescribed medicine by Dr. Robert H. Archer circa Dec 1804 (Rx Book, 1802-1804, p. 67); "Mr. Marche" was treated by Dr. Archer in Baltimore before 1822 [no dates or details were given] (Dr. Archer's "Alphabet to Ledger H" is his booklet [filed in the Archives of the Historical Society of Harford County] that contains his index to Ledger H [which is missing] for his patients in Baltimore before 1822 and Harford County after 1822, according to a notation by Dr. George W. Archer.)

Marford, John, son-in-law to William Robinson, was treated by Dr. John Archer in Dec 1790 (Ledger F, p. 163)

Marford, Thomas, was treated by Dr. John Archer in Sep 1788 (Ledger F, p. 181)

Marshall, John, was visited by Dr. John Archer who treated him in Sep 1779 and his wife in Oct 1779 (Ledger D, p. 21, spelled his name Marshal noted "debt forgiven as before") [John Marshall was a Revolutionary War veteran.]

Marshall, John, was treated by Dr. Robert H. Archer in Baltimore before 1822 [no dates or details were given] (Dr. Archer's "Alphabet to Ledger H" is his booklet [filed in the Archives of the Historical Society of Harford County] that contains his index to Ledger H which is missing] for his patients in Baltimore before 1822 and in Harford County after 1822, according to a notation by Dr. George W. Archer.)

Martin, ---- [blank], at Ring Factory [on Winters Run, west of Bel Air], was visited by Dr. Matthew J. Allen who treated his wife in Jul, Aug and Sep 1848 (p. 90)

Martin, Charles, "lives at Elkridge and works in iron factory," was visited by Dr. Matthew J. Allen who treated his son for a wound by applying two stitches and four strips and other treatment at the request of Mr. Griffin in Sep 1847 (p. 64)

Martin, Edward, was treated by Dr. John Archer in Jun 1775 (Ledger B, p. 98) [Edward Martin was a Revolutionary War veteran.]

Martin, Mr. &ca (sic), was treated by Dr. Robert H. Archer after 1822 [no dates or details were given] (Dr. Archer's "Alphabet to Ledger H" is his booklet [filed in the Archives of the Historical Society of Harford County] that contains his index to Ledger H [which is missing] for his patients in Baltimore City before 1822 and in Harford County after 1822, according to a notation by Dr. George W. Archer.)

Martin, Mrs., was treated by Dr. Robert H. Archer in Jul 1822 (p. 10; Ledger F, p. 58)

Martin, Rev., at Slate Ridge, was visited by Dr. John Archer who treated his family at various times between 1796 and 1800 (Ledger I, which is missing, was abstracted by Dr. George W. Archer circa 1890; his notes are in Archives of the Historical Society of Harford County folder "Archer, G. W. Coll. – Ledgers and Day Books")

Martin, Robert, was visited by Dr. John Archer who treated him and a child in July 1802 (Ledger F, p. 142)

Martin, Samuel (reverend), was prescribed medicine by Dr. Robert H. Archer on 31 Jul 1829 (Rx Book, 1825-1851, p. 96)

Martin, Widow, was visited by Dr. John Archer who treated her daughter in Aug 1776 (Ledger C, p. 56, noted "debt forgiven by order of testator")

Martin, William, was treated by Dr. John Archer in Feb 1774, Jun 1775, Mar 1778, Aug 1779 and Apr 1793 (Ledger B, p. 31, transferred to Ledger C, p. 105, transferred to Ledger D, p. 8, transferred to Ledger F, p. 151) [continued in Ledger I, which is missing]; see John Cosley, q.v.

Mason, John, near Little Falls, Lee's Mill [David Lee's Jerusalem Mill on Little Gunpowder River], was treated by Dr. John Archer in 1788 (Ledger F, p. 310)

Mason, Mrs., was treated by Dr. Robert H. Archer in Baltimore before 1822 [no dates or details were given] (Dr. Archer's "Alphabet to Ledger H" is his booklet [filed in the Archives of the Historical Society of Harford County] that contains his index to Ledger H [which is missing] for his patients in Baltimore before 1822 and in Harford County after 1822, according to a notation by Dr. George W. Archer.)

Massey, Aquila (silversmith), was visited by Dr. John Archer who inoculated Caroline Johns, James Massey and James Hart in 1795 and treated him [Aquila] in 1796 (Ledger F, p. 369)

Massey, Aquila, see Isaac Massey, q.v.

Massey, Aquila, Jr., was treated by Dr. Robert H. Archer in Apr 1827 (p. 223)

Massey, Isaac, was visited by Dr. John Archer who treated him and his wife in Sep 1788 and him and son Aquila at various times between 1796 and 1798, and was visited by Dr. James Archer who treated his wife eleven times between Nov 1805 and Feb 1806 (Dr. John Archer's Ledger F, p. 55, spelled his name Massy [account continued in Ledger G, which is missing] (Dr. James Archer's Ledger, p. 16; Dr. John Archer's Ledger I, which is missing, was abstracted by Dr. George W. Archer circa 1890 and spelled his name Massy; his notes are in the Archives of the Historical Society of Harford County folder "Archer, G. W. Coll. – Ledgers and Day Books")

Massey, J., see Negro Harry, q.v.

Massey, James, see Aquila Massey, q.v.

Massey, John, was visited by Dr. Robert H. Archer who treated an infant in 1845 and John and his wife in 1851 [exact dates were not given] (Document filed in the Archives of the Historical Society of Harford County folder "Archer, Robert H., 1775-1857 – Receipts" and noted on 4 Oct 1856 that the bill had not been paid and the doctor was sending Mr. Jackson to collect payment.)

Massey, Mr., see Mrs. Leage, q.v.

Mathens, Widow Sr. (sic), was treated by Dr. John Archer in Jan 1790 (Ledger F, p. 178) [account continued in Ledger G, which is missing]

Mathers, Michael, was treated by Dr. John Archer in April 1791 (Ledger F, p. 246) [account continued in Ledger H, which is missing] [Michael Mather was a Revolutionary War veteran.]

Mathers, Michael, was treated by Dr. Robert H. Archer in Baltimore before 1822 [no dates or details were given] (Dr. Archer's "Alphabet to Ledger H" is his booklet [filed in the Archives of the Historical Society of Harford County] that contains his index to Ledger H [which is missing] for his patients in Baltimore before 1822 and in Harford County after 1822, according to a notation by Dr. George W. Archer.)

Matson, Mrs. (widow), at Slate Ridge Meeting House, was treated by Dr. John Archer in 1788 and the last entry in 1804 indicated "gone to Baltimore" (Ledger F, p. 254)

Matthews, Bennett (captain), was visited by Dr. John Archer who treated a negro in May 1774. Negro Dinah and a negro infant in Aug 1774, negroes Dick, Sal and Phillis in Sep 1774 and mentioned Mrs. Dellam [Dallam]; treated his wife in Sep 1775, him in Oct 1775, a child in Nov 1775, him [Bennett] in Jul 1779 and Feb 1780, a negro in Jul 1780, him in Oct 1780 and Oct 1781 and Dec 1782, and inoculated 4 of his family, "vizt., Betsy Horton, Negro Harry, Jacob & Flora" in Dec 1782; dressed his finger in Feb 1783 and treated him in Apr 1783, a negro and Miss Gittings in Jul 1783, his wife in Aug and Sep 1785 and him in Jul 1789 (Ledger B, p. 53, spelled his name Bennet Mathews; Ledger D, pp. 1, 72, listed him as Capt. Bennet Mathews; Ledger F, p. 186, spelled his name Benit Matthews) [account continued in Ledger G, which is missing] [Bennett Matthews was a Revolutionary War veteran.]; see Ann Dallam and Mrs. Dallam (widow), q.v.

Matthews, Bennett, son of John, was treated by Dr. John Archer in Feb 1790 (Ledger F, p. 327, spelled his name Bennet Mathews) [account continued in Ledger G, which is missing]

Matthews, Carvil, see Nancy Matthews, q.v.

Matthews, Fanny, Miss, daughter of John, was treated by Dr. John Archer in Oct 1790 (Ledger F, pp. 105, 210, spelled her name Mathews)

Matthews, Ignatius (reverend), was visited by Dr. John Archer who treated him at times between Nov 1772 and Jul 1775, a negro boy and a girl in Mar 1772, a negro in Jun 1772, Rev. Mr. Dedricks in Oct 1774, Negro Betty in Jun 1775, Negro Davy in Apr 1777 and him [Ignatius] in Jul 1777 (Ledger B, p. 90, and Ledger C, p. 29, both spelled his name Mathews)

Matthews, James, was visited by Dr. John Archer who treated him at times before 1772 and to 14 Sep 1773, Negro Belind (sic) in Dec 1772 and Sep 1773, Negro Jem (sic) in Sep 1774, Negro Jim (sic) in May 1777 and Mar 1778, a negro woman in Jul 1777, Negro Belinda in Sep 1777, him [James] in Oct 1777, a negro in Aug 1778, him [James] in Apr 1780, May 1781 and Jun 1781, a negro in Aug 1781, "---- at Jos. Brownley's" in Oct 1781, a negro in Feb and Mar 1782 and Negro Jacob in Jul 1782 (Ledger B, p. 59; Ledger C, p. 90; Ledger D, p. 126 [account continued in Ledger E, which is missing] [James Matthews was a Revolutionary War veteran.]

Matthews, John (Mr. Finney's overseer), was visited by Dr. Robert H. Archer who treated an infant in Feb 1827 (pp. 215, 216, spelled his name Mathews)

Matthews, John, see Bennett Matthews and Fanny Matthews, q.v.

Matthews, Levin, was treated by Dr. John Archer in 1791 and the account was paid by R. Matthews in 1802 (Ledger F, p. 252) [Levin Matthews was a Revolutionary War veteran.]

Matthews, Nancy, Miss, was treated by Dr. John Archer in 1793 and 1795 and her account also mentioned Carvil Matthews (Ledger F, pp. 30, 36); see Parker Lee, q.v.

Matthews, R., see Levin Matthews, q.v.

Matthews, Roger, was treated by Dr. John Archer in Feb 1787 and Apr 1801 and his account also mentioned F. Holland in 1787 (Ledger F, pp. 99, 210) [Roger Matthews was a Revolutionary War veteran.]; see Thomas Chancy, q.v.

Matthews, William, was prescribed medicine for his child by Dr. Robert H. Archer on 26 Nov 1802 and for his wife on 24 Jan 1803 (Rx Book, 1802-1804, pp. 26, 30, spelled his name Mathews)

Maulsby, David (carpenter), in Belle Air (sic), was visited by Dr. John Archer who treated his son Morris in 1787 and him [David] in 1794 (Ledger F, p. 96, stated "this man has gone to Baltimore County, Va." (sic) and misspelled his name Malsby) [account continued in Ledger I, which is missing]; David was visited by Dr. James Archer who treated his wife in Mar and Nov 1806 by bleeding her and prescribing various medicines (p. 17)

Maulsby, Betsey, see Mrs. Maulsby, q.v.

Maulsby, Edith, see Mrs. Maulsby, q.v.

Maulsby, I. D. [1781-1839], was visited by Dr. Alonzo Preston who treated him at various times between 1821 and 1826 [no details were given] and his wife and son William in 1825 (p. 26) [Israel David Maulsby was a War of 1812 veteran.]

Maulsby, Mrs., widow of Morris, was visited by Dr. John Archer who treated her and daughters Edith and Betsey at times between 1796 and 1799 (Ledger I, which is missing, was abstracted by Dr. George W. Archer circa 1890; his notes are in the Archives of the Historical Society of Harford County folder "Archer, G. W. Coll. – Ledgers and Day Books")

Maulsby, Morris, appeared on a list of debts dated 26 Dec 1822 and titled "A List of Allen's Claims" that were due and payable to Dr. Richard N. Allen for services rendered [no dates were given] by him to said Maulsby (Document filed in Archives of the Historical Society of Harford County folder "R. N. Allen"); see David Maulsby and Mrs. Maulsby, q.v.

Maulsby, W., was treated by Dr. Alonzo Preston in 1826 (p. 86)

Maulsby, William, was treated by Dr. John Archer in Sep 1791 (Ledger F, p. 266) [account continued in Ledger H, which is missing]

Maxwell, Jacob, on Gunpowder Neck, was treated by Dr. John Archer in 1788 (Ledger F, p. 260)

Maxwell, Robert, was visited by Dr. John Archer, Jr. who treated him and his wife in Nov 1816 and mentioned Gen. John Steele "paid cash" on 18 Jul 1817 (p. 31)

May, James (blacksmith), was treated by Dr. John Archer in Mar 1775 (Ledger B, p. 13)

Maybury, Francis, was visited by Dr. John Archer who treated him before 1772 [no details given], his wife in Aug 1772 and Oct 1773, Nicholas Sinnet in Oct 1772, a child in Jan 1773 and him [Francis] in Nov 1774 (Ledger B, p. 55)

McAdow, Andrew, see James McAdow, q.v.

McAdow, James, was treated by Dr. John Archer in July 1776 (Ledger C, p. 61, noted "Andrew McAdow refuses to pay this acct. that his father assumed"); see John McAdow, q.v.

McAdow, John, was visited by Dr. John Archer who treated him before 1772 [no details were given], his wife in Nov 1773 and Jun 1775, and mentioned "to James McAdow, Ledger C, fol. 61, £3.2" in 1776 (Ledger B, p. 41); John McAdo (sic) was visited by Dr. Archer who treated him in May and Jul 1780, Aug and Sep 1782, and May, Aug and Sep 1783, and his son in Oct 1783 (Ledger D, p. 66) [account continued in Ledger E, which is missing]

McAdow, John, was visited by Dr. John Archer who treated him and wife in 1789 (Ledger F, p. 26) [John McAdow was a Revolutionary War veteran.]

McAdow, Mr., see James W. Williams, q.v.

McAlaster, James, was visited by Dr. John Archer who treated his sons George and Nehemiah in 1795 (Ledger I, which is missing, was abstracted by Dr. George W. Archer circa 1890; his notes are in Archives of the Historical Society of Harford County file "Archer, G. W. Coll. – Ledgers and Day Books"); see James McCallaster, q.v.

McArdle, Fergus, was treated by Dr. John Archer in Jun 1775 (Ledger B, p. 34)

McAtee, ----, see Thomas Butler and also see Macatee, q.v.

McAtee, George, was treated by Dr. John Archer in Jan 1788 (Ledger F, p. 189)

McAteer, John (pedlar), was treated by Dr. John Archer in 1794 [no dates were given] (Ledger I, which is missing, was abstracted by Dr. George W. Archer circa 1890; his notes are in the Archives of the Historical Society of Harford County folder "Archer, G. W. Coll. – Ledgers and Day Books")

McBride, John, was visited by Dr. John Archer who treated him and his mother in Dec 1777 and him in Jan 1779 (Ledger C, p. 79) [John McBride was a Revolutionary War veteran.]

McCafferty, Mr., "near Jeffrey," was treated by Dr. Robert H. Archer in 1828 (Ledger F, p. 13)

McCall, John, near Ashmore's Mill, was visited by Dr. John Archer who treated a child in Nov 1774 (Ledger B, p. 21) [John McCall was a Revolutionary War veteran.]

McCalla, Mrs. (widow), near William Ashmore's, was treated by Dr. John Archer in Feb 1787 (Ledger F, p. 207)

McCallaster, James, was treated by Dr. John Archer in Jul 1795 and his security was John McCoy (Ledger F, p. 245); see James McAlaster, q.v.

McCandless, Alexander (Slate Ridge), was treated by Dr. John Archer in Aug 1772 and Jul 1775 (Ledger B, p. 41)

McCandless, George, was treated by Dr. John Archer in 1786 and was prescribed medicine by Dr. Robert H. Archer on 18 Feb 1801 (Ledger F, p. 290; Rx Book, 1796-1801, p. 34)

McCandless, Hetty, see James McCandless, q.v.

McCandless, J., see Robert Gordon, q.v.

McCandless, James, was visited by Dr. John Archer who treated his son twice in Oct 1772 and four times in Jan 1775, him [James] in Jan and Feb 1775, him in Feb 1778, a child in May 1779, him [James] in Apr, Aug and Sep 1782, and daughters Hetty and Sally in Sep 1788 (Ledger B, p. 31; Ledger C, p. 103, noted "debt forgiven by order of testator" [account continued in Ledger E, which is missing]; Ledger F, p. 79); see Thomas King, q.v.

McCandless, James, was prescribed medicine by Dr. Robert H. Archer on 5 Mar 1801 and 24 Mar 1803 (Rx Book, 1796-1801, p. 39; Rx Book, 1802-1804, p. 38)

McCandless, Robert, was prescribed medicine by Dr. Robert H. Archer on 12 Mar 1801 (Rx Book, 1796-1801, p. 45)

McCandless, Ruth (widow), was treated by Dr. John Archer in Oct 1788 and Jun 1789 (Ledger F, p. 194, and p. 258 listed her as Ruthia)

McCandless, Sally, see James McCandless, q.v.

McCandless, William, was visited by Dr. John Archer who treated a child in Mar 1777, him in Aug, Sep and Oct 1777 and May, Aug and Sep 1778 and Feb and Nov 1780, him and a child in 1795 and him in 1796 and 1797 (Ledger C, p. 74; Ledger F, p. 310; Ledger I, which is missing, was abstracted by Dr. George W. Archer circa 1890; his notes are in the Archives of the Historical Society of Harford County file "Archer, G. W. Coll. – Ledgers and Day Books"); see Negro Rose and Mrs. Lemon, q.v.

McCann, Arthur, was visited by Dr. John Archer who treated him and a negro in Apr 1780 (Ledger D, p. 58, misspelled his first name Arthew and noted "debt forgiven as before") [Arthur McCann (weaver) was a Revolutionary War soldier who enrolled in the county militia in 1775 and Arthur McCann (miller) was a patriot who took the Oath of Allegiance and Fidelity in 1778.]

McCann, John, was treated by Dr. John Archer in Jul 1775 (Ledger B, p. 6) [John McCann was a Revolutionary War veteran.]

McCann, Mr. T., see ---- Kenley, q.v.

McCann, Mrs., near Dublin, was visited by Dr. Robert H. Archer who treated a child in Sep 1822 and her in Apr and May 1824 (pp. 19, 22, 105, 106; Ledger F, p. 81, noted "supposed to be insolvent"); see Daniel Chipman, q.v.

McCantie, James, was visited by Dr. John Archer in 1787 who treated his stepdaughter for a head wound (Ledger F, p. 302)

McCarnicle, George, was treated by Dr. Matthew J. Allen in Feb, Mar, Jun, Jul and Sep 1844 and Feb and Aug 1845 (p. 32 spelled his name Carnicle and p. 40, spelled his name McCarnicle)

McCartey, Owen, at James Webster's, was treated by Dr. John Archer in Feb 1787 (Ledger F, p. 196)

McCaskey, William, was treated by Dr. John Archer in Nov 1794 (Ledger F, p. 118)

McCaslin, David, was visited by Dr. John Archer who treated a child in Aug 1780 and him in Jul 1781 and Feb 1782 (Ledger D, p. 84, noted "debt forgiven as before")

McCausland, George (major), was visited in 1822 by Dr. Robert H. Archer who treated him and son Jefferson "Jeff" several times between 16 Sep 1822 and 22 Oct 1822; Mrs. George McCausland (widow) was treated by Dr. Archer in Mar 1824 (pp. 20-23; Ledger F, pp. 82, 94, 95) [George McCausland was a War of 1812 veteran.]

McCausland, Jefferson, see George McCausland, q.v.

McCausland, Robert, was visited by Dr. Robert H. Archer who treated his wife in Aug 1825 (Ledger F, p. 110)

McCay, John, at James Moores', was treated by Dr. John Archer in Oct 1786 (Ledger F, p. 219); see John McCrackin, q.v.

McChanney, William, see Michael Adkinson, q.v.

McCherry, Stephen, was treated by Dr. John Archer in Sep 1777 and Jul 1780 (Ledger C, p. 58)

McClaskey, Alexander, was visited by Dr. John Archer who treated him and his family in 1797 (Ledger I, which is missing, was abstracted by Dr. George W. Archer circa 1890; his notes are in the Archives of the Historical Society of Harford County folder "Archer, G. W. Coll. – Ledgers and Day Books")

McClaskey, George, was prescribed medicine by Dr. Robert H. Archer on 4 Nov 1802 (Rx Book, 1802-1804, p. 24)

McClaskey, Joseph, was treated by Dr. John Archer in Mar 1780 (Ledger D, p. 53, noted "Settled") [Joseph McClaskey was a Revolutionary War veteran.]

McClaskey, William [c1790-1844], was treated by Dr. Robert H. Archer in Sep 1821 and was also mentioned by Dr. Archer in a non-medical matter in 1827 (p. 235; Ledger F, p. 13) [William McClaskey was a War of 1812 veteran.]

McCleary, Mr., was visited by Dr. Robert H. Archer who treated his child in Mar 1823 (p. 57; Ledger F, p. 148)

McClellan, Robert, was prescribed medicine by Dr. Robert H. Archer on 22 Feb and 20 Apr 1803 and for his wife on 26 Aug 1803 (Rx Book, 1802-1804, pp. 40, 54, and p. 33 noted "Take this up immediately."); Robert was treated by Dr. Archer in Baltimore before 1822 [no dates or details were given] (Dr. Archer's "Alphabet to Ledger H" is his booklet [filed in the Archives of the Historical Society of Harford County] that contains his index to Ledger H [which is missing] for his patients in Baltimore before 1822 and Harford County after 1822, according to a notation by Dr. George W. Archer.)

McClerey, William, near Quaker Meeting in Pennsylvania, was treated by Dr. John Archer in Aug 1788 (Ledger F, pp. 175, 298)

McClintock, Matthew, was visited by Dr. John Archer who treated him at various times between Sep 1772 and June 1779, his son in Jan 1773 and July 1774, Eacy Taylor in July 1774, his [Matthew's] wife in May 1779, him in Aug 1779 and Mar 1780 ("hamorrhoid"), his wife in Dec 1781, him in Jul and Nov 1782, his wife in Jan 1783, him in Jul 1783 and him and his wife in Oct 1788 (Ledger B, p. 50; Ledger D, p. 9, listed his as Marthew MClintick Senr.) [account continued in Ledger E, which is missing]; Ledger F, p. 61; Ledger C, p. 39, titled "Mathew McClintock's Estate alias Susannah McClintock" stated "October 27, 1790, To the assessment on the lot at the Cross Roads paid to Robert Amoss, Collector, for 1783 and 1788) [account continued in Ledger G, which is missing] [Matthew McClintock was a Revolutionary War veteran.]; see James Little and James Harris, q.v.

McClintock, Matthew, Jr., was visited by Dr. John Archer who treated him in Jul 1774 and Feb 1775, mentioned sundries charged to his father's account in 1774, and treated his wife, Ned Morgan and Edward Morgan in Jan 1777, his wife in Sep 1777, him in Jan 1778, Nancy McFadden and an infant in Apr 1778, his wife in Jul and Oct 1778, him in Dec 1778 and Jul 1779, a child in Aug 1779 and inoculated two children in Feb 1782 (Ledger B, p. 61; Ledger C, p. 17; Ledger D, p. 81, noted "debt forgiven as before")

McClintock, Mrs., was prescribed medicine by Dr. Robert H. Archer on 29 May 1799 (Rx Book, 1796-1801, p. 16); Mrs. McClintick (sic) was treated by Dr. Archer in Baltimore at some time before 1822 [no dates or details were given] (Dr. Archer's "Alphabet to Ledger H" is his booklet [filed in the Archives of the

Historical Society of Harford County] that contains his index to Ledger H [which is missing] for his patients in Baltimore before 1822 and Harford County after 1822, according to a notation by Dr. George W. Archer.)

McClintock, Susanna or Susannah, see Matthew McClintock and James Harris, q.v.

McClure, ----, see John Hanna, q.v.

McClure, John, was visited by Dr. Alonzo Preston who treated a child in 1826 and noted "assumed to pay acct. against Smith" for $5.00 plus his child's account for $1.50 which he paid "by work" on 17 Oct 1826 (p. 60, spelled his name McLure) [John McClure was a Revolutionary War veteran.]

McClure, Nathaniel, was treated by Dr. John Archer in Nov 1781 and Feb 1784 (Ledger D, p. 92, spelled his name McLure and noted "debt forgiven as before")

McClure, Robert, was treated by Dr. John Archer in Jul 1774, Jun 1775 and May 1778 (Ledger B, p. 56; Ledger C, p. 50, noted "debt forgiven by order of testator")

McClure, William, was treated by Dr. John Archer five times in Sep 1772 and six times between Feb 1774 and Jul 1775; recorded separately as William McClure & Company in the ledger when the doctor treated his servant in May 1773, Andrew [son] in Jun 1773, Honora [daughter] in Jul 1773 and him between Aug 1773 and Jan 1774 and circa 1776-1777 [no dates were given] (Ledger B, pp. 82, 84; Ledger C, p. 53, noted "debt forgiven by order of testator") [William McClure was a Revolutionary War veteran.]

McCollock, Richard, near John Barkley's, was treated by Dr. John Archer circa 1787 [no date given] (Ledger F, p. 335)

McCollock, William, in Bel Air, was visited by Dr. John Archer who treated him and his family at various times between 1797 and 1803 (Ledger I, which is missing, was abstracted by Dr. George W. Archer circa 1890; his notes are in the Archives of the Historical Society of Harford County folder "Archer, G. W. Coll. – Ledgers and Day Books")

McComas, ---- [blank], was treated by Dr. Robert H. Archer in Baltimore before 1822 [no dates or details given] (Dr. Archer's "Alphabet to Ledger H" is his booklet [filed in the Archives of the Historical Society of Harford County] that contains his index to Ledger H [which is missing] for his patients in Baltimore before 1822 and Harford County after 1822, according to a notation by Dr. George W. Archer.)

McComas, Aaron [1761-1845], near Bush [i. e., Bush Town], was treated by Dr. John Archer in Jan and Mar 1787 (Ledger F, pp. 156, 228) [Aaron McComas was a Revolutionary War veteran.]

McComas, Alexander, see Richard McCoy, q.v.

McComas, Aquila, was treated by Dr. John Archer in Mar 1773 (Ledger B, p. 93)

McComas, Benjamin, was treated by Dr. John Archer in Oct 1778 (Ledger C, p. 110) [Benjamin McComas was a Revolutionary War veteran.]

McComas, Deborah, was listed in Dr. John Archer's ledger circa 1773, but no entries were made in her account (Ledger B, p. 60, spelled her name M'Comus)

McComas, James [1735-1791] (colonel), was treated by Dr. John Archer in Jun 1790 (Ledger F, p. 232) [James McComas was a Revolutionary War veteran and a signer of the Bush Declaration on March 22 1775.]

McComas, John, was visited by Dr. John Archer who treated a child in Oct 1782 (Ledger D, p. 10, noted "debt forgiven as before") [John McComas, of Daniel, and John McComas, of William, were both Revolutionary War veterans.]

McComas, John (bricklayer), was treated by Dr. John Archer in Oct 1774 (Ledger B, p. 35, spelled his name M'Comus)

McComas, John (doctor), was visited by Dr. John Archer who treated his wife in Apr 1781, a child in Oct 1782 and him and a young woman [name not given] in Aug 1784 (Ledger D, p. 10, noted "debt forgiven as before")

McComas, Mary, see Negro Jessee, q.v.

McComas, Preston [1781-1837], was visited by Dr. Alonzo Preston who treated him at various times between 1822 and 1825 [no dates or details were given] and treated his wife and child in 1825 (p. 51, noted the "assumption [of the $11 medical bill] in presence of Benjn. R. Bond – paid in wood") [Preston McComas was a War of 1812 veteran.]

McComas, William, was treated by Dr. John Archer in Jun 1786 and Feb 1787 (Ledger F, pp. 47, 340) [William McComas was a Revolutionary War veteran.]; see John Barnet, q.v.

McCormick, Elizabeth, was treated by Dr. John Archer in Sep 1773 (Ledger B, p. 70)

McCowan, ---- [blank], Ring Factory [on Winters Run, west of Bel Air], was treated by Dr. Matthew J. Allen eight times in Sep 1847 (p. 65)

McCoy, David, near James Barnett's, was treated by Dr. John Archer in May 1787 (Ledger F, p. 287)

McCoy, John, see James McCallaster, q.v.

McCoy, Michael, at Josias William Dallam's near Abingdon, was treated by Dr. John Archer in Nov 1788 (Ledger F, p. 264)

McCoy, Richard, cooper(?), stepson of Alexander McComas, was treated by Dr. John Archer in Jan 1791 (Ledger F, p. 224)

McCoy, William, "cordmaker," was treated by Dr. John Archer in Aug 1784 (Ledger F, p. 248)

McCrackin (McCackin?), Captain, son-in-law to Thomas Smith, was treated by Dr. John Archer in Jan 1791 (Ledger F, p. 314)

McCrackin, John, was visited by Dr. John Archer who treated him in Jan 1791 and his sister [name was not given] and his daughters Patty and Katy in 1797 and 1798 (Ledger F., p. 138 [account continued in Ledger H, which is missing]; Ledger I, which is missing, was abstracted by Dr. George W. Archer circa 1890; his notes are in the Archives of the Historical Society of Harford County file "Archer, G. W. Coll. – Ledgers and Day Books" and spelled his name McCracken)

McCrackin, Katy, see John McCrackin, q.v.

McCrackin, Patty, see John McCrackin, q.v.

McCrackin, William [1745-c1835], "trans fluis" at John McCay's [i.e., "across the water," meaning he lived across the Susquehanna River in Cecil County], was treated by Dr. John Archer in Oct 1799 (Ledger F, p. 334) [William McCracken or McCrackin was a Revolutionary War veteran.]

McCrail, Patrick, was treated by Dr. John Archer in Jun 1784(?) [year unclear] (Ledger D, p. 6, noted he paid £0.4.6 by cash, but then stated "debt forgiven as before"); see John Cretin and Patrick McGrill, q.v.

McCubbins (McGibbons?), Mrs. (widow), on Bennett Wheeler's place, was treated by Dr. John Archer in 1793 (Ledger F, p. 241)

McCulloch, William, was prescribed medicine by Dr. Robert H. Archer on 19 Nov 1804 and 5 Dec 1804 and medicine for his child on 29 Nov 1804 (Rx Book, 1802-1804, pp. 61, 65, 66)

McCullough, John, at Port Deposit [in Cecil Co.], was treated by Dr. John Archer, Jr. in Oct 1819 and also mentioned apprentice Boyd and H. Boyd in Jun 1819 and William Burk in Jul 1819 (p. 73)

McCullough, William, was prescribed medicine by Dr. Robert H. Archer on 5 Sep 1796 (Rx Book, 1796-1801, p. 9) [William McCullough was a Revolutionary War veteran.]

McCurdy, Elenor, Mrs., was treated by Dr. John Archer in Sep 1787 (Ledger F, p. 351)

McDannal, Widow, was visited by Dr. John Archer who treated a daughter and inoculated 5 of her family in March 1776 and treated a daughter in Sep 1777 (Ledger C, p. 32, noted "debt forgiven by order of testator")

McDannal, ---- [blank], near E. Flagan's, was visited by Dr. John Archer who treated a child in May 1785 (Ledger D, p. 18, noted "debt forgiven as before")

McDonnal, Archibald, was treated by Dr. John Archer in July 1775 (Ledger B, p. 82)

McDonnel, Peggy, Miss, was treated by Dr. Robert H. Archer in Baltimore before 1822 [no dates or details were given] (Dr. Archer's "Alphabet to Ledger H" is his booklet [filed in the Archives of the Historical Society of Harford County] that contains his index to Ledger H [which is missing] for his patients in Baltimore before 1822 and Harford County after 1822, according to a notation by Dr. George W. Archer.)

McElderry, Thomas, was prescribed medicine for a negro by Dr. Robert H. Archer on 7 Aug 1802 and 27 Dec 1802, medicine for Thomas' child on 9 May 1803 and medicine for Thomas in 1804 [exact date was not given] (Rx Book, 1802-1804, pp. 10, 28, 42, 69)

McFadden, ---- [blank], was visited by Dr. Alonzo Preston who treated his daughter Eliza in Feb 1825 (p. 28)

McFadden, Ann, see William McFadden, q.v.

McFadden, Charles, was treated by Dr. John Archer in Mar 1787 (Ledger F, p. 374, spelled his name McFaddin)

McFadden, Daniel, was treated by Dr. John Archer in Dec 1790 (Ledger F, p. 118, spelled his name Danniel McFaddin)

McFadden, Eliza, see ---- McFadden, q.v.

McFadden, Jenny, see Mrs. McFadden, q.v.

McFadden, John (tailor), was visited by Dr. Robert H. Archer who treated his wife in Dec 1827 (p. 258)

McFadden, John [1787-1864], was visited by Dr. Alonzo Preston who treated a child in 1826 and 1827 and John's wife in Feb 1828 (p. 83, noted the bill totaled $4.00 and "This acct. settled by acct. in bar.") [John McFadden was a War of 1812 veteran.]; see William McFadden, Jr.

McFadden, John B., see Michael Gilbert, q.v.

McFadden, Mary, see William McFadden, q.v.

McFadden, Mrs. (widow), was visited by Dr. John Archer who treated her daughter Jenny in 1794 and 1795 and also noted "Cr. by ferriage" (Ledger I, which is missing, was abstracted by Dr. George W. Archer circa 1890; his notes are in Archives of the Historical Society of Harford County file "Archer, G. W. Coll. - Ledgers and Day Books")

McFadden, Nancy, see Nancy McFadian and Matthew McClintock, Jr., q.v.

McFadden, Samuel, was treated by Dr. John Archer in April 1787 (Ledger F, p. 200) [Samuel McFadden was a Revolutionary War veteran.]

McFadden, Tom, see William McFadden, q.v.

McFadden, William [c1765-1842], was visited by Dr. John Archer who treated him and his daughter Mary in 1789 and him and his children Ann and Tom at various times between 1797 and 1799 (Ledger F, p. 28 [account continued in Ledger G, which is missing]; Ledger I, which is missing, was abstracted by Dr. George W. Archer circa 1890; his notes are in Archives of the Historical Society of Harford County folder "Archer, G. W. Coll. – Ledgers and Day Books"); William McFaddon was visited by Dr. Robert H. Archer who treated Negro Herman in 1824 (p. 121)

McFadden, William, Jr. [1794-1830s], was visited by Dr. Alonzo Preston who treated his wife in Apr 1827 (p. 88, noted "Paid on this acct. by John McFadden, $1.00") [William McFadden was a War of 1812 veteran.]

McFadian, Nancy, was treated by Dr. John Archer in March 1782 (Ledger D, p. 125, noted "debt forgiven as before")

McFadon, John, was prescribed medicine by Dr. Robert H. Archer on 2 Jul 1803 and 14 Dec 1804 and for his brother [name not given] on 25 Nov 1804 (Rx Book, 1802-1804, pp. 46, 63, 64, 66) [John McFadon, merchant in Baltimore, was a Revolutionary War veteran.]; see Mrs. Bates, q.v.

McFadon, William, was prescribed medicine by Dr. Robert H. Archer on 5 Sep 1802 and medicine for his wife on 23 Jun 1803 and for his child on 6 Jul 1803 (Rx Book, 1802-1804, pp. 18, 45, 47); he was treated by Dr. Archer in Baltimore before 1822 [no dates or details were given] (Dr. Archer's "Alphabet to Ledger H" is his booklet [filed in the Archives of the Historical Society of Harford County] that contains his index to Ledger H [which is missing] for his patients in Baltimore City before 1822 and in Harford County after 1822, according to a notation by Dr. George W. Archer.)

McField, Daniel (schoolmaster), was visited by Dr. John Archer who inoculated 2 of his children in Feb 1777 and treated him in Jul and Sep 1782 (Ledger C, p. 85)

McGaa, George, below Spesutia Church [St. George's P. E. Church in Perryman], was treated by Dr. John Archer in Dec 1789 (Ledger F, p. 367)

McGaa, John, son of Robert, was treated by Dr. John Archer in Mar 1788 (Ledger F, p. 283)

McGaa, Robert, see John McGaa and Benedict Hall, q.v.

McGaughlin, --- [blank], Havre de Grace, was treated by Dr. John Archer in 1797 (Ledger I, which is missing, was abstracted by Dr. George W. Archer circa 1890; his notes are in the Archives of the Historical Society of Harford County folder "Archer, G. W. Coll. – Ledgers and Day Books")

McGaw, James, near Widow Wheelers, in the Barrens [area in the northwest part of the county near Pennsylvania], was treated by Dr. John Archer in 1798 (Ledger I, which is missing, was abstracted by Dr. George W. Archer circa 1890; his notes are in Archives of the Historical Society of Harford County folder "Archer, G. W. Coll. – Ledgers and Day Books")

McGaw, James, at Union, was treated by Dr. Robert H. Archer in Oct 1825 and also mentioned Dr. Bristor and John Kirk's administrator. (Ledger F, p. 33); see Robert Blackburn, q.v.

McGaw, John [1797-1863] (late deputy sheriff), was treated by Dr. Robert H. Archer in consultation with Dr. Preston in 1825 (p. 152; Ledger F, p. 117) [John McGaw was a War of 1812 veteran.]

McGaw, Mrs. (widow), at Union, was visited by Dr. Robert H. Archer in Aug 1825 who treated her child in consultation with Dr. Preston (p. 153; Ledger F, p. 124); see Michael Clark, q.v.

McGee, Mrs., was treated by Dr. John Archer in July 178 (sic) [year incomplete, probably 1780 or 1781] (Ledger D, p. 53, noted "debt forgiven as before")

McGibbons (McCubbins?), Mrs. (widow), on Bennett Wheeler's place, was treated by Dr. John Archer in Nov 1793 (Ledger F, p. 241)

McGill, John, was prescribed medicine by Dr. Robert H. Archer on 10 Aug 1802 (Rx Book, 1802-1804, p. 11)

McGill, William, was visited by Dr. John Archer who treated his wife in June 1775, him in Dec 1777 and Sep 1778, and him, his wife and child in Mar 1789 (Ledger B, p. 34; Ledger C, p. 79, noted part paid "by yr. dividend to the poor of Boston, 3/6½;" Ledger F, p. 336)

McGirr, Arthur, "near X Roads," was visited by Dr. John Archer who treated him and his family at various times in 1797 and 1798 (Ledger I, which is missing, was abstracted by Dr. George W. Archer circa 1890; his notes are in the Archives of the Historical Society of Harford County folder "Archer, G. W. Coll. – Ledgers and Day Books")

McGlaughlin, Daniel, "brother-in-law to Johns," was treated by Dr. John Archer in 1794 (Ledger I, which is missing, was abstracted by Dr. George W. Archer circa 1890; his notes are in Archives of the Historical Society of Harford County file "Archer, G. W. Coll. - Ledgers and Day Books")

McGlaughlin, Daniel, was treated by Dr. Robert H. Archer in Baltimore before 1822 [no dates or details were given] (Dr. Archer's "Alphabet to Ledger H" is his booklet [filed in the Archives of the Historical Society of Harford County] that contains his index to Ledger H [which is missing] for his patients in Baltimore before 1822 and Harford County after 1822, according to a notation by Dr. George W. Archer.)

McGlaughlin, James, "storekeeper for Enoch Churchman," was treated by Dr. John Archer at various times between 1795 and 1798 (Ledger I, which is missing, was abstracted by Dr. George W. Archer circa 1890; his notes are in the Archives of the Historical Society of Harford County file "Archer, G. W. Coll. – Ledgers and Day Books")

McGlaughlin, John, near Trappe, was treated by Dr. John Archer from 1794 to 1804 (Ledger I, which is missing, was abstracted by Dr. George W. Archer circa 1890; his notes are in Archives of the Historical Society of Harford County folder "Archer, G. W. Coll. – Ledgers and Day Books")

McGlaughlin, Joseph, was visited by Dr. John Archer who treated him and his family at various times in 1797 and 1798 (Ledger I, which is missing, was abstracted by Dr. George W. Archer circa 1890; his notes are in the Archives of the Historical Society of Harford County folder "Archer, G. W. Coll. – Ledgers and Day Books"); see George McLaughlin, q.v.

McGonigal, Daniel, was visited by Dr. Matthew J. Allen who treated a child five times in Jan 1845 (p. 42, noted "paid to A. J. Greme in full"); see Augustus J. Greme, q.v.

McGonigal, Roland, was treated by Dr. Robert H. Archer in Baltimore before 1822 [no dates or details were given] (Dr. Archer's "Alphabet to Ledger H" is his booklet [filed in the Archives of the Historical Society of Harford County] that contains his index to Ledger H [which is missing] for his patients in Baltimore before 1822 and Harford County after 1822, according to a notation by Dr. George W. Archer.)

McGough, James (merchant), at Broad Creek, was treated by Dr. John Archer in 1795 (Ledger I, which is missing, was abstracted by Dr. George W. Archer circa 1890; his notes are in Archives of the Historical Society of Harford County file "Archer, G. W. Coll. - Ledgers and Day Books")

McGough, Miles, was treated by Dr. John Archer in Aug 1779 and Mar and May 1783 (Ledger D, p. 8, noted "debt forgiven as before")

McGowan, Mrs., was prescribed medicine twice by Dr. Robert H. Archer in Oct 1804 (Rx Book, 1802-1804, pp. 59, 60)

McGrill, Patrick, was visited by Dr. John Archer who treated him in May 1781 and Apr 1783, a child in Dec 1783 or 1784, and him [Patrick] in Sep and Dec 1785 (Ledger D, p. 20, noted "debt forgiven as before"); see Patrick McCrail, q.v.

McGuire, John, near C. Town [Coop Town], was treated by Dr. John Archer in May and June 1785 (Ledger D, p. 4, noted "debt forgiven as before")

McGuire, Philip, was treated by Dr. John Archer in Jun 1775 (Ledger B, p. 98) [Philip McGuire was a Revolutionary War veteran.]

McIlhainey, Michael, was treated by Dr. Robert H. Archer in Baltimore before 1822 [no dates or details were given] (Dr. Archer's "Alphabet to Ledger H" is his booklet [filed in the Archives of the Historical Society of Harford County] that contains his index to Ledger H [which is missing] for his patients in Baltimore before 1822 and Harford County after 1822, according to a notation by Dr. George W. Archer.)

McIlroy, James, student at Mears' School, was treated by Dr. John Archer in Jun 1795 (Ledger I, which is missing, but it was abstracted by Dr. George W. Archer circa 1890; his notes are in the Archives of the Historical Society of Harford County folder "Archer, G. W. Coll. – Ledgers and Day Books"); see Alexander Mears, q.v.

McJilton, Frances, see William McJilton, q.v.

McJilton, William, in Darlington, was treated by Dr. Robert H. Archer in Oct 1822 (p. 30, misspelled his name as McGilton) and who treated a child in Sep 1825 and his daughter Frances in May 1827 (pp. 160, 224; Ledger F, p. 103)

McKenless, William, see Negro Rose, q.v.

McKenney, Christianna, alias Lancaster, at Mr. Dorsey's, was treated by Dr. John Archer in Sep 1787 (Ledger F, p. 15, spelled her name McKenny); see Christianna Lancaster, q.v.

McKenney, Delia, see John McKenney, q.v.

McKenney, Fanny, see John McKenney, q.v.

McKenney, John, was prescribed medicine by Dr. Robert H. Archer on 29 Dec 1796 (Rx Book, 1796-1801, p. 10)

McKenney, John, was visited by Dr. Robert H. Archer who treated his wife in June 1825 and he was treated at times between 1824 and 1828 by Dr. Alonzo Preston who treated daughter Fanny several times in 1826, daughter Delia several times in 1826 and 1827, Josua (sic) in 1826, and Matilda "in partu" [in childbirth] on 26 Mar 1827; also vaccinated some black children in June 1827, treated his father and a boarder in Jun 1832 and also mentioned Thomas Lochary; John was treated in Aug 1838 and his wife in Oct 1839 by Dr. Robert Archer in consultation with Dr. Munnikhuysen (Dr. Archer, p. 136; Dr. Preston, pp. 36, 76; Dr. Archer, Ledger F, p. 73, spelled his name McKenney) [John McKenny or McKenney was a War of 1812 veteran.]

McKenney, Josua (sic), see John McKenney, q.v.

McKenney, Matilda, see John McKenney, q.v.

McLaughlin, see McGlaughlin, q.v.

McLaughlin, Catherine, Mrs., "near Pesuia Church" [Spesutia or St. George's P. E. Church], was treated by Dr. John Archer in Jun 1786 (Ledger F, p. 290)

McLaughlin, Daniel, was treated by Dr. John Archer in Aug and Nov 1772 (Ledger B, pp. 3, 8)

McLaughlin, George, was visited by Dr. John Archer who treated him many times between Aug 1772 and May 1775, son George in Aug 1773, son Joseph in Mar 1773 (sewed a wound in his head), son John or Johnny in Apr 1773 (opened his knee in May 1773 and incised an ulcer in his leg in June 1773), his [George's] wife in Feb 1774 and May 1775, his mother in May 1774, him in Nov 1776, his wife in Jan 1777, him in Jan and Jul 1777, John in Sep 1777, a child in Jul 1778, him in Oct 1778, son George in Aug 1779, him [George] at times between Mar 1780 and Dec 1781, him in Jul 1782, wife in Dec 1782, son Robert in Feb 1783, son George in Jul 1788, and him and a daughter in Aug 1790 (Ledger B, p. 48; Ledger C, pp. 7-8, stated "debt forgiven by order of testator;" Ledger D, p. 70, illegibly misspelled his name [account continued in Ledger E, which is missing]; Ledger F, p. 2, p. 19 misspelled his name as McGlaughlin) [account continued in Ledger H, which is missing] [George McLaughlin was a Revolutionary War veteran.]

McLaughlin, George, was visited by Dr. Robert H. Archer who treated his wife in Sep 1822 (p. 20; Ledger F, p. 83)

McLaughlin, George, Jr., was treated by Dr. John Archer in Jan 1787 (Ledger F, p. 175)

McLaughlin, James, appeared on a list of debts dated 26 Dec 1822 and titled "A List of Allen's Claims" that were due and payable to Dr. Richard N. Allen for services rendered [no dates] by him to the said McLaughlin (Document filed in Historical Society of Harford County Archives folder "R. N. Allen"); James was visited by Dr. Alonzo Preston who treated his wife during the night of 29 Jan 1826 (p. 66); see James McGlaughlin, q.v.

McLaughlin, John (pedagogue), was treated by Dr. John Archer in Sep 1790 (Ledger F, p. 206)

McLaughlin, John or Johnny, see George McLaughlin and John McGlaughlin, q.v.

McLaughlin, Joseph, see George McLaughlin and Joseph McGlaughlin, q.v.

McLaughlin, Mickey, was treated by Dr. Robert H. Archer in Mar and Apr 1823 and Aug 1824 (pp. 61, 118; Ledger F, p. 153) [Michael "Mickey" McLaughlin was a War of 1812 veteran.]

McLaughlin, Mr. (schoolmaster), at William Smithson's, was treated by Dr. Robert H. Archer in Nov 1825 and in May and Jun 1827 (pp. 167, 168, 169, 230, 231; Ledger F, p. 150) [The Smithson-Webster Springhouse, better known as the DH Springhouse, is a two-story, coursed ashlar stone structure built by David Hopkins in 1816. The second story was a classroom and McLaughlin was the teacher. The building still stands majestically on the north side of Sandy Hook Road.]

McLaughlin, Robert, was treated by Dr. John Archer in Feb 1780 (Ledger D, p. 41, noted "debt forgiven as before") [Robert McLaughlin was a Revolutionary War veteran.]

McLaughlin, Samuel (mason), Havre de Grace, was visited by Dr. John Archer who treated him and his family in 1797 (Ledger I, which is missing, was abstracted by Dr. George W. Archer circa 1890; his notes are in the

Archives of the Historical Society of Harford County folder "Archer, G. W. Coll. – Ledgers and Day Books")

McMath, Mr., see Walter Billingslea, q.v.

McMath, Samuel, was treated by Dr. John Archer in 1797 and he noted in his ledger that William McMath was his executor in 1802 (Ledger I, which is missing, was abstracted by Dr. George W. Archer circa 1890; his notes are in the Archives of the Historical Society of Harford County folder "Archer, G. W. Coll. – Ledgers and Day Books"); see William McMath, q.v.

McMath, William, was treated by Dr. John Archer at various times between 1795 and 1803 and also treated Benjamin Crockett, Samuel McMath, John Clark and Mrs. McMath in 1803 (Ledger F, p. 328, 342) [William McMath was a Revolutionary War veteran.]; see Samuel McMath, q.v.

McMillion, Mrs., was prescribed medicine ("strengthening pills" and "laxative pills") by Dr. Robert H. Archer on 25 Nov 1802 and other medicine on 24 Feb 1803 (Rx Book, 1802-1804, pp. 25, 34)

McMullen, Jo., was visited by Dr. John Archer, Jr. who treated him in Oct 1815 and him and his daughter in Sep 1821 (p. 31; Ledger F, p. 9, spelled his name McMullin)

McMullen, Robert (pedagogue), at S. Gover's, was treated by Dr. John Archer in 1794 (Ledger I, which is missing, was abstracted by Dr. George W. Archer circa 1890; his notes are in the Archives of the Historical Society of Harford County folder "Archer, G. W. Coll. – Ledgers and Day Books") [Dr. George W. Archer's own notes indicated Robert McMullen had a family.]

McMullen, Samuel, was visited by Dr. Robert H. Archer who treated his wife "in partu" [in childbirth] on 25 Nov 1822 in consultation with Dr. LeBarron (p. 39, noted in the margin of the ledger was "preternatural presentation;" Ledger F, p. 125, noted "supposed to be insolvent")

McMullen, T., see Thomas Huggins & Co., q.v.

McNabb, ---- [blank], "at X Roads," was visited by Dr. Robert H. Archer who treated him in August 1822 and mentioned, and possibly treated, a son [not named] in October 1822 (Ledger F, p. 68)

McNabb, James, was treated by Dr. John Archer in Jan 1792 (Ledger F, p. 103); he appeared on a list of debts dated 26 Dec 1822 and titled "A List of Allen's Claims" that were due and payable to Dr. Richard N. Allen for services rendered [no dates were given] to said McNabb (Document filed in Historical Society of Harford County Archives folder "R. N. Allen"); James McNabb, near Harmer's above Dublin, was visited by Dr. Robert H. Archer who treated a child in Jan 1823 (p. 50; Ledger F, p. 140, noted he was "considered too poor to pay") [James McNabb was a Revolutionary War veteran.]

McNabb, John, at Mount Pleasant, was visited by Dr. John Archer who treated him in Sep 1781 and his wife in Oct and Nov 1781 (Ledger D, p. 77, noted "debt forgiven as before"); John McNabb [residence not stated] was treated by Dr. Archer in Dec 1787 and Mar 1791 (Ledger F, p. 67) [account continued in Ledger H, which is missing]; John McNabb "over the river" [i.e ., over the Susquehanna in Cecil County] was treated by Dr. Archer in 1797 and 1798 (Ledger I, which is missing, was abstracted by Dr. George W. Archer circa 1890; his notes are in the Archives of the Historical Society of Harford County folder "Archer, G. W. Coll. – Ledgers and Day Books")

McNamara, Joseph, soldier near Broad Creek, was treated by Dr. John Archer in Oct 1790 (Ledger F, pp. 145, 256) [Joseph McNamara was a Revolutionary War veteran.]

McOwen, Francis, "at ye Priest's place," was treated by Dr. John Archer in 1795 (Ledger I, which is missing, was abstracted by Dr. George W. Archer circa 1890; his notes are in the Archives of the Historical Society of Harford County file "Archer, G. W. Coll. – Ledgers and Day Books")

McQuiston, Joseph, was treated by Dr. John Archer in Aug 1773 (Ledger B, p. 30)

McSwine [McSwain], David, was visited by Dr. John Archer who treated him in Jul 1780, his wife in Apr 1782 and him in Sep 1782 and Jul 1785 (Ledger D, p. 80, spelled his name McSwine and noted "debt forgiven as before") [David McSwain was a Revolutionary War veteran.]

McVay, Dorcas, was treated by Dr. John Archer in Jul 1785 (tooth extraction) (Ledger D, p. 54, noted "debt forgiven as before")

McVay, John (weaver), was visited by Dr. John Archer who treated him and a child in Apr 1786 and him in May 1791 (Ledger F, pp. 71, 212) [account continued in Ledger H, which is missing]

McVey, John, was visited by Dr. Matthew J. Allen who treated his wife twenty-one times between 5 Jun 1847 and 19 Dec 1847 (pp. 53, 60) [The following statement was written on a separate page dated 24 Nov 1853 that was inserted in the back of Dr. Allen's ledger. The letter, addressed to Major Bond, was signed by I. Day and stated "I have just returned after 3 days ride to look up the Drs. of Dr. Allen and the following is the result."

It mentioned several patients, including this one: "John McVey says that he will pay $5 within 10 days & if not he would pay nothing at all – as his wife had but one arm. I promised it should be in full, he is old & is not worth 1 cent."]

Mead, Benjamin, "at Gun. P. Neck" [Gunpowder Neck], was treated by Dr. John Archer in Jun 1787 (Ledger F, p. 308)

Mears, Alexander [schoolmaster], was visited by Dr. John Archer who treated "pupil Phedemon" in Jun 1795, "pupil Goodwin" in Aug 1795 and his [Alexander's] brother in Sep 1795 (Ledger I, which is missing, was abstracted by Dr. George W. Archer circa 1890; his notes are in the Archives of the Historical Society of Harford County folder "Archer, G. W. Coll. – Ledgers and Day Books"); see James McIlroy, q.v.

Meek, Andrew, was visited by Dr. John Archer who treated him and Barney [no relationship was indicated] in Nov 1776 and him [Andrew] in Oct 1777 (Ledger C, p. 46) [Andrew Meek was a Revolutionary War veteran.]

Meeks, Martha (widow), was treated by Dr. John Archer in Sep and Oct 1779 and Oct 1781 (Ledger D, p. 18, noted "debt forgiven as before")

Meratty, Peter, was treated by Dr. John Archer in Oct 1781 (Ledger D, p. 81, noted "debt forgiven as before")

Merrican, ----, see Robert Nesbitt, q.v.

Merryman, John, was prescribed medicine by Dr. Robert H. Archer on 9 Aug 1802 (Rx Book, 1802-1804, p. 10)

Merryman, Samuel, was treated by Dr. Robert H. Archer in Baltimore before 1822 [no dates or details were given] (Dr. Archer's "Alphabet to Ledger H" is his booklet [filed in the Archives of the Historical Society of Harford County] that contains his index to Ledger H [which is missing] for his patients in Baltimore before 1822 and Harford County after 1822, according to a notation by Dr. George W. Archer.)

Metcalf, James, at Mrs. Dorsey's, was treated by Dr. Matthew J. Allen in Oct and Nov 1847 and Mar 1848 (p. 67)

Meyers, C., Mr., was prescribed medicine by Dr. Robert H. Archer on 11 Mar 1801 (Rx Book, 1796-1801, p. 42)

Michael, Belsher [1728-1795], was treated by Dr. John Archer in October 1781 (Ledger D, p. 83, noted "debt forgiven as before") [Balsher Michael, of Hall's Cross Roads, now Aberdeen, was a veteran of the French and Indian War and also a veteran of the Revolutionary War.]

Michael, William [c1776-1857], was visited by Dr. Robert H. Archer who treated him in Sep 1822 and Negro Pie in June 1825 (pp. 16, 136; Ledger F, p. 73)

Michel, J., see John Trago, q.v.

Mifflin, Mary, Mrs., was treated by Dr. Robert H. Archer seven times in Jan 1823 in consultation with Dr. Worthington and at various times through 16 Mar 1823; her medical bill was paid by Joshua Husband on 23 Sep 1823 (pp. 45, 46, 47, 48, 50; Ledger F, p. 133); see Mrs. Mifflin, q.v.

Mifflin, Mrs., mother of Joshua Husbands, was visited by Dr. John Archer who treated her son Samuel in 1797 (Ledger I, which is missing, was abstracted by Dr. George W. Archer circa 1890; his notes are in the Archives of the Historical Society of Harford County folder "Archer, G. W. Coll. – Ledgers and Day Books"); see Mrs. Mary Mifflin, q.v.

Mifflin, Samuel, see Mrs. Mifflin, q.v.

Mildew, Aquila, was prescribed medicine for his wife and child by Dr. Robert H. Archer on 5 Aug 1802 (Rx Book, 1802-1804, p. 8)

Millburn, Mary, was treated by Dr. John Archer in Aug 1781 (Ledger D, p. 63, noted "debt forgiven as before")

Miles, Joshua, near Cooptown, was treated by Dr. John Archer in Dec 1787 (Ledger F, p. 73) [Joshua Miles was a Revolutionary War veteran.]

Miles, Thomas, was treated by Dr. John Archer in Nov and Dec 1781 and Jan, Feb, Apr and Jun 1782 (Ledger D, p. 100) [Thomas Miles was a Revolutionary War veteran.]

Miller, see Israel Morris, q.v.

Miller, Adeline, Miss, was treated by Dr. Robert H. Archer in Oct 1825, July 1826, Mar, Apr and June 1827 and July and Aug 1828 (pp. 161, 192, 217, 218, 219, 220, 236, 288, 289; Rx Book, 1825-1851, p. 87); see Peggy Stump, q.v.

Miller, Ann (Cecil Co.), was listed in Dr. John Archer's ledger circa 1773, but no entries were made in her account (Ledger B, p. 53)

Miller, Dr., was consulted by Dr. John Archer in 1787 (Ledger F, p. 51); see Joseph P. Ryland, q.v.

Miller, H., see Peggy Stump, q.v.

Miller, James (Jimmy), see Thomas Miller, q.v.

Miller, John, was treated by Dr. Robert H. Archer in Baltimore before 1822 [no dates or details were given] (Dr. Archer's "Alphabet to Ledger H" is his booklet [filed in the Archives of the Historical Society of Harford County] that contains his index to Ledger H [which is missing] for his patients in Baltimore City before 1822 and in Harford County after 1822, according to a notation by Dr. George W. Archer.)

Miller, Joseph, was visited by Dr. John Archer who treated his wife in Oct 1779, him in Nov 1779, Sep and Nov 1780 and May and June 1781, his wife in Nov 1781, him in Dec 1781 and Apr 1782 ("hamorrhoid"), his wife in May 1782, him in Feb 1783 and his wife in Nov and Dec 1783 (Ledger D, p. 30 [initially gave the appearance that his name was McCiller, but the fancifully handwritten MC is actually just the letter M] [account continued in Ledger E, which is missing]

Miller, Joseph (fuller), was treated by Dr. John Archer in Oct 1788 and him and his family between 1794 and 1808 (Ledger F, p. 174) [account continued in Ledger G, which is missing] (Ledger I is also missing, but was abstracted by Dr. George W. Archer circa 1890; his notes are in Historical Society of Harford County Archives folder "Archer, G. W. Coll. - Ledgers and Day Books")

Miller, Joseph, see Negro Roger, Widow Yeates, Suckey Chew, John Wilson and Thomas Smith, q.v.

Miller, Margaret (widow), was visited by Dr. John Archer who inoculated five of her family in 1777 [exact date was not given] (Ledger C, p. 50, noted "debt forgiven by order of testator")

Miller, Mary (widow), was visited by Dr. John Archer who treated her and daughter Patsy in Dec 1781 (Ledger D, p. 106, noted partly paid in 1783 "by an order on Joseph Davis" and partly paid "by cash recd. of Henry Waters" in Apr and May 1784, but then noted "debt forgiven as before")

Miller, Miss, see Mrs. Stump and Peggy Stump, q.v.

Miller, Mrs., see William Finney, q.v.

Miller, Nancy (Ann), see Thomas Miller, q.v.

Miller, Patsy, see Mary Miller, q.v.

Miller, Samuel (Sammy), see Thomas Miller, q.v.

Miller, Samuel, of Thomas, was treated by Dr. John Archer in May 1782 (Ledger D, p. 9, noted "debt forgiven as before") [Samuel Miller was a Revolutionary War veteran.]

Miller, Thomas, was visited by Dr. John Archer who treated his children Samuel (Sammy), Nancy (Ann), James (Jimmy) in Nov 1772 and him [Thomas] from Apr to Jun 1774 (Ledger B, p. 51)

Miller, William, see John Farmer, q.v.

Miller, William, near Darlington, was treated by Dr. Robert H. Archer in Sep 1826 (p. 199)

Miller, William, was visited by Dr. Robert H. Archer who treated his wife 14 times from 4 Feb to 21 Mar 1823, a child in May and Jun 1823, and his wife in Jun 1823; mentioned Monohan's Smith Shop in Oct 1822 (pp. 51-58; Ledger F, p. 114) [William Miller was a War of 1812 veteran]

Miller, William F. [1791-1840], was visited by Dr. Robert H. Archer who treated his wife and child in Jun 1823, his wife in Jun and Jul 1826 and a child in Apr and May 1828 (pp. 81, 83, 191, 192, 270, 274) [William Franklin Miller was a War of 1812 veteran.]; see William Welch, q.v.

Mills, Robert, was visited by Dr. John Archer who treated him before 1772 [no details were given], in Apr 1777, his wife in Jul 1777 and him and "Johan" in Sep 1777 (Ledger B, p. 52; Ledger C, p. 36, contained an account in Robert's name in 1777 that mentioned only his wife, but then crossed it out and noted "debt forgiven by order of testator;" Ledger C, p. 60, noted "assumption of Robert Allen's account" in Nov 1777 and the balance of "debt forgiven by order of testator")

Mitchael, Jno., see Benedict Edward Hall, q.v.

Mitchel, Johannem, see William Coale, q.v.

Mitchell, Aquila, was treated by Dr. John Archer in Jan 1788 (Ledger F, p. 116)

Mitchell, Bernard, was visited by Dr. Alonzo Preston who treated him and his wife six times in Sep 1828 (p. 103, noted "10th Aug 1830 paid in full. W. B. B." [referring to Dr. William B. Bond]

Mitchell, Edward, see Elijah Mitchell, q.v.

Mitchell, Elijah, was visited by Dr. James Archer who treated his son Edward five times in July 1806 for dysentery; visited by Dr. Robert H. Archer who treated a child at Mrs. Martin's, his wife and daughter Kitty in Sep 1822, son Elijah in Oct 1822, son Gerard in Dec 1822, and his [Elijah's] wife in Apr 1823, and him [Elijah] in Oct 1825 (Dr. James Archer, p. 18; Dr. Robert H. Archer, pp. 16, 25, 26, 42, 62, 162; Ledger F, pp. 67, 91); see John Mitchell and Robert Mitchell, q.v.

Mitchell, Elisha, was visited by Dr. Matthew J. Allen who treated his wife five times and rendered obstetrical services [childbirth] to her on 30 Apr 1845 and treated a child in Aug 1845 and his wife in Sep 1845 (p. 35, noted part of bill was paid in Sep 1848 and part was paid in May 1852)

Mitchell, Frederick [1775-1851], was visited by Dr. Robert H. Archer who treated his wife in Jun and Jul 1826 and he was treated by Dr. Alonzo Preston in Jan and Aug 1827 (Dr. Archer, pp. 191, 194; Dr. Preston, p. 75) [Frederick Mitchell was a War of 1812 veteran.]

Mitchell, Gerard, see Elijah Mitchell, q.v.

Mitchell, Howell, appeared on a list of debts dated 26 Dec 1822 and titled "A List of Allen's Claims" that were due and payable to Dr. Richard N. Allen for services rendered [no dates or details were given] by him to said Mitchell (Document filed in the Archives of the Historical Society of Harford County folder "R. N. Allen"); Howell Mitchell (blacksmith), in Bel Air, was treated by Dr. Robert H. Archer in Apr 1825 consultation with Dr. Forwood (p. 130; Ledger F, p. 107, noted he was "insolvent") [Howell Mitchell was a War of 1812 veteran.]

Mitchell, James, see Sarah Mitchell, q.v.

Mitchell, Johanna, see William Coale, q.v.

Mitchell, John, was treated by Dr. Robert H. Archer in Nov 1822 (pp. 35, 37, 38)

Mitchell, John, was treated by Dr. Matthew J. Allen eight times between 20 Jun and 8 Jul 1845 (p. 50 spelled his name Mitchel and noted that the $11.75 medical bill was "forgiven" [forgiven])

Mitchell, John (millwright), was visited by Dr. John Archer who treated him in Feb 1782 and Jun 1783, his wife in Jul 1783, him in Aug 1783, him, his wife and child in 1788 and him in May 1793 (Ledger D, p. 118, mistakenly listed him as Mitchel John, millright) [continued in Ledger E, which is missing]; Ledger F, p. 132, listed him as Jno. Mitchel, millwright) [continued in Ledger H, which is missing] [Three men named John Mitchell served in the Revolutionary War.]

Mitchell, John, of Elijah, was treated by Dr. Robert H. Archer nine times between 2 Nov and 2 Dec 1822 (p. 34; Ledger F, p. 116)

Mitchell, Joseph (blacksmith), was visited by Dr. John Archer, Jr. who treated him in Jul 1816 and his wife in Sep 1818 (p. 52, listed his name as Jo. Mitchill)

Mitchell, Kent, see Elenor Robison, q.v.

Mitchell, Kitty, see Elijah Mitchell, q.v.

Mitchell, Micajah [deputy sheriff], was visited by Dr. John Archer who treated him in Apr 1782, Oct 1782 and Jun 1783, his wife, a negro and "T: Lee" in Jul 1783, his wife in Sep 1783, him in May 1784, Jun 1785, Oct 1785 and Sep 1789 (Ledger D, p. 3, listed him as Cage Mitchel and noted he assumed the bill of William Montgomery and paid it on 24 Jun 1785 [account continued in Ledger E, which is missing]; Ledger F, p. 222, indicated Mitchell's bill was assumed by Samuel Webb) [Micajah "Cage" Mitchell was a Revolutionary War veteran.]; see Samuel Webb, James Ford, Harmon Pritchard and Stephen Pritchard (Pritchet), q.v.

Mitchell, Mr., was visited by Dr. Robert H. Archer who treated his wife in Aug 1822 and a child in Aug 1827 (pp. 13, 243, 244)

Mitchell, Mr., "at Watson's X Roads," was treated by Dr. Robert H. Archer in Sep 1826 (p. 201)

Mitchell, Robert (Rob), was treated by Dr. Robert H. Archer in Aug 1827 (p. 243)

Mitchell, Robert, of Elijah, was treated by Dr. Robert H. Archer seven times in July and Aug 1823 and again in Aug 1827 (pp. 84, 85, 85a; Ledger F, p. 68)

Mitchell, Sarah, widow of James, was visited by Dr. John Archer who treated her in Jun 1785 and her and a child in Sep 1788 (Ledger D, p. 122; Ledger F, pp. 6, 198)

Mitchell, William, was treated by Dr. John Archer in Apr 1780 (Ledger D, p. 55, noted the "debt forgiven as before")

Mitten, Jobe, was treated by Dr. Alonzo Preston in 1827 (p. 88)

Moffitt, James, was visited by Dr. Matthew J. Allen who treated his son in Jan and Feb 1844, him [James] in Feb 1844, him and his wife and Marg.(?) in Mar 1844, his wife in Apr 1844 and Jan and Feb 1845 (pp. 30, 43) [The following statement was written on a separate page dated 24 Nov 1853 that was inserted in the back of Dr. Allen's ledger. The letter, addressed to Major Bond, was signed by I. Day and stated "I have just returned after 3 days ride to look up the Drs. of Dr. Allen and the following is the result." It mentioned several patients, including this one: "Jas. Moffett (sic) says he will pay $10 in March next & if paid then I promised should be in full, being poor."]; see Negro Isabella, q.v.

Mohon, John, was visited by Dr. John Archer who treated his wife in Dec 1781 and Apr 1783, inoculated Polly Mohon in 1782, and treated him in Feb 1785, his wife in Sep 1785, him in Nov 1785 and him and a child in 1788 (Ledger D, p. 102, noted "debt forgiven as before;" Ledger F, p. 76) [account continued in Ledger G, which is missing]

Mohon, John, was treated by Dr. Matthew J. Allen three times in Jun 1845 (p. 48, noted the bill was paid "by cash for Samuel Webster" on 4 Oct 1848)

Mohon, Polly, see John Mohon, q.v.

Mohon, William (blacksmith), was visited by Dr. John Archer who treated his wife in Apr 1782 and him in Feb 1783 and Jul 1786 (Ledger D, p. 1, noted "debt forgiven as before;" Ledger F, p. 373)

Molly, Miss, see John Paca, q.v.

Molton, Matthew, see Negro Gamboe, q.v.

Monday, John (negro), was treated by Dr. Robert H. Archer in Baltimore before 1822 [no dates or details were given] (Dr. Archer's "Alphabet to Ledger H" is his booklet [filed in the Archives of the Historical Society of Harford County] that contains his index to Ledger H [which is missing] for his patients in Baltimore before 1822 and Harford County after 1822, according to a notation by Dr. George W. Archer.)

Monk, Francis [c1785-1837], was visited by Dr. Robert H. Archer who treated his son in June 1825 and a negro "in partu" [in childbirth] on 5 Jun 1826 in consultation with Dr. Allen (pp. 137, 189; Ledger F, p. 153) [Francis E. Monks was a War of 1812 veteran.]

Monk, Mr., a merchant in Abingdon, was treated by Dr. John Archer in June 1791 (Ledger F, p. 205) [Capt. John Monk (Monks), also known as John Clark Monk (1760-1827) was entombed in a vault in St. George's Church Cemetery and his coffin suspended above the ground by chains. He was memorialized in song as the Swinging Sailor of Perryman by the rock band Captain Quint.]

Monk, Richard, see William Monk, q.v.

Monk, William, brother of Richard, was treated by Dr. John Archer in March 1786 (Ledger F, p. 70)

Monks, Edward, see James Monks, q.v.

Monks, James, was visited by Dr. Matthew J. Allen who treated a child in Jun, Jul and Aug 1847, son Edward in Aug 1847 and a child eleven times between 7 Aug and 27 Sep 1847 (pp. 56, 61, noted the medical bill was paid in judgment "by cash to W. H. Dallam" in Feb and Jul 1851)

Monks, John, or John Clark Monk, see Mr. Monk, q.v.

Monohan, Arthur, was treated by Dr. John Archer in Dec 1779 (Ledger D, p. 39, spelled his name Arthew Monohon) [Arthur Monohan was a Revolutionary War veteran.]

Monohan, Barnard, was treated by Dr. John Archer in Sep 1793 (Ledger F, p. 289, spelled his name Monohon) [account continued in Ledger I, which is missing]

Monohan, John [c1753-1833], was visited by Dr. John Archer who treated him in Jun 1780 and Mar 1784(?) and an infant in Jul 1784 (Ledger D, p. 72, spelled his name Monohon and noted "debt forgiven as before") [John Monohan was a Revolutionary War veteran.]

Monohan, Martin, was visited by Dr. James Archer who treated his daughter in May 1806 with a "blister to side" and various pills (p. 19, misspelled his name as Menahon)

Monohan, Mr., see William Miller and also Monohon, q.v.

Monohan, Thomas, was treated by Dr. John Archer in Oct 1781 and Dec 1789 (Ledger D, p. 90, spelled his name Monahon and noted "debt forgiven as before;" Ledger F, p. 159; he was also visited by Dr. James Archer who treated him in Oct 1806 "by bleeding" and prescribing various pills (p. 20) [continued in Ledger H, which is missing] [Thomas Monohan was a Revolutionary War veteran.]

Monohon, see John Ellis and also see Monohan, q.v.

Monro, Widdow (sic), was treated by Dr. John Archer in Aug 1781 (Ledger D, p. 60, noted "debt forgiven as before")

Montgomery, Aquilla (a yellow man), was visited by Dr. Alonzo Preston who treated his wife "in partu" [in childbirth] on 17 Jan 1825 (p. 21)

Montgomery, John (weaver), was treated by Dr. John Archer in Oct 1772 and eighteen times between 12 Jan 1773 and 30 Nov 1773 (Ledger B, p. 57)

Montgomery, John, at Slate Ridge, was visited by Dr. John Archer who treated him in Sep 1777 and a child in Jun 1778 (Ledger C, p. 95)

Montgomery, John [1765-1828], was visited by Dr. John Archer who treated him in 1787 and him and his daughter Sally at various times between 1795 and 1798; ledger also mentioned William Montgomery in 1808

(Ledger F, p. 133; Ledger I, which is missing, was abstracted by Dr. George W. Archer circa 1890; his notes are in the Archives of the Historical Society of Harford County folder "Archer, G. W. Coll. – Ledgers and Day Books")

Montgomery, Sally, see John Montgomery, q.v.

Montgomery, Thomas [1792-1837], appeared on a list of debts dated 26 Dec 1822 and titled "A List of Allen's Claims" that were due and payable to Dr. Richard N. Allen for services rendered [no dates were given] to said Montgomery (Document filed in the Archives of the Historical Society of Harford County folder "R. N. Allen") [Thomas Montgomery was a War of 1812 veteran.]

Montgomery, William, was visited by Dr. John Archer who treated him in Sep 1778 and William Caskey's wife in Nov 1782 (Ledger C, p. 122); see John Montgomery and Micajah Mitchell, q.v.

Mooberry, ---- [blank], criminal, Harford Co. jail, was treated by Dr. Alonzo Preston from 23 May to 26 May 1825 (p. 38)

Mooberry, William, was treated by Dr. John Archer in 1788 (Ledger F, p. 351) [William Mooberry was a Revolutionary War veteran.]

Mooney, John, Ring Factory [on Winters Run, west of Bel Air], was visited by Dr. Matthew J. Allen who treated him several times in Dec 1847, his wife in Aug 1848 and him in Sep 1848 (p. 69)

Moore, Ann (widow), Bel Air, was visited by Dr. John Archer who treated her and children Polly, Nelly and "J." in 1795 and 1796 (Ledger I, which is missing, was abstracted by Dr. George W. Archer circa 1890; his notes are in the Archives of the Historical Society of Harford County file "Archer, G. W. Coll. – Ledgers and Day Books") [Dr. George Archer's own note indicated "This was the mother of Jason," so the child listed as "J." was most likely him.]; see Jason Moore, q.v.

Moore, Charles, was treated by Dr. John Archer in Sep 1796 (Ledger F, p. 27)

Moore, Edward, at Josias Wheeler's, was treated by Dr. John Archer in Jan 1791 (Ledger F, p. 311)

Moore, J., see Jon Harwood, q.v.

Moore, James (weaver), was visited by Dr. John Archer who treated him in Jun, Jul, Aug and Sep 1773 and Nov 1774, his wife in Mar 1774, a child in Jun and Jul 1774, him in Nov 1774, a son and daughter in Jun and Aug 1781, an infant in Nov 1781, his wife in Aug 1782, a daughter in Nov 1782, him in Feb 1783 and a child in Jun 1783; inoculated 6 of his family in Feb 1782 (Ledger B, p. 58; Ledger D, p. 34, noted "debt forgiven as before") [James Moore (1742-1798) and James Moore (c1748-c1794) were both veterans of the Revolutionary War.]

Moore, Jason [c1790-1830], in Bel Air, was treated by Dr. John Archer in 1797 (Ledger I, which is missing, was abstracted by Dr. George W. Archer circa 1890 who noted ["son of widow Ann Moore]" and his notes are in Archives of the Historical Society of Harford County file "Archer, G. W. Coll. – Ledgers and Day Books"); Jason Moore was visited by Dr. Robert H. Archer who treated his wife in March 1823 in consultation with Dr. Forwood (p. 56; Ledger F, p. 144) [Jason Moore was a War of 1812 veteran and later served as the county sheriff.]; see Ann Moore, q.v.

Moore, John, appeared on a list of debts dated 26 Dec 1822 and titled "A List of Allen's Claims" that were due and payable to Dr. Richard N. Allen for services rendered [no dates were given] by him to said Moore (Document filed in Archives of the Historical Society of Harford County folder "R. N. Allen") [John Moor or Moore was a Revolutionary War veteran.]

Moore, John (surveyor, Baltimore Co.), near Aquila Hall's, Esq., was treated by Dr. John Archer in 1787 (Ledger F, p. 375)

Moore, Joseph, was visited by Dr. John Archer, Jr. who treated a child in Aug 1816 and mentioned Skipwith Coale in Nov 1817 (p. 58)

Moore, Nelly, see Ann Moore, q.v.

Moore, Polly, at Mrs. Dickson's, was treated by Dr. John Archer in Jun 1782 (Ledger D, p. 113, noted "debt forgiven as before"); see Ann Moore, q.v.

Moore, Susan, Miss, Bel Air, was treated by Dr. John Archer in 1797 and 1798 (Ledger I, which is missing, was abstracted by Dr. George W. Archer circa 1890; his notes are in the Archives of the Historical Society of Harford County file "Archer, G. W. Coll. – Ledgers and Day Books") [Dr. George W. Archer noted "she had children in spite of the Miss!"]; see Henry Chamberlaine, q.v.

Moore, Thomas (weaver), was treated by Dr. John Archer in July 1775 (Ledger B, p. 47)

Moore, Thomas, at Sarah Wilson's, was treated in Aug 1789 by Dr. John Archer (Ledger F, p. 149, spelled his name Moor)

138

Moore, William, at Slate Ridge, was treated by Dr. John Archer in Jan 1791 (Ledger F, p. 302)

Moore, William, near John Cox, was treated by Dr. John Archer in Oct 1786 (Ledger F, p. 109)

Moores, Aquila Paca [1792-1853] was treated by Dr. Robert H. Archer in Dec 1823 and mentioned John Cloman in Jan 1829 (Ledger F, p. 83, listed him as A. P. Moores); see Mary Moores, q.v.

Moores, Dr., was consulted by Dr. John Archer at various times in 1789 and 1791 (Ledger F, p. 135); see John Moores and Parker Moores, q.v.

Moores, James, see Mary and Parker Moores. John McCay, Prush A. Bond and Mrs. Moores, q.v.

Moores, James (collector), was treated by Dr. Robert H. Archer in Dec 1822 and also mentioned John Moores, dec'd., and William Hanna, dec'd., in Dec 1824 (Ledger F, p. 131)

Moores, James (tailor), was treated by Dr. John Archer in 1788 and mentioned Viney Buckingham (Ledger F, pp. 197, 240) [account continued in Ledger G, which is missing]

Moores, James (tanner), was visited by Dr. John Archer who treated him many times between Jan 1773 and Feb 1774, his wife in Feb 1773 and Oct 1774, a negro in Apr 1773, a child in Sep 1774, negroes Betsey and Pegg in Sep and Oct 1774, and James, his wife, two daughters and Negro Pegg in Oct 1774; inoculated James' family in Feb 1776 and treated him in Jul 1776, Jammy Moores in Dec 1776, Carolin in Apr 1777, him in Jul 1779, an infant in Feb 1778, him in Nov 1778 and Feb 1779, his daughter and Miss Horton in Apr 1779, him in Aug 1779, a negro in Oct 1779 and Feb 1780, him in Feb, Mar and Jun 1780, a negro in Jul 1780, him [James] in Dec 1780, his wife in Jan 1781, him in Feb and Mar 1781, a negro in Mar 1781, him [James] in Apr 1781, daughter Sally in Aug 1781, John in May 1782, J. N. in Jul 1782, daughter in Aug 1782, Will Campbell in Feb 1783, Negro Grace in Jul 1783, and him [James] in Nov 1791; also mentioned John Moores in 1801 (Ledger B, p. 49; Ledger C, p. 28, noted "paid in depreciated Congress money" on 11 Feb 1779; Ledger D, pp. 51, 81, noted that part of the bill was paid and then noted "debt forgiven as before") [account continued in Ledger E, which is missing]; Ledger F, p. 135) [James Moores (tanner) was a Revolutionary War veteran.]

Moores, James (weaver), was visited by Dr. John Archer who treated him in March 1779, a child in June 1780 and him [James] in Apr 1781 (Ledger C, p. 29)

Moores, James, of James, was treated by Dr. John Archer in Dec 1793 (Ledger F, p. 350) [account continued in Ledger I, which is missing]

Moores, James Lee, was visited by Dr. Robert H. Archer who treated Negro Ned in May and June 1825 and prescribed medicine for him on 23 May and 25 Jul 1825 (pp. 132-133, 137; Rx Book, 1825-1851, pp. 78, 82)

Moores, Jammy, see James Moores (tanner), q.v.

Moores, John [1757-1823], was treated by Dr. Robert H. Archer in Aug 1823 in consultation with Dr. Preston and Dr. Moores (p. 90; Ledger F, p. 51); see James Moores (tanner), James Moores (collector) and Mrs. Moores, q.v.

Moores, Mary, was visited by Dr. Alonzo Preston who treated her at various times between 1823 and 1828, Clarissa in 1823, Ned in 1825, Elizabeth and Hannah in 1826, James Bond in 1827, "Mrs. P. M." [probably Mrs. Parker Moores] in 1827, a child in 1827, and a black girl and Isaac in 1828 (pp. 27, 104, noting "Recd. The above balance in full" and followed by "April 1st 1833, Wm. B. Bond. The above acct. properly chargeable to J. & A. P. Moores so says Jas. Moores.")

Moores, Mr., see Peter Hanlin and Robert Hunt, q.v.

Moores, Mrs., widow of John, was treated by Dr. Robert H. Archer three times in May 1825, five times in Feb 1828 and three times in July 1828; also treated Negro Ned in May 1825 and noted that James Moores paid her medical bill in full on 5 Dec 1829 (pp. 264, 265, 266, 286, 287; Ledger F, p. 144)

Moores, Parker, was treated at various times between 1824 and 1827 by Dr. Alonzo Preston who also treated Samuel Gover on 17 Jul 1827; Parker was treated on 30 Sep and 1 Oct 1827 by Dr. Robert H. Archer in consultation with Dr. Preston and Dr. Moores and the last treatment to Parker was on 3 Oct 1827 by Dr. Preston, followed by an undated note, probably made by Dr. William B. Bond, stating, "Settled the above acct. [for $22] with James Moores, admr. of P. Moores, after deducting this amt. from P. Moores acct. there remained a balance from Dr. Preston's estate of $33.01¼." (Dr. Preston, p. 35; Dr. Archer, p. 248)

Moorn, John, was murdered in 1778: "State of Maryland, Harford County, to wit: The Jurors for the State that now is for the body of Harford County aforesaid upon their oath present that Joseph Jarvis, late of Harford County, laborer, not having the fear of God before his eyes but being moved and seduced by the instigation of the Devil on the twentieth day of February in the year of our Lord one thousand seven hundred and seventy eight with force and arms and so forth at Harford County aforesaid and within the jurisdiction of this

Court in and upon one John Moorn in the peace of God and of the said State then and there being, feloniously and in the fury of his mind did make an assault and *(sic)* the said Joseph Jarvis by repeated stricks *(sic)* with his fists in and upon the said John Moorn under his left breast then and there did in the fury of his mind feloniously strick *(sic)* and bruise, giving unto the said John Moorn under his left breast one mortal wound and bruise – of which said mortal wound and bruise – the said John Moorn then and there instantly died [at Lower Cross Roads in the house occupied by William Bodesman]; and so the Jurors aforesaid upon their oath aforesaid do say that the said John Moorn, Joseph Javis *(sic)* the said John Moorn in manner and form aforesaid then and there feloniously and in the fury of his mind did kill and slay against the form of the ---- [four illegible words] made and proved and against the peace, government and dignity of the State … Indict. – Manslaughter. A True Bill. Benjamin B. Norris, foreman." (File 3.00(12) in the Court Records Department of the Historical Society of Harford County)

Mootrie, Libby, was treated by Dr. Robert H. Archer in Baltimore before 1822 [no dates or details were given] (Dr. Archer's "Alphabet to Ledger H" is his booklet [filed in the Archives of the Historical Society of Harford County] that contains his index to Ledger H [which is missing] for his patients in Baltimore before 1822 and Harford County after 1822, according to a notation by Dr. George W. Archer.)

Morarty, Daniel, was visited by Dr. John Archer who treated him in Mar 1773 and his son Matthew in Jul 1774 (Ledger B, p. 45)

Morarty, Matthew, see Daniel Morarty, q.v.

Morgan, see Samuel Palmer, q.v.

Morgan, C., Mrs., widow of William, was visited by Dr. John Archer who treated her and daughters Polly and Peggy at times between 1795 and 1798 (Ledger I, which is missing, was abstracted by Dr. George W. Archer circa 1890; his notes are in the Archives of the Historical Society of Harford County folder "Archer, G. W. Coll. – Ledgers and Day Books")

Morgan, Cassy, see William Morgan, q.v.

Morgan, Edward, was visited by Dr. John Archer who treated him in Sep and Oct 1777 and Nov 1778, his wife in Apr 1781 and him in Jul 1782 (Ledger C, p. 85, noted that part of the bill was paid "by making a cooler for the large still" and balance of "debt forgiven by order of testator;" Ledger D, p. 45, noted "debt forgiven as before") [Edward Morgan was a Revolutionary War veteran.]; see Robert Morgan and Matthew McClintock, Jr., q.v.

Morgan, Edward, of William, was treated by Dr. John Archer at various times between 1797 and 1804 (Ledger I, which is missing, was abstracted by Dr. George W. Archer circa 1890; his notes are in the Archives of the Historical Society of Harford County folder "Archer, G. W. Coll. – Ledgers and Day Books")

Morgan, Hamilton, was treated by Dr. James Archer in March 1806 (p. 21); he also appeared on a list of debts dated 26 Dec 1822 and titled "A List of Allen's Claims" that were due and payable to Dr. Richard N. Allen for services rendered [no dates given] to said Morgan (Document filed in Historical Society of Harford County Archives folder "R. N. Allen"); see Robert Morgan, q.v.

Morgan, Hillen, see James Lee Morgan, q.v.

Morgan, James Lee, was visited by Dr. Robert H. Archer who treated son Hillen in Apr 1823, his wife in May 1823 and infant in Jun 1825; he was visited by Dr. Matthew J. Allen who treated his wife in Jul 1847 (Dr. Archer, pp. 65, 74, Ledger F, pp. 152. 159; Dr. Allen's ledger, p. 59; Dr. Archer's "Alphabet to Ledger H" is his booklet [filed in the Archives of the Historical Society of Harford County] that contains his index to Ledger H [which is missing] for his patients in Baltimore City before 1822 and in Harford County after 1822, according to a notation by Dr. George W. Archer.)

Morgan, John, was treated by Dr. John Archer in Jan 1790 and also mentioned his brother William in 1788 (Ledger F, p. 329) [account continued in Ledger G, which is missing]

Morgan, Lurena, see Robert Morgan, q.v.

Morgan, Ned, see Matthew McClintock, Jr., q.v.

Morgan, Peggy, see C. Morgan, q.v.

Morgan, Peggy, at E. Gilbert's, was treated by Dr. Robert H. Archer in Sep 1825 (Ledger F, p. 58)

Morgan, Polly, see C. Morgan, q.v.

Morgan, Robert [1755-1820s], was visited by Dr. John Archer who treated him in Apr 1780, a negro in Apr 1781, a negro and a child in May 1781, him in Dec 1781, an infant in Feb 1783, him in Jul and Dec 1783 and in Mar 1791 and also inoculated his children Sarah, Hamilton, Lunna [Lurena], Ed: [Edward] and William, and negroes Hannah, Phillis, Bill, Betsy, Pliny, Ned, Grace, Hector, Ben, Sin:, Mary, Priss and Mich (Ledger D,

p. 58, noted "debt forgiven as before;" Ledger F, p. 241) [account reportedly continued in Ledger H, which is missing, but the index to that ledger is extant, yet Robert is not listed] [Robert Morgan was a Revolutionary War veteran and a signer of the Bush Declaration on March 22, 1775.]; see Edward Lee, q.v.

Morgan, Rulough, was treated by Dr. John Archer in Feb 1791 (Ledger F, p. 205)

Morgan, Sarah, see Robert Morgan, q.v.

Morgan, Wakeman, was treated by Dr. Matthew J. Allen in Jun 1848 (p. 85)

Morgan, Widow, was visited by Dr. John Archer who inoculated 4 of her family in Jan 1776 (Ledger C, p. 18)

Morgan, William, see Edward Morgan, John Morgan, Robert Morgan and William Scotton, q.v.

Morgan, William [1744-1795], was visited by Dr. John Archer who treated his negroes in Oct 1772, him in Aug 1774, his family in Nov 1775, a negro boy "at widow Morgan's" in Feb 1776, a daughter in Apr 1778, him [William] in Jul, Aug, Sep and Nov 1780 and Apr and May 1781, his wife in Sep 1781, a negro in Feb 1782, a negro in Mar 1783, him [William] in May 1783, Negro Violet "obstetricand" [pregnant] on 12 Jul 1783, him [William] and a child in 1789 and him and daughter Cassy in 1795 (Ledger B, p. 60; Ledger C, p. 4; Ledger D, p. 85 [account continued in Ledger E, which is missing]; Ledger F, p. 1) [account continued in Ledger G, which is missing]; Ledger I, which is missing, but abstracted by Dr. George W. Archer circa 1890, noted Thomas Chew was his executor); Dr. George Archer's notes are in the Archives of the Historical Society of Harford County folder "Archer, G. W. Coll. – Ledgers and Day Books") [William Morgan was a Revolutionary War veteran and a signer of the Bush Declaration on March 22, 1775.]

Morrice, John, near J. Bond's, was treated by Dr. John Archer in Sep 1773 (Ledger B, p. 23)

Morris, Israel, was visited by Dr. John Archer who treated Miller (sic) in Mar 1782, him [Israel] in Apr, Jun, Jul and Nov 1782, an infant and Jacob Hayns in Feb 1783, his [Israel's] wife and a child in Jul 1784, son(?) in Oct 1784, and him [Israel] and daughter Sucky in Dec 1791 (Ledger D, p. 129, spelled his name Morriss [account continued in Ledger E, which is missing]; Ledger F, p. 203); see Mr. Cole, Nicholas Grossman and Negro Dick, q.v.

Morris, James, was visited by Dr. Matthew J. Allen who treated his son in Jul 1852 (p. 97, noted that the $2 medical bill was paid "by wife making 1 pr. pantaloons")

Morrice, John, see John Morris, q.v.

Morris, Sucky, see Israel Morris, q.v.

Morris, William, was treated by Dr. Robert H. Archer in Baltimore before 1822 [no dates or details were given] (Dr. Archer's "Alphabet to Ledger H" is his booklet [filed in the Archives of the Historical Society of Harford County] that contains his index to Ledger H [which is missing] for his patients in Baltimore before 1822 and Harford County after 1822, according to a notation by Dr. George W. Archer.)

Morrison, David, was visited by Dr. Alonzo Preston who treated his wife "in partu" [in childbirth] on 31 (sic) Nov 1826 and a child [unnamed] in Feb, May, Aug and Nov 1827 (pp. 78, 95, noted he was "insolvent and removed")

Morrison, Dougal, near Slate Ridge, was treated by Dr. John Archer in Jan 1775 (Ledger B, p. 60)

Morrison, George (Rev.), was treated by Dr. Robert H. Archer between 14 May and 14 Jul 1825 "in consultation with Drs. Davidge, Archer, Forwood and Wilson when shot by Smith" (and noted that Samuel E. Smith paid the medical bill in Feb 1826); Dr. Archer treated his [George's] wife in Jun 1824 in consultation with Dr. Forward and in Sep 1824; George was treated in Feb 1825 by Dr. Alonzo Preston who also treated his wife at times between 1823 and 1825 (Dr. Archer, pp. 98, 131-137, 140, 143; Ledger F, p. 89; Dr. Preston, p. 28) [Rev. George Morrison was shot by James Smith and the Harford County Criminal Court Docket, August Term, 1825, p. 172, indicated the case was sent for trial in Baltimore County.]

Morrison, Hannah, was inoculated by Dr. John Archer in Apr 1779 (Ledger C, p. 87, misspelled her first name as Hanna and noted "debt forgiven by order of testator")

Morsel, James, was treated by Dr. Jacob A. Preston in Aug 18— [page torn] and the bill was paid in Aug 1832 (Document filed in Historical Society of Harford County Archives folder titled "Preston, Dr. Jacob A.")

Mortimer, see William Brown, q.v.

Morton, Nathaniel, was prescribed medicine for his child by Dr. Robert H. Archer on 6 Aug and 18 Sep 1802 (Rx Book, 1802-1804, pp. 4, 9); he was treated by Dr. Robert H. Archer in Baltimore before 1822 [no dates or details given] (Dr. Archer's "Alphabet to Ledger H" is his booklet [filed in the Archives of the Historical Society of Harford County] that contains his index to Ledger H [which is missing] for his patients in Baltimore before 1822 and in Harford County after 1822, according to a notation by Dr. George W. Archer.)

Mosier, Mr., was prescribed medicine by Dr. Robert H. Archer on 18 Mar 1801 (Rx Book, 1796-1801, p. 49)

Moulton, John, was treated by Dr. John Archer in Mar 1787 (Ledger F, p. 220)

Mr. ---- [blank], son-in-law of Mrs. Laughrey, was visited by Dr. Robert H. Archer who treated a child in Aug 1823 (p. 89)

Muckelmurry, Mrs. (widow), was treated by Dr. John Archer in May 1781 (Ledger D, p. 22, noted "debt forgiven as before")

Mullen, Patrick, was treated by Dr. John Archer in Sep 1774 and May to Jul 1778 (Ledger B, p. 29; Ledger C, p. 110, spelled his name Mullein and noted "debt forgiven by order of testator") [Patrick Mullen was a Revolutionary War veteran.]

Mullen, William, at Patrick Hanlin's, was treated by Dr. John Archer in Aug 1778 (Ledger C, p. 119, spelled his name Mullein)

Mun, John, "brother-in-law to Whiteford," was treated by Dr. John Archer in 1788 (Ledger F, p. 331)

Munnikhuysen, Jacob, was treated by Dr. Robert H. Archer in Apr 1823 in consultation with Dr. Moores (p. 68; Ledger F, p. 4, listed him as J. Munichuysen)

Murdock, William [near] Sias Billingsley, Jr., was treated by Dr. John Archer in Jul and Aug 1779 (Ledger C, p. 54, noted "debt forgiven by order of testator")

Murphy, Henry, was visited by Dr. John Archer who treated his wife in Nov 1781, him in Jul and Aug 1782 and Feb and Mar 1783, and him, his wife and child in Oct 1789 (Ledger D, p. 93, had "Newtown" written after his name and noted "debt forgiven as before;" Ledger F, p. 306 did not)

Murphy, Timothy, was visited by Dr. John Archer who treated him and his wife in Jan 1787 (Ledger F, p. 306)

Murphy, William, was treated by Dr. John Archer in Jul 1787 (Ledger F, p. 193)

Murray, Alexander, was visited by Dr. John Archer who treated him and "Ellice Ellice" (by dressing his eye and ear) in Dec 1772, him [Alexander] in Jul 1780, Sep 1781, Sep 1785 ("hamorrhoid") and in Mar 1786 (Ledger B, p. 43; Ledger D, p. 76, noted "debt forgiven as before;" Ledger F, p. 56, spelled his name Murry)

Murray, James, was murdered in 1774: "Harford County to wit: The Jurors for the Right Honourable the Lord Proprietary that now is the body of Harford County upon their oath do present that Elizabeth Roberts of Harford County, spinster, not having the fear of God before her eyes but being moved and seduced by the instigation of the Devil on the Twenty seventh day of December in the year Seventeen hundred and Seventy four with force and arms at the County aforesaid in and upon one James Murry in the peace of God and of the Lord Proprietary then and there being feloniously and in the fury of her mind did make an assault and that the said Elizabeth Roberts with a certain drawn knife of the value of twenty pounds of tobaco *(sic)* which she the said Elizabeth Roberts in her right hand then and there had and held in and upon the right side of the belly near the short ribbs *(sic)* of him the said James Murry ---- [three sentences lined out and rewritten] ---- then and there in the fury of her mind feloniously did strike with the knife aforesaid in and upon the said right side --- [page torn] --- near the short ribs of him the said James Murry make a mortal wound of the bredth *(sic)* of one inch and depth of two inches which said mortal wound he the said James Murry instantly died. And the jurors foresaid upon their oath aforesaid do say that the said Elizabeth Roberts the *(sic)* said James Murry in manner and form aforesaid then and there feloniously and in the fury of her mind did kill and slay against the peace of said Lord Proprietor his good rules and government." (File 1.46.1 in the Court Records Department of the Historical Society of Harford County)

Murray, James (tailor), at White House [near Fallston], was treated by Dr. John Archer in 1797 (Ledger I, which is missing, was abstracted by Dr. George W. Archer circa 1890 and listed him as Jas. Murry; Dr. George W. Archer's notes are in Archives of the Historical Society of Harford County file "Archer, G. W. Coll. – Ledgers and Day Books")

Murray, John, was visited by Dr. John Archer who treated him in Aug 1781, his wife in Jan 1783 and him in Feb, Mar and May 1783 (Ledger D, p. 61) [continued in Ledger E, which is missing]

Myers, Henry, at Ring Factory [on Winters Run, west of Bel Air], was visited by Dr. Matthew J. Allen who treated his wife in Sep 1847, rendered obstetrical services on 31 Dec 1847 with Dr. E. Bond, and treated her for hemorrhoids in Jan 1848 (p. 65)

Myers, Jacob, was treated by Dr. Robert H. Archer in Sep 1815 (Ledger F, p. 2)

Myers, Mrs., was prescribed medicine by Dr. Robert H. Archer on 17 Aug 1802 and 2 Apr 1803 and medicine for her child on 19 Aug 1802 (Rx Book, 1802-1804, pp. 14, 15, 38)

Myres, Jacob, was treated by Dr. Robert H. Archer in Baltimore before 1822 [no dates or details] (Dr. Archer's "Alphabet to Ledger H" is his booklet [filed in the Archives of the Historical Society of Harford County] that contains his index to Ledger H [now missing] for his patients in Baltimore before 1822 and Harford County after 1822, according to a notation by Dr. George W. Archer.)

Myres, Philip, was treated by Dr. Robert H. Archer in Baltimore before 1822 [no dates or details were given] (Dr. Archer's "Alphabet to Ledger H" is his booklet [filed in the Archives of the Historical Society of Harford County] that contains his index to Ledger H [which is missing] for his patients in Baltimore before 1822 and Harford County after 1822, according to a notation by Dr. George W. Archer.)

Neal, Nancy, was visited by Dr. John Archer who treated her and children [no names were given] in Mar 1781 (Ledger D, p. 124, noted "debt forgiven as before")

Neal, Thomas, ---- by John [wording illegible due to stained page], was treated by Dr. John Archer in Mar and Apr 1781 (Ledger D, p. 128, noted "debt forgiven as before")

Negro ---- [blank], owned by Thomas Jeffery, was prescribed medicine by Dr. Robert H. Archer on 22 May 1796 (Rx Book, 1796-1801, p. 5)

Negro ---- [blank], belonging to Dr. Harris, was treated by Dr. Robert H. Archer in Baltimore before 1822 [no dates or details given] (Dr. Archer's "Alphabet to Ledger H" is his booklet [filed in the Archives of the Historical Society of Harford County] that contains his index to Ledger H [which is missing] for his patients in Baltimore City before 1822 and in Harford County after 1822, according to a notation by Dr. George W. Archer.)

Negro ---- [blank], near Gorsuch, was treated by Dr. Robert H. Archer in Baltimore before 1822 [no dates or details given] (Dr. Archer's "Alphabet to Ledger H" is his booklet [filed in the Archives of the Historical Society of Harford County] that contains his index to Ledger H [which is missing] for his patients in Baltimore before 1822 and Harford County after 1822, according to a notation by Dr. George W. Archer.)

Negro Abe, see Benedict Edward Hall, q.v.

Negro Abigail, at Capt. Sear's, B. Town [i. e., Bush Town or Harford Town], was treated by Dr. John Archer in 1786 and 1791 (Ledger F, pp. 160, 233)

Negro Abram's child died on 2 May 1846 ("True Book, 1845, 46, 47" filed in Archives of Historical Society of Harford County folder "Archer, Dr. Robert H., 1775-1857, Day Book, 1845-47") and Negro Abraham was visited by Dr. Matthew J. Allen who treated his wife in Jun 1848 (p; 88); see Abram Cooper, q.v.

Negro Adam, at C. H. Lee's Quarters, was treated by Dr. John Archer in Dec 1788 (Ledger F, p. 78)

Negro Amanda, was treated by Dr. Matthew J. Allen in Mar 1848 (tooth extraction) (p. 75)

Negro Amy, see George Davidson, q.v.

Negro Andrew, see Smith & Giles and John Forwood, of Jacob, q.v.

Negro Anne, see John Paca, q.v.

Negro Anny, see John Paca, q.v.

Negro Anthony, see John Paca, q.v.

Negro Antony, see Reed & Vanbibber, q.v.

Negro Aquilla, see William Woolsey, q.v.

Negro Archy, see Aquila Paca, q.v.

Negro Barney, see John Forwood, of Jacob, q.v.

Negro Beck, see George Gale, q.v.

Negro Beck, was prescribed medicine for her child by Dr. Robert H. Archer on 12 Mar 1803 (Rx Book, 1802-1804, p. 35)

Negro Belind or Belinda, see James Matthews, q.v.

Negro Ben, see Robert Morgan, George Gale, Ann Gale, Levin Gale, Nathaniel W. S. Hays and Negro Gamboe, q.v.

Negro Benjamin, see Negro Dundee, q.v.

Negro Betsey, see James Moores, q.v.

Negro Betsy, see Robert Morgan, q.v.

Negro Bett, see Aquila Paca, q.v.

Negro Betta, Josias hus [?], was treated by Dr. John Archer in Feb and Mar 1781 (Ledger D, p. 124, noted "visit & delivering" on 23 Feb 1781 and "debt forgiven as before")

Negro Betty, see Ignatius Matthews, Margaret Gale and Reed & Vanbibber, q.v.

Negro Bidy, see Edward Hall, q.v.

Negro Bill, see Robert Morgan and John Forwood, of Jacob, q.v.

Negro Bob, see Bob Howard, Jane Guyton, Thomas Huggins, Levin Gale, Samuel Lee and Reed & Vanbibber, q.v.

Negro Bob (painter), was treated by Dr. John Archer, Jr. in Dec 1816 (p. 44)

Negro Boyce, was treated by Dr. Robert H. Archer in Baltimore before 1822 [no dates or details were given] (Dr. Archer's "Alphabet to Ledger H" is his booklet [filed in the Archives of the Historical Society of Harford County] that contains his index to Ledger H [which is missing] for his patients in Baltimore before 1822 and Harford County after 1822, according to a notation by Dr. George W. Archer.)

Negro Cam, see John Forwood, of Jacob, q.v.

Negro Captain, see Reed & Vanbibber, q.v.

Negro Caroline, see John Dallam and Reed & Vanbibber, q.v.

Negro Cass, who belongs to Robert Bryerly, was treated by Dr. John Archer in Feb 1795 (Ledger F, p. 80); also spelled Cas, see John Forwood, of Jacob, q.v.

Negro Charles, was visited by Dr. John Archer, Jr. who treated him in Jun 1816 and Negro Richard in Aug 1816 (p. 56); see Nathaniel Chew, Reuben H. Davis, Joseph Parker, Edward Hall and James Amos, Jr., q.v.

Negro Charls *(sic)*, was treated by Dr. John Archer five times in Aug 1782 (Ledger D, p. 55, noted "debt forgiven as before")

Negro Charlotte, see Levin Gale, q.v.

Negro Clare, see John F. Wheeler, q.v.

Negro Cleniss, was visited by Dr. Alonzo Preston who treated his wife in Apr 1825 (p. 20)

Negro Cloe, see Aquila Paca and Isaac Pennington, q.v.

Negro Corbin, see Bennett Love, q.v.

Negro Cudger, see Thomas Hall, q.v.

Negro Cupid, see James White Hall, q.v.

Negro D., see Nathaniel Chew, q.v.

Negro Dan, see Cecil Furnace, q.v.

Negro Daniel, was treated by Dr. John Archer, Jr. in May 1815 and Jun 1816 (pp. 9, 34); see Mathew Cain, Thomas Huggins and T. Huggins & Co., q.v.

Negro Darby, see Archer Hays, q.v.

Negro Darcas, see Aquila Paca, q.v.

Negro David, freed by Isaac Webster, was treated by Dr. John Archer in Dec 1790 (Ledger F, p. 132)

Negro Davy, see Ignatius Matthews, Edward Hall and James White Hall, q.v.

Negro Deb, see Richard Wilmott, q.v.

Negro Dermest (Dermett?), see Ann Scott, q.v.

Negro Dick, at Freeborn Brown's, freed by Israel Morris, was treated by Dr. John Archer in Aug 1787 (Ledger F, p. 348)

Negro Dick, at Mount Felix, was visited by Dr. John Archer who treated him and his wife in Sep 1787 (Ledger F, p. 11)

Negro Dick, see Samuel Daugherty and George Davidson, q.v.

Negro Dina, see James White Hall, q.v.

Negro Dinah, "belongs to Robert Bryerly," was treated by Dr. John Archer in 1795 (Ledger F, p. 80)

Negro Dorsey, see Ann Gale, q.v.

Negro Duke, see Benedict Edward Hall, Betsey Lee and Amos Garrett, q.v.

Negro Duke, freed by Joseph Hopkins, was treated by Dr. John Archer in Apr 1796 (Ledger F, p. 122) [account continued in Ledger I, which is missing]

Negro Dundee, at Cumberland Forge, was visited by Dr. John Archer who treated him and son Benjamin in Dec 1790 (Ledger F, p. 126)

Negro Eli, see James White Hall, q.v.

Negro Elizabeth, see John Dallam, q.v.

Negro Emma, see Charlotte Cherry and Hannah Lee, q.v.

Negro Emmory, see Emmory Dead, q.v.

Negro Essex, see William Brown, q.v.

Negro Esther, see John Paca, q.v.

Negro Eveline, see Reed & Vanbibber, q.v.

Negro Fan, see Aquila Paca and John Paca, q.v.

Negro Faney, see Thomas Hall, q.v.

Negro Fanie, see Ann Gale, q.v.

Negro Fanny, see George Gale, q.v.

Negro Fanny, daughter of John, was treated by Dr. John Archer in Jul 1787 (Ledger F, p. 363)

Negro Flora, see Bennett Matthews, q.v.

Negro Forester, was treated by Dr. Matthew J. Allen in Mar 1845 (p. 45); see Parker Hall Lee, q.v.

Negro Frank, see Ephraim Litle, q.v.

Negro Gamboe, was murdered in 1793: "Harford County, State of Maryland. An inquisition taken this twentieth day of April in the year of our Lord one thousand Seven hundred and Ninety three before me Bennet Bussey one of the coroners for the County and State aforesaid on the land of Matthew Molton – over the body of a certain Negro Gamboe then and there lying dead by the oath of good and lawful men of the County and State aforesaid … who on their oaths do say that a certain Negro man named Ben not having the fear of God before his eyes on the nineteenth day of April in the year of our Lord seventeen hundred and ninety three in the County aforesaid, and then and there murder the said Negro Gamboe with a falling ax did strike giveing *(sic)* to the said Negro Gamboe one mortal wound of which said mortal wound the said Negro Gamboe then and there in less then one hour died and so the Jury aforesaid on their oaths do say that the said Negro Ben did murder the said Negro Gamboe aforesaid." (Court Records file 18.16(15) A in the Court Records Department of the Historical Society of Harford County)

Negro George, freed by Mrs. Husbands, was visited by Dr. John Archer who treated him and his son Ned in Jan 1791 (Ledger F, p. 180)

Negro George, see Philip Thomas, Henry Ruff, William Webb, John Paca, Nathaniel W. S. Hays and Aquila Hall, q.v.

Negro Georgeanne, see George Gale, q.v.

Negro Grace, see Robert Morgan and James Moores, q.v.

Negro Hagar, see Aquila Paca, Edward Hall and Richard Wilmott, q.v.

Negro Hagar, "belongs to Robert Bryerly," was treated by Dr. Archer in Feb 1795 (Ledger F, p. 80)

Negro Hagar, freed by William Talbott, was visited by Dr. John Archer who treated him and a child in Aug 1786 (Ledger F, p. 13)

Negro Hagar, was treated by Dr. John Archer in Apr 1788 (Ledger F, p. 301)

Negro Hannah, see John Paca, Mrs. Guyton, Robert Morgan, Nathaniel Hays and Edward Hall q.v.

Negro Harriet or Harriot, see Ann Bond, Ann Gale, James White Hall and Mrs. Greme, q.v.

Negro Harriet, was treated by Dr. Robert H. Archer in Oct 1822 (p. 28)

Negro Harrison, see Reed & Vanbibber, q.v.

Negro Harry, see John Paca, Daniel Richardson, Benedict Hall and Bennett Matthews, q.v.

Negro Harry, at J. Massey's, was treated by Dr. John Archer in Sep 1788 (Ledger F, p. 90)

Negro Harry, freed by Mrs. Richardson, was treated by Dr. John Archer in Apr 1789 and mentioned his son Jim (Ledger F, p. 295)

Negro Hector, see Robert Morgan, q.v.

Negro Heny, see John Cretin, q.v.

Negro Herman, see William McFadden, q.v.

Negro Hetty, see Nathaniel W. S. Hays, q.v.

Negro Horace, see Reed & Vanbibber, q.v.

Negro Isaac, see Aquila Paca and Philip Thomas, q.v.

Negro Isabella, near J. Moffit's, was visited by Dr. Matthew J. Allen who treated a child in Mar 1845 (p. 46)

Negro Jack, freed by Barnard Preston, was treated by Dr. John Archer in Oct 1787 (Ledger F, p. 303)

Negro Jack, see Margaret Gale and Ruthen Garretson, q.v.

Negro Jacob, see Freeborn Brown, Bennett Matthews, William Cox, Jr., Parker Hall Lee, Capt. John Hall and Thomas Hall, q.v.

Negro Jacob, "tanner by H. Watters," was visited by Dr. James Archer who treated him five times in Nov and Dec 1806 by "bleeding, blistering and various medicines" for typhus fever (p. 22)

Negro Jacob, freed by Col. Hall, was treated by Dr. John Archer in Sep 1786 (Ledger F, p. 308)

Negro Jacob, freed by Mrs. Cox, was treated by Dr. John Archer in Aug 1787 (Ledger F, p. 305)

Negro Jacob, was visited by Dr. Robert H. Archer who treated him and wife in July 1822 and May 1825, an unnamed free woman and a child named Si (pp. 8, 9, 131; Ledger F, p. 52)

Negro Jane, see Charlotte Preston and James W. Williams, q.v.

Negro Jeffry or Jeffrey, was treated by Dr. John Archer in Mar 1783 and Mar 1787 (Ledger D, p. 17, noted "debt forgiven as before;" Ledger F, p. 226); see James White Hall, q.v.

Negro Jehu, was visited by Dr. John Archer who treated him in Jun 1778, a child in Apr 1781 and negroes [no names given] in Jun 1781 (Ledger C, p. 94); see "Negroe Son: of Jehu," q.v.

Negro Jem, see James Matthews, q.v.

Negro Jene, see Archer Hays, q.v.

Negro Jenny, see Margaret Gale, q.v.

Negro Jerry, see James White Hall, q.v.

Negro Jesse, see Mrs. Isabella Hall, q.v.

Negro Jessee, was murdered in 1841: "State of Maryland, Harford County, to wit: An Inquisition taken at the house of Thomas W. Hall in the County and State aforesaid on the second day of September in the year of our Lord one thousand Eight Hundred and forty one before me Richard F. Hollis one of the Justices of the said State for the County aforesaid did upon the view of the body of Negro Jessee, the slave of Mary McComas, then and there lying dead upon the Oaths of … good and lawfull (sic) men of the County aforesaid who being sworn upon the Holly (sic) Evangely of Almighty God and charged to inquire when, where and how and after what manner the said Negro Jessee, the slave of Mary McComas, of said County came to his death do say upon there (sic) oaths that the said Negro Jessee, slave of Mary McComas, came to his death by a blow inflicted on the head by Negro Jacob, slave of George W. Hall. In witness whereof as well the aforesaid Justice of the Peace as the Jurors aforesaid have to this Inquisition put there hands and seals on the day and year aforesaid and at the place aforesaid. Richard F. Hollis, Justice of the Peace … Received and Recorded the 4th day of September 1841 in Liber H. D. No. 25, folio, 168, one of the Land Record Books of Harford County." ("Slavery Inquisitions" file in the Archives Department of the Historical Society of Harford County)

Negro Jim, freed by Philip Cole, was treated by Dr. John Archer in Oct 1788 (Ledger F, p. 279)

Negro Jim, see Nat Cooper (negro), Ann Scott, Negro Harry, James Matthews, Capt. John Hall, and Reed & Vanbibber, q.v.

Negro Jinny &ca (sic), was treated by Dr. Robert H. Archer in Baltimore before 1822 [no dates or details given] (Dr. Archer's "Alphabet to Ledger H" is his booklet [filed in the Archives of the Historical Society of Harford County] that contains his index to Ledger H [which is missing] for his patients in Baltimore before 1822 and Harford County after 1822, according to a notation by Dr. George W. Archer.); see George Gale, q.v.

Negro Jo or Joe, see Aquila Paca, Archer Hays, James Lee, Jr. and James White Hall, q.v.

Negro Joe, near Mount Felix, was visited by Dr. John Archer who treated him and his mother-in-law [name not given] in Aug 1788 (Ledger F, p. 4)

Negro John, see Mrs. Greme, William Albert, Negro Fanny, Negro Joshua, George Gale and Ann Gale, q.v.

Negro John &ca (sic), was treated by Dr. Robert H. Archer in Baltimore before 1822 [no dates or details were given] (Dr. Archer's "Alphabet to Ledger H" is his booklet [filed in the Archives of the Historical Society of Harford County] that contains his index to Ledger H [which is missing] for his patients in Baltimore before 1822 and Harford County after 1822, according to a notation by Dr. George W. Archer.)

Negro John, died in 1830: An inquisition taken at Joseph Trimble's farm on 7 Apr 1830 determined that "Negro John came to his death by intemperance and exposure in a very inclement night on the 25th March last." (Document in the Archives of the Historical Society of Harford County file "Inquisitions – Unknown Persons")

Negro Joseph, see Archer Hays, q.v.

Negro Joshua, see John Magness, q.v.

Negro Joshua, son of John, was treated by Dr. John Archer in Jan 1786 (Ledger F, p. 35)

Negro Juda, see Ann Gale, q.v.

Negro Jude, see Margaret Gale, q.v.

Negro Judie, see James W. Williams, q.v.

Negro June, see James W. Williams, q.v.

Negro Juniper, see Edward Hall, q.v.

Negro Juno, Frederick Street [Baltimore City], was prescribed medicine by Dr. Robert H. Archer on 3 Aug 1802 (Rx Book, 1802-1804, p. 7)

Negro Leah, see M. Gale, q.v.

Negro Little Mary, see Reed & Vanbibber, q.v.

Negro Lloyd, see Ann Gale, q.v.

Negro Louis, see Reed & Vanbibber, q.v.

Negro Louisa, see Henry Ruff, q.v.

Negro Lucy, see Edward Hall, q.v.

Negro Lyd, see Nathaniel Chew, q.v.

Negro Lydia, was treated by Dr. Robert H. Archer in Baltimore before 1822 [no dates or details were given] (Dr. Archer's "Alphabet to Ledger H" is his booklet [filed in the Archives of the Historical Society of Harford County] that contains his index to Ledger H [which is missing] for his patients in Baltimore before 1822 and Harford County after 1822, according to a notation by Dr. George W. Archer.)

Negro Mane(?), see John Forwood, of Jacob, q.v.

Negro Manuel, see Mrs. Isabella Hall, q.v.

Negro Margaret, freed by John Peacock, was treated by Dr. John Archer in May 1789 and mentioned her daughter in 1786 [name not given] in 1786 (Ledger F, p. 123)

Negro Margaret, was prescribed medicine by Dr. Robert H. Archer on 4 Aug 1802 (Rx Book, 1802-1804, p. 7)

Negro Marhea, see Negro Moll and Reed & Vanbibber, q.v.

Negro Maria, see Richard Lee, Isabella Hall, George Davidson, James White Hall and Jane Cain, q.v.

Negro Martin, see Reed & Vanbibber, q.v.

Negro Mary, see Robert Morgan and Reed & Vanbibber, q.v.

Negro Matilda, see Parker H. Lee, q.v.

Negro Mich, see Robert Morgan, q.v.

Negro Milcha, see James White Hall, q.v.

Negro Milley, see James W. Williams, q.v.

Negro Minerva, see Michael Gilbert and Reed & Vanbibber, q.v.

Negro Minta, see Jane Cain, q.v.

Negro Moll, "Marhea's daughter," was treated by Dr. John Archer in Jul 1782 (Ledger D, p. 15, noted "debt forgiven as before")

Negro Mortimer, see James White Hall, q.v.

Negro Nan, see Aquila Paca, q.v.

Negro Nance, see Edward Hall, q.v.

Negro Nancy, see Peggy Stump and Edward Hall, q.v.

Negro Nat, see William Brown, Patrick Cretin, and Cecil Furnace, q.v.

Negro Ned, freed by E. Barnes, was treated by Dr. John Archer in Feb 1789 (Ledger F, p. 317)

Negro Ned, see John Cavenaugh, Isaac Guyton, Negro George, James Lee Moores, Robert Morgan, James W. Williams, Isabella Hall and Mrs. Moores q.v.

Negro Neddy, see Thomas Hall, q.v.

Negro Nell, see James Lee, Jr., q.v.

Negro Nelly, see Henrietta Wheeler, q.v.

Negro Neoma, see John Forwood, of Jacob, q.v.

Negro Nero, at Mr. Keech's, was treated by Dr. Matthew J. Allen in Jul, Aug and Sep 1848 (p. 88)

Negro Newbury, was treated by Dr. Robert H. Archer in Baltimore before 1822 [no dates or details were given] (Dr. Archer's "Alphabet to Ledger H" is his booklet [filed in the Archives of the Historical Society of Harford County] that contains his index to Ledger H [which is missing] for his patients in Baltimore before 1822 and Harford County after 1822, according to a notation by Dr. George W. Archer.)

Negro Nicholas, see John Paca and George Gale, q.v.

Negro Ophelia, see Reed & Vanbibber, q.v.

Negro Orange, "belongs to William Smith," was treated by Dr. John Archer in Dec 1788 (Ledger F, p. 78); see John Henderson, q.v.

Negro Patience, "freed by Robert Hawkins, at Fany Jehu's," was treated by Dr. John Archer in Aug 1787 (Ledger F, p. 370)

Negro Patty, was prescribed medicine by Dr. Robert H. Archer on 12 Mar 1801 (Rx Book, 1796-1801, p. 46); Negro Patty &ca (sic), was treated by Dr. Archer in Baltimore before 1822 [no dates or details] (Dr. Archer's "Alphabet to Ledger H" is his booklet [filed in the Archives of the Historical Society of Harford County] that contains his index to Ledger H [which is missing] for his patients in Baltimore before 1822 and Harford County after 1822, according to a notation by Dr. George W. Archer.)

Negro Patty, see Archer Hays, q.v.

Negro Paul, belonging to John Patrick, was visited by Dr. John Archer who inoculated three children in Feb 1782 (Ledger D, p. 36, noted "debt forgiven as before")

Negro Peg, see Philip Thomas, q.v.

Negro Pegg, see James Moores, q.v.

Negro Perry, see Levin Gale, q.v.

Negro Peter, see Thomas Hall and James W. Williams, q.v.

Negro Peter, was treated by Dr. John Archer in May 1790 (Ledger F, p. 196)

Negro Phil, see Henry Chamberlaine, q.v.

Negro Phillip, see Edward Hall, q.v.

Negro Phillis, see James Phillips and Robert Morgan, q.v.

Negro Pie, see William Michael, q.v.

Negro Pliny, see Robert Morgan, q.v.

Negro Pol, see John Forwood, of Jacob, q.v.

Negro Polydore, near Coxes ferry, was treated by Dr. John Archer in Oct 1782 (Ledger D, p. 122, noted "debt forgiven as before"); An inquisition taken at Belle View, the farm of Dr. Elijah Davis, on 1 Jul 1818 determined that "Negro Polydore [the slave of Dr. Elijah Davis] came to his death by a wound in the head inflicted by a certain Aquila Ayres." (Document in the Archives of the Historical Society of Harford County file "Inquisitions – Unknown Persons")

Negro Pompey, freed by James Rigbie, was treated by Dr. John Archer in Mar 1788 (Ledger F, p. 11)

Negro Pompy (or Pompey), was murdered in 1825: "Maryland, Harford County: An Inquisition taken at Harfordtown in the County aforesaid on the 18th day of April 1825 before William Allen one of the Justices for said County acting as Coroner with the view of the body of Negro Pompy then & there lying dead upon the Oaths of … good & lawful (sic) [men] of Harford County aforesaid who being sworn on the Holy Evangells of Almighty God & affirmed and charged to inquire how & after what manner the said Pompy came to his death do say upon their Oaths & Affirmation that said Pompy came to his death by an inflamation (sic) of his bowels (sic) occationed (sic) by a severe kicking given him by Jem Hollond. In witness whereof as well the aforesaid Justice acting as Coroner as the Jurors aforesaid have to this Inquisition putt (sic) their hands & seals on the day & year aforesaid & at the place aforesaid. William Allen, Justice of the Peace acting as Coroner. Inquisition of Negro Pompey. Received and Recorded the sixth day of June Eighteen hundred and Twenty five in Liber H. D. No. 2, folio 197, one of the land record books of Harford County Court." ("Slavery Inquisitions" file in the Archives Department of the Historical Society of Harford County)

Negro Primus, was prescribed medicine for his wife by Dr. Robert H. Archer on 5 Sep 1796 (Rx Book, 1796-1801, p. 8)

Negro Priss, see Robert Morgan, q.v.

Negro Rache, see James W. Williams, q.v.

Negro Rachel, was treated by Dr. John Archer in Aug 1782 (Ledger D, p. 60, noted "debt forgiven as before")

Negro Rachel, freed by Jacob Giles, was treated by Dr. John Archer in Mar 1788 (Ledger F, p. 363)

Negro Rachel, see Black Rachel, James W. Williams, Garretson Archer (or Archer Garretson) and William Silver, q.v.

Negro Rebecca, was prescribed medicine by Dr. Robert H. Archer on 25 Nov 1804 (Rx Book, 1802-1804, p. 64)

Negro Rebecca, see George Gale, q.v.

Negro Richard, was treated by Dr. John Archer, Jr. in Jul 1815 (p. 19); see Levin Gale, Aquila Paca and Negro Charles, q.v.

Negro Riller, see Benedict Edward Hall, q.v.

Negro Robert, see Levin Gale and Reed & Vanbibber, q.v.

Negro Rock Run Tom, was treated by Dr. John Archer in Mar 1788 (Ledger F, p. 159)

Negro Roger, freed by Joseph Miller, was treated by Dr. John Archer in Mar 1790 (Ledger F, p. 144)

Negro Rose, was murdered in 1775: "Harford County, ss: An Inquisition … Taken at Col. Thomas White's Quarter in the County of Harford aforesaid the 8th day of March Seventeen hundred and Seventy five … View of the body of a negro girle (sic) named Rose belonging to a certain William McKanless of the County aforesaid then and there lying dead upon the Oath of good and lawful men of the County aforesaid who being Sworn and Charged to Enquire where, when and after what manner the said Negro girle *(sic)* Rose came to her Death do say upon their Oath that William McKanless, master of the said Negro girl Rose did Voluntarily of his own Mallace *(sic)* forethought *(sic)* beat her in the Head with the Butt end of a Waggon whipp and whipping her Sundry times with Hickory switches of which said Beating with the Wagon whip and the hickorys *(sic)* aforesaid the said William McKenless *(sic)* then & there feloniously give to the said Negro girle *(sic)* Rose she the said Negro girle *(sic)* Rose died on the fifth day of this Inst. So the said William McKenless then and their *(sic)* feloniously killed and murdered the said Negro girle *(sic)* Rose against the Peace of said Lord Proprietary his Good Rule & Government. In Witness Whereof as well the aforesaid Magistrates as the Jurors aforesaid have to this Inquisition Put their hands & Seals on the Day and year aforesaid and at the Place aforesaid." (Document 1.46.2 in the Court Records Department of the Historical Society of Harford County)

Negro Rose, see John Paca, q.v.

Negro Rumney, see Edward Hall, q.v.

Negro Rute, see Moses Ruth, Sr., q.v.

Negro Sal, see Freeborn Brown, Capt. John Hall and John Forwood, of Jacob, q.v.

Negro Sall, see Richard Wilmott and James Phillips, q.v.

Negro Sally, see George Gale, q.v.

Negro Sam, see Freeborn Brown, James Phillips, Paca Smith, Thomas Hall, Benedict Hall, Edward Hall, Nathaniel W. S. Hays and John Forwood, q.v.

Negro Sam, freed by Skipwith Coale, was treated by Dr. John Archer in Aug 1791 (Ledger F, p. 302)

Negro Sam, on James Walker's place, freed by Col. T. White, was treated by Dr. John Archer in 1790 (Ledger F, p. 145)

Negro Sam &ca *(sic)*, was treated by Dr. Robert H. Archer in Baltimore before 1822 [no dates or details were given] (Dr. Archer's "Alphabet to Ledger H" is his booklet [filed in the Archives of the Historical Society of Harford County] that contains his index to Ledger H [which is missing] for his patients in Baltimore before 1822 and Harford County after 1822, according to a notation by Dr. George W. Archer.)

Negro Samuel, see Elizabeth Bussey, q.v.

Negro Sarah, freed by William Scott at Mount Felix, was visited by Dr. John Archer who treated her and a child in Oct 1789 (Ledger F, p. 11)

Negro Scott, see Reed & Vanbibber, q.v.

Negro Sharlotte, see Reed & Vanbibber, q.v.

Negro Sharper, see Richard Dallam, q.v.

Negro Shelah, see William Webb, q.v.

Negro Si, see Negro Jacob, q.v.

Negro Simon &ca *(sic)*, was treated by Dr. Robert H. Archer in Baltimore before 1822 [no dates or details were given] (Dr. Archer's "Alphabet to Ledger H" is his booklet [filed in the Archives of the Historical Society of Harford County] that contains his index to Ledger H [which is missing] for his patients in Baltimore before 1822 and Harford County after 1822, according to a notation by Dr. George W. Archer.)

Negro Sin, see Robert Morgan, q.v.

Negro Sophia, see John Forwood, of Jacob, q.v.

Negro Spinner, see Edward Flanagan, q.v.

Negro Stephen, see John Cavenaugh, Parker Hall Lee and Peggy Stump, q.v.

Negro Suck, see John Paca, q.v.

Negro Sue, see John Paca, q.v.

Negro Susan, see Aquila Giles and Reed & Vanbibber, q.v.

Negro Tim, see Josias Bailey, q.v.

Negro Tom, see Aquila Paca, Margaret Gale, James White Hall and Reed & Vanbibber, q.v.

Negro Tony, see Enoch Churchman, q.v.

Negro Troilus, see Benedict Edward Hall, q.v.

Negro Tyrone, see George Steuart, q.v.

Negro Valentine, freed by Jacob Giles, was visited by Dr. John Archer who treated him in Apr 1791 and also inoculated a grandchild (Ledger F, p. 208)

Negro Violet, was prescribed medicine by Dr. Robert H. Archer circa Dec 1804 (Rx Book, 1802-1804, p. 67)

Negro Wash, see Mrs. Brown, q.v.

Negro Welton, see John Forwood, of Jacob, q.v.

Negro Wesley, see Nathaniel W. S. Hays, q.v.

Negro Will, freed by Nat. Johns, was treated by Dr. John Archer in Apr 1788 (Ledger F, p. 8)

Negro Will, was treated by Dr. John Archer as noted in John Scarff's acct. in 1792 (Ledger F, p. 262)

Negro William, see George Davidson, q.v.

"Negroe Son: of Jehu," was treated by Dr. John Archer in Jul and Sep 1780 (Ledger D, p. 77, noted "debt forgiven as before")

Neil, Henry (weaver), at Philip Quinlan's, was treated by Dr. J. Archer in Jun 1786 (Ledger F, p. 319)

Neile, Francis (doctor), was treated by Dr. John Archer in Mar 1798 (Ledger F, p. 143)

Neilson, Joseph, at Ring Factory [on Winters Run, west of Bel Air], was visited by Dr. Matthew J. Allen who treated his wife in Apr, May, Jul, Aug and Sep 1848 (p. 81)

Nelson, John, son-in-law to H. Vansickle, was treated by Dr. John Archer in Oct 1789 (Ledger F, p. 206) [account continued in Ledger G, which is missing]

Nesbitt, Robert (schoolmaster), was visited by Dr. John Archer who treated daughters Caroline and Charlotte and "scholars Merrican and (probably) Killan" between 1794 and 1799 [dates were not given]; Robert was prescribed medicine by Dr. Robert H. Archer on 8 May 1796 and for his brother [name not given] on 14 Aug 1802 (Rx Book, 1796-1801, p. 4; Rx Book, 1802-1804, p. 12; Ledger I, which is missing, was abstracted by Dr. George W. Archer circa 1890; his notes are in the Archives of the Historical Society of Harford County folder "Archer, G. W. Coll. – Ledgers and Day Books")

Nevill, Cassandra, Mrs., was treated by Dr. Robert H. Archer in Apr 1824 (p. 102; p. 103 spelled her name Neville)

Nevill, John [1787-1861], was treated by Dr. Robert H. Archer in Oct 1822 in consultation with Dr. Worthington; Mr. Nevill, at Elberton [near Darlington] and Rigdon (sic) were treated in Aug 1823 (pp. 28, 32, 89; Ledger F, p. 97) [John Nevill was a War of 1812 veteran.]

Nevill, Mrs., see Mr. Jones and William Nevill, q.v.

Nevill, Simon, near William Ashmore's, was treated by Dr. John Archer in Feb 1788 (Ledger F, p. 159, spelled his name Nevil)

Nevill, William [1783-1822], near Dublin, was treated twice by Dr. Robert H. Archer in Oct 1822; Mrs. Nevill, widow of William, paid the $6.27 account in full on 21 May 1824 (pp. 26, 30, 32, 106; Ledger F, p. 95) [William Nevill or Neville was a War of 1812 veteran.]

Newberry, Joseph, was visited by Dr. John Archer who treated him and a child in Aug 1789 (Ledger F, p. 377)

Nichols, ---- [blank], L.L.D., was treated by Dr. John Archer in Aug 1798 (Ledger I, which is missing, was abstracted by Dr. George W. Archer circa 1890; his notes are in the Archives of the Historical Society of Harford County folder "Archer, G. W. Coll. – Ledgers and Day Books")

Nicholson, Mary, was prescribed medicine for a child on 16 Mar 1803 by Dr. Robert H. Archer (Rx Book, 1802-1804, p. 36)

Nicholson, Mrs., was prescribed medicine by Dr. Robert H. Archer on 6 Mar 1801 (Rx Book, 1796-1801, p. 40)

Nickle, J., see John G. Allen, q.v.

Nickleson, James, near Widow Stinson, was visited by Dr. John Archer who treated him and child in Feb 1791 (Ledger F, p. 119)

Nicoll, Warren L., see Thomas Jenkins, q.v.

Nindes, Isaac, see William Lawrence, q.v.

Norris, Alexander, was visited by Dr. John Archer who treated him in Mar and Apr 1780 and sister Sucky in Aug 1782 (Ledger D, p. 55) [account continued in Ledger E, which is missing]

Norris, Amanda, see Sophia Norris, q.v.

Norris, Amelia, see Elizabeth Norris, q.v.

Norris, Aquila [1754-1825], was prescribed medicine for his wife on 6 Jun 1803 by Dr. Robert H. Archer (Rx Book, 1802-1804, p. 43) and he was treated by Dr. Archer in Baltimore before 1822 [no dates or details were given] (Dr. Archer's "Alphabet to Ledger H" is his booklet [filed in the Archives of the Historical Society of Harford County] that contains his index to Ledger H [which is missing] for his patients in Baltimore before 1822 and Harford County after 1822, according to a note by Dr. George W. Archer.) [Aquila Norris, of Edward, was a Revolutionary War veteran.]

Norris, Benjamin, was treated by Dr. John Archer in Oct 1781 and noted that his brother was his security (Ledger D, p. 82, noted "debt forgiven as before"); see John Norris, q.v.

Norris, Benjamin, was visited by Dr. John Archer who treated an infant in May 1781 and him in Oct 1781, Apr 1782 and Sep 1783; his account also mentioned Benjamin's "assumption of father's account" in Apr 1776 (Ledger C, p. 44)

Norris, Benjamin, was prescribed medicine for his child by Dr. Robert H. Archer on 8 Jul 1803 (Rx Book, 1802-1804, p. 49)

Norris, Benjamin (tavern keeper), in Bel Air, was visited by Dr. John Archer who treated him, his wife and children in 1787 (Ledger F, p. 44. indicated he was "poor and died insolvent")

Norris, Benjamin B. [1745-1790], was visited by Dr. John Archer who treated him and a child in 1788 (Ledger F, p. 332) [Benjamin Bradford Norris was a Revolutionary War veteran and a signer of the Bush Declaration on March 22, 1775.]; see Elizabeth Norris and John Moorn, q.v.

Norris, Betsey, see John Norris (tanner), q.v.

Norris, Col., see John Reese, q.v.

Norris, Daniel [1728-1804], was treated by Dr. John Archer in Aug 1796 (Ledger F, p. 190) [Daniel Norris was a Revolutionary War veteran.]

Norris, Dr., see Henry Smith, q.v.

Norris, E., Miss, see William Wann, Jr., q.v.

Norris, Edward, was prescribed medicine by Dr. Robert H. Archer on 7 Oct 1802 (Rx Book, 1802-1804, p. 6)

Norris, Elizabeth, widow of B. B., [Benjamin Bradford Norris], was visited by Dr. John Archer who treated her and daughter "Mille" [Milly, i.e, Amelia] and son Bradford [Benjamin Bradford, Jr.] at various times between 1796 and 1799 (Ledger I, which is missing, was abstracted by Dr. George W. Archer circa 1890; his notes are in the Archives of the Historical Society of Harford County folder "Archer, G. W. Coll. – Ledgers and Day Books")

Norris, Elizabeth, was prescribed medicine for her child by Dr. Robert H. Archer on 14 Aug 1802 and 16 Aug 1802 (Rx Book, 1802-1804, pp. 13, 14)

Norris, George A., was treated by Dr. Robert H. Archer twenty-nine times between 20 May 1828 and 22 Jul 1828 at which time the doctor noted he was "moribund" [i. e., near death] (pp. 276-286)

Norris, Jacob [1753-1807], in Belle Aire [Bel Air], was visited by Dr. John Archer who treated him, his wife and daughter Sophia in Mar 1792 (Ledger F) [account continued in Ledger H, which is missing] [Jacob Norris was a Revolutionary War veteran.]

Norris, James, "on the Mountain" [an area between Joppa-Magnolia and Fallston near Mountain Christian Church], was treated by Dr. John Archer in Oct 1780 and Mar 1783 (Ledger D, p. 101, noted "debt forgiven as before") [James Norris, of James, was a Revolutionary War veteran.]; see Sarah Norris, q.v.

Norris, John, was visited by Dr. John Archer who treated his brother Benjamin in Mar 1778 and him [John] in Oct 1778 (Ledger C, p. 40)

Norris, John (cooper), in Harford Town, was treated by Dr. John Archer in 1781 (Ledger F, p. 20)

Norris, John (tanner), son of John, was visited by Dr. John Archer who treated him in 1789 and him and daughter Betsey at times between 1795 and 1797 (Ledger F [account continued in Ledger H which is missing]; Ledger I, which is missing, was abstracted by Dr. George W. Archer circa 1890; his notes are in the Archives of the Historical Society of Harford County file "Archer, G. W. Coll. – Ledgers and Day Books") [John Norris, of John, was a Revolutionary War veteran.]

Norris, John C., see Robert Sanders (Saunders), q.v.

Norris, Joseph, was treated by Dr. John Archer in Jan 1774 and Jun 1775 (Ledger B, p. 62)

Norris, Lloyd [1779-1804], was treated by Dr. Robert H. Archer in Baltimore before 1822 [no dates or details were given] (Dr. Archer's "Alphabet to Ledger H" is his booklet [filed in the Archives of the Historical Society of Harford County] that contains his index to Ledger H [which is missing] for his patients in Baltimore before 1822 and Harford County after 1822, according to a notation by Dr. George W. Archer.)

Norris, Luther, see Ruthen Garretson, q.v.

Norris, Luther A., was visited by Dr. Alonzo Preston who treated him at times between 1823 and 1825 and Julius and a black girl and Mrs. K. and a child and A. Calwell in 1825; Luther Norris paid part of his medical bill with a silver watch worth $10.50 and also paid $1.00 cash for opium; Henry Preston paid $5.00 in his behalf (pp. 7, 8) [His full name was Luther Augustus Norris.]

Norris, Mille or Milly, see Elizabeth Norris, q.v.

Norris, Mrs. (widow), was treated by Dr. Robert H. Archer in Baltimore before 1822 [no dates or details given] (Dr. Archer's "Alphabet to Ledger H" is his booklet [filed in the Archives of the Historical Society of Harford County] that contains his index to Ledger H [which is missing] for his patients in Baltimore before 1822 and Harford County after 1822, according to a notation by Dr. George W. Archer.)

Norris, Otho [c1790-1829], was visited by Dr. Alonzo Preston who treated him at various times between 1823 and 1825 [no details were given], his wife "in partu" [in childbirth] on 23 Oct 1825 and a black woman also in 1825 (pp. 33, 53) [Otho Norris was a War of 1812 veteran who served in the U. S. Navy and was lost at sea aboard the USS Hornet in 1829]

Norris, Robert, was treated by Dr. Matthew J. Allen in Aug and Sep 1847 (p. 63)

Norris, Sarah, at James Norris' near the Black Horse, Baltimore Co., was treated by Dr. John Archer in May 1780 (Ledger D, p. 65, noted "debt forgiven as before")

Norris, Sophia, was visited by Dr. Alonzo Preston who treated her in 1825 and daughter Amanda fifteen times from 15 Jul to 30 Jul 1825 (p. 14, noted that the medical bill of $29.00 was paid in full by William Norris, of Baltimore, and initialed "WBB") [referring to Dr. William B. Bond]; see Jacob Norris, q.v.

Norris, Sucky, see Alexander Norris, q.v.

Norris, Susanna (widow), was treated by Dr. John Archer circa 1776 [date illegible] (Ledger C, p. 40)

Norris, Thomas [1756-1818], was treated by Dr. John Archer in Jan 1781 (Ledger D, p. 114, noted "debt forgiven as before") [Thomas Norris was a Revolutionary War veteran.]

Norris, William [1749-1837], was treated by Dr. John Archer in Aug and Oct 1778 and Aug 1779 and him, his wife and a child in 1792 (Ledger C, p. 103; Ledger F, p. 27) [William Norris was a Revolutionary War veteran.]

Norton, Stephen, was treated by Dr. John Archer in Sep 1781 (Ledger D, p. 81, noted "debt forgiven as before")

Nully, John, was treated by Dr. Thomas Archer at various times before Dec 1804 as noted in a complaint filed by the doctor who stated, in part, that "as a physician … performed and bestowed in and about the visiting of prescribing and furnishing and physic to and for the said John … labouring and languishing under divers diseases, maladies and disorders ..." and he had not been paid for his services. (Court Records File 39.24.4C at the Historical Society of Harford County)

Nutterwell, Daniel, was visited by Dr. John Archer who treated him in Dec 1776, Jan 1777, Jun 1779, Aug 1780, Apr and Aug 1781 and Mar and Apr 1782 and his wife in Mar 1782 (Ledger C, p. 77, spelled his name Nutawell and noted he had paid part with the balance of "debt forgiven by order of testator"); Ledger D, p. 6, noted "debt forgiven as before") [account continued in Ledger E, which is missing] [Daniel Nutterwell was a Revolutionary War veteran.]

Nutterwell, Minta, was treated by Dr. John Archer in March 1786 (Ledger F, p. 258, spelled her name Nutawell)

O'Daniel, Edward, see John O'Daniel, q.v.

O'Daniel, John, was visited by Dr. Robert H. Archer who treated him and his wife in Sep 1822 in consultation with Dr. Preston and treated a child in May 1823 and a child in Jan 1826 in consultation with Dr. Preston; John was also treated at times between 1821 and 1825 by Dr. Alonzo Preston who treated his family [no names were given] twice in 1825 and Edward O'Daniel four times; John was also prescribed medicine for a child by Dr. Robert H. Archer on 17 Dec 1825 (Dr. Preston, p. 55, spelled his name O'Dannel; Dr. Archer, pp. 19, 75, 174, Ledger F, p. 79; Archer's Rx Book, 1825-1851, p. 85)

O'Donal, James, at Widow Baker's, was treated by Dr. John Archer in 1786 (Ledger F, p. 70)

O'Donnal, Constus, was treated by Dr. John Archer in 1789 and his security was Martin Baker (Ledger F, p. 245)

O'Hara, Kane, was treated by Dr. John Archer in Feb 1773 (Ledger B, p. 85)

O'Neil, Henry, was treated by Dr. Robert H. Archer in Baltimore before 1822 [no dates or details were given] (Dr. Archer's "Alphabet to Ledger H" is his booklet [filed in the Archives of the Historical Society of Harford County] that contains his index to Ledger H [which is missing] for his patients in Baltimore before 1822 and Harford County after 1822, according to a notation by Dr. George W. Archer.)

O'Neill, Henry (butcher), at Darlington, was prescribed medicine for his wife by Dr. Robert H. Archer on 26 Jul 1799 and his child on 24 Oct 1799, and visited by Dr. Archer who treated his child in Jan 1824 in consultation with Dr. Worthington and also in Mar 1824, his wife in Aug 1824 and him in Sep 1825 (pp. 97, 101, 160; Ledger F, p. 85; Rx Book, 1796-1801, pp. 24, 26)

O'Neill, John (tailor), was treated by Dr. John Archer on 14 Jul 1773 (Ledger B, p. 97, listed him as "John O'Neile, taylor")

O'Neill, John [1768-1838], "at ferry" [referring to Lower Ferry, now Havre de Grace], was treated by Dr. John Archer, Jr. in Nov 1817 (p. 79) [John O'Neill was a War of 1812 veteran.]

Ogle, Charles, "at the Canal" [i. e., Tidewater Canal that ran parallel to the Susquehanna River from Havre de Grace north into Pennsylvania], was treated by Dr. John Archer in Dec 1787 and also mentioned his housekeeper [name not given] and Jacob Cuddy (Ledger F, p. 337)

Oliver, James, "near Spesutia" [i. e., St. George's (Old Spesutia) Episcopal Church in Perryman], was treated by Dr. John Archer in Mar 1786 (Ledger F, p. 126); see Charles Thompson, q.v.

Omel, Isaac (carpenter), was treated by Dr. John Archer in Mar 1774 (Ledger B, p. 99)

Onion, Thomas, see William Green, q.v.

Orr, Thomas &ca (sic), was treated by Dr. Robert H. Archer in Baltimore before 1822 [no dates or details were given] (Dr. Archer's "Alphabet to Ledger H" is his booklet [filed in the Archives of the Historical Society of Harford County] that contains his index to Ledger H [which is missing] for his patients in Baltimore before 1822 and Harford County after 1822, according to a notation by Dr. George W. Archer.)

Orrick, Charles, was treated by Dr. Robert H. Archer in Baltimore before 1822 [no dates or details were given] (Dr. Archer's "Alphabet to Ledger H" is his booklet [filed in the Archives of the Historical Society of Harford County] that contains his index to Ledger H [which is missing] for his patients in Baltimore before 1822 and Harford County after 1822, according to a notation by Dr. George W. Archer.)

Osborn, see Osburn, q.v.

Osborn, Amos S., "near Log meeting," was visited by Dr. Robert H. Archer who treated his wife "in partu" [in childbirth] on 6 May 1827 and rendered obstetrical services on 8 May 1827 (p. 224)

Osborn, Benjamin, was visited by Dr. John Archer who treated him in Apr 1781, his wife in Aug 1795 in consultation with Dr. Lee, his wife in Dec 1785, and him, his wife and infant in Jul 1788 (Ledger D, p. 15, spelled his name Osburn and transferred the account to Ledger F, p. 43, where he spelled the name Osborn) [account continued in Ledger G, which is missing] [Benjamin Osborn was a Revolutionary War veteran.]

Osborn, Cyrus, experienced mental issues before 12 Mar 1818 when Chief Judge Walter Dorsey ordered the following, in part: "Whereas Edward Courtney, administrator of Jonas Courtney, by his petition to the Judges of Harford County Court, hath stated that Cyrus Osborn of said county has been for some time past of an unsound mind (often insane with lucid intervals) that he has a title in fee to a valuable real and personal property which without the interposition of the said Court must go to loss and ruin, as he is from mental disarrangement wholly incompetent to manage the property or to take care of same." The Judge ordered that Cyrus Osborn be examined by twelve good and lawful men and inquire of his state of mind. On 29 May 1818 Dr. Jacob A. Preston led the inquisition which made this determination: "That we have attentively heard the testimony of Clark Hollis, James White and Sarah Osborn (the wife of the said Cyrus Osborn) as witnesses sworn before us and have examined also the said Cyrus Osborn in person and confidently believe him to be incapable from mental insanity of taking care either of himself or his property." (Court Records file 60.06.11 in the Historical Society of Harford County)

Osborn, Frances, Miss, was visited by Dr. Robert H. Archer who treated her at times between 25 Jul 1822 and 1 Aug 1822 and also treated niece Dever (sic) in July 1822 (p. 10; Ledger F, p. 57)

Osborn, James, see James Osburn, q.v.

Osborn, Miss, see Mr. Hollis, q.v.

Osborn, S., see Michael Scott, q.v.

Osborn, Samuel G. [1752-c1794], was treated by Dr. John Archer in Apr 1782 (Ledger D, p. 126, listed him as Samuel G. Osburn and noted "debt forgiven as before") [Samuel Groome Osborn was a Revolutionary War veteran.]

Osborn, Sangster(?), see William Osborn, q.v.

Osborn, Sarah, see Cyrus Osborn, q.v.

Osborn, William, at B. R. Neck [Bush River Neck], was visited by Dr. John Archer who treated him and his children in 1788, but only named one person, Sangster(?) [unclear] (Ledger F, p. 376) [account continued in Ledger G, which is missing] [William Osborn and William Osbourn were both Revolutionary War veterans.]

Osborne, James, was visited by Dr. John Archer who treated him and his wife in 1790 (Ledger F, p. 22) [account continued in Ledger H, which is missing]

Osborne, Mr., was prescribed medicine for his child on 4 Feb 1801 by Dr. Robert H. Archer (Rx Book, 1796-1801, p. 32)

Osborne, William, was prescribed medicine by Dr. Robert H. Archer on 22 Feb 1803 (Rx Book, 1802-1804, p. 33); he was treated by Dr. Robert H. Archer in Baltimore before 1822 [no dates or details were given] (Dr. Archer's "Alphabet to Ledger H" is his booklet [filed in the Archives of the Historical Society of Harford County] that contains his index to Ledger H [which is missing] for his patients in Baltimore before 1822 and Harford County after 1822, according to a notation by Dr. George W. Archer.)

Osburn, Benjamin, see Benjamin Osborn, q.v.

Osburn, James, was treated by Dr. John Archer in Aug 1779 (Ledger D, p. 5)

Osburn, James, Sr., was treated by Dr. John Archer in Nov 1779 and Feb 1784 (Ledger D, p. 34)

Otly, John, was treated by Dr. John Archer in Jul and Sep 1780 (Ledger D, p. 81, noted "debt forgiven as before")

Owens, Benjamin, deceased, Cecil Co., was noted by Dr. Robert H. Archer as having been paid $10 cash by his widow on 30 Sep 1823 and the balance was forgiven; Benjamin and his wife were treated by Dr. John Archer, Jr. in Mar 1817, son Samuel in Feb 1819, an unnamed child in Dec 1819, and wife in Sep 1820; Dr. Robert H. Archer treated son Samuel and daughters Sally and Hannah in 1822 (Dr. John Archer, Jr. p. 94; Dr. Robert H. Archer, Ledger F, p. 32); see Thomas Huggins & Co., q.v.

Owens, Edward, was treated by Dr. Robert H. Archer in Baltimore before 1822 [no dates or details were given] (Dr. Archer's "Alphabet to Ledger H" is his booklet [filed in the Archives of the Historical Society of Harford County] that contains his index to Ledger H [which is missing] for his patients in Baltimore before 1822 and Harford County after 1822, according to a notation by Dr. George W. Archer.)

Owens, Hannah, see Benjamin Owens, q.v.

Owens, John, was prescribed medicine for his child by Dr. Robert H. Archer on 19 Mar 1803 (Rx Book, 1802-1804, p. 36)

Owens, John (captain), was visited by Dr. John Archer, Jr. who treated his wife in Sep 1815 and Oct 1820 and a child in Oct 1820 (p. 27)

Owens, M., Miss, was prescribed medicine by Dr. Robert H. Archer circa Dec 1804 (Rx Book, 1802-1804, p. 68)

Owens, Sally, see Benjamin Owens, q.v.

Owens, Samuel, see Benjamin Owens, q.v.

Owings, Mrs., in Abingdon, was visited by Dr. John Archer who treated her and a daughter in 1789 (Ledger F, p. 134)

Paca, Aquila [1738-1788] (esquire), was visited by Dr. John Archer who treated him at times between 1772 and July 1775, a negro wench, a man, a boy and Negro Darcas in 1772, a negro child, a stepson, a son, Negro Cloe, a negro [unnamed], Negro Archy, and James Jones in 1773, an infant and Negro Cloe in Jan 1774, Negro Fan in Apr and Jun 1774, Negro Sam in Aug 1774, Negro Rich or Richard in Aug 1774, a negro at Otter Point Quarter, Negro Isaac and Negro Nan in Oct 1774, Negro Tom and Negro Nan in Nov 1774, Negro Jo and Negro Hagar in Dec 1774, J. Hagg and William Phrisby in Feb 1775, Billy Paca in May 1775, William Paca in Jun 1775, a negro in Feb 1776, Negro Rich and Negro Hagar in Jan 1777, a negro wench in Apr 1777, him [Aquila] in Jul 1778, Paul Shields in Aug 1778, him [Aquila] in Sep 1778, a negro in May 1779, a negro in Jul 1779, him [Aquila] in Oct 1779, a negro in Aug 1780, him [Aquila] in Oct 1780 and Feb 1781, a negro in Jan 1782, Aug 1783 and Oct 1784, inoculated Negro Bett in Oct 1784 and treated him [Aquila] in Feb 1788 in consultation with Dr. Hall [Aquila died later that month]; his account further mentioned that £15 was paid "to boarding your stepson Mr. William Prisby (sic) 1 year" [no date was given] and noted that a significant part of Aquila Paca's medical bill (over £165) was paid by William Paca's bond (Ledger B, pp. 63, 71, 76, 78, 79; Ledger C, p. 23; Ledger D, pp. 29, 71, 77) [Aquila Paca was a Revolutionary War veteran and a signer of the Bush Declaration on March 22, 1775.]; see James Phillips, q.v.

Paca, Aquila, Jr., was visited by Dr. John Archer who treated his brother James Paca in Nov 1780, Mar 1781 and May 1782 and him in Jan and Feb 1783 (Ledger D, p. 105) [account continued in Ledger E, which is missing] [Aquila Paca, Jr. was a Revolutionary War veteran.]

Paca, Billy, see Aquila Paca, q.v.

Paca, James, see Aquila Paca, Jr., q.v.

Paca, James [1754-1828], was treated by Dr. John Archer in Oct 1781 (Ledger D, p. 78, noted "debt forgiven as before" and later noted the bill was paid in cash by William Wilson on 21 Oct 1801) [James Paca was a Revolutionary War veteran.]

Paca, John [1712-1786] (captain and esquire), was visited by Dr. John Archer who treated negroes George and Anne in Apr 1773, Nicholas in Sep 1773, Suck and Hannah in Apr 1774, infant Sue in May 1774, Esther in

Sep 1774, an infant in Mar 1775, Negro Rose and a negro child in Mar 1777, a negro child in Apr 1777, Anny in May 1777, old Negro Fan and her child and Anthony and young Fan and a negro child and Hannah in July 1777, Miss Molly [daughter] and a negro infant in Sep 1777, Negro Harry and Negro Esther in Dec 1777, Negro Hannah in Jan 1778, and him [John] in Sep and Dec 1778, Jan 1779, Aug 1781 (in consultation with Dr. Henderson) and Jun and Dec 1782 (Ledger B, pp. 64, 89; Ledger C, p. 88) [account continued in Ledger E, which is missing] [John Paca was a militia captain in 1735 and a Revolutionary War patriot in 1778; his son William Paca was a Signer of the Declaration of Independence on July 4, 1776.]

Paca, Molly, see John Paca, q.v.

Paca, William, see Aquila Paca and John Paca, q.v.

Paca, William, was visited by Dr. Matthew J. Allen who rendered obstetrical services to his wife on 14 Dec 1847 and treated a child in Jan and Feb 1848, his wife in Feb, Apr, Mary and Jun 1848, a child and him [William] in Jun 1848 and a child in Sep and Oct 1848 (pp. 69, 94) [The following statement was written on a separate page dated 24 Nov 1853 that was inserted in the back of Dr. Allen's ledger. The letter, addressed to Major Bond, was signed by I. Day and stated "I have just returned after 3 days ride to look up the Drs. of Dr. Allen and the following is the result." It mentioned several patients, including this one: "Wm. Peaca (sic) says he won't pay all the judgt. I have directed him to call on you to settle which he promises to do."]

Pace, Jane, see Harford County for Pensioners, q.v.

Palmer, Samuel, at Morgan's Mill on Broad Creek, was visited by Dr. John Archer who treated a child in May 1785 (Ledger D, p. 19, noted "debt forgiven as before")

Pannell, Edward, was visited by Dr. Robert H. Archer who treated his wife and rendered obstetrical services [childbirth] in the night of 22 Oct 1822 (p. 31, spelled his name Pannel)

Pannell, Emily, see James Pannell, q.v.

Pannell, James [1784-1864], was visited by Dr. Robert H. Archer who treated his wife in Oct 1822, daughter Sarah ten times in Sep and Oct 1823 and in Dec 1824 and Sep and Oct 1825, his wife in Dec 1824 and Sep 1825, a child in Aug 1825, daughter Emily three times in Jul 1825 and Sep 1825, son James in Sep 1825, wife in Apr 1827, George Glasgow in May 1827 and Aug 1828, daughter Eliza four times in Nov 1827, daughter Sarah eight times between 14 Feb and 1 Mar 1828 and in May 1828, and D. Glasgow and daughter Jane Pannell in Aug 1828 (pp. 91-96, 124, 139, 153, 157, 226, 252, 253, 254, 263, 264, 265, 275, 292, 294; Ledger F, p. 109; Dr. Robert H. Archer's "Alphabet to Ledger H" is his booklet [filed in the Archives of the Historical Society of Harford County] that contains his index to Ledger H [which is missing] for his patients [no dates or details given] in Baltimore before 1822 and Harford County after 1822, according to a notation by Dr. George W. Archer.); see Elizabeth Glasgow, q.v.

Pannell, Jane, see James Pannell, q.v.

Pannell, Sarah, see James Pannell, q.v.

Park, Mrs. (widow), near John Whiteford in the Barrens [an area in the northwest part of the county near Pennsylvania], was treated by Dr. John Archer in Jan 1791 (Ledger F, p. 273)

Parker, Edward, near Upper Cross Roads, was treated by Dr. J. Archer in Feb 1787 (Ledger F, p. 47)

Parker, Eliza, see Robert Parker, q.v.

Parker, Hetty, see Joseph Parker, q.v.

Parker, John, was visited by Dr. John Archer who treated him in Apr 1780 and Aug and Sep 1781 and his wife in May and Jul 1783 (Ledger D, p. 60, noted "debt forgiven as before")

Parker, John, Mrs., see Ephraim Litle, q.v.

Parker, Joseph, was visited by Dr. Robert H. Archer who treated daughters Hetty and Mary in June 1825 in consultation with Dr. Forwood, him [Joseph] at various times from July to Sep 1825, Negro Charles at times from July to Nov 1825, and daughter Hetty in May 1826 (pp. 138, 142, 149, 153, 168, 187; Ledger F, p. 134)

Parker, Mary, see Joseph Parker, q.v.

Parker, Mrs. &ca (sic), was treated by Dr. Robert H. Archer in Baltimore before 1822 [no dates or details were given] (Dr. Archer's "Alphabet to Ledger H" is his booklet [filed in the Archives of the Historical Society of Harford County] that contains his index to Ledger H [which is missing] for his patients in Baltimore before 1822 and Harford County after 1822, according to a notation by Dr. George W. Archer.)

Parker, Robert, in Baltimore, was visited by Dr. Robert H. Archer who treated his daughter Eliza seven times in Sep 1823 and again in Sep 1826 (pp. 92-96, 100, 199; Ledger F, p. 66)

Parker, William, at Jeremiah Heaton's, was visited by Dr. John Archer who treated him and wife in 1788 (Ledger F, p. 273) [William Parker was a Revolutionary War veteran.]

Parks, Andrew, was prescribed medicine for his child by Dr. Robert H. Archer on 30 Dec 1802 and 22 Feb 1803 and medicine for himself on 12 Mar 1803 (Rx Book, 1802-1804, pp. 28, 33, 35); he was treated by Dr. Archer in Baltimore before 1822 [no dates or details given] (Dr. Archer's "Alphabet to Ledger H" is his booklet [filed in the Archives of the Historical Society of Harford County] that contains his index to Ledger H [which is missing] for his patients in Baltimore before 1822 and Harford County after 1822, according to a notation by Dr. George W. Archer.)

Parran, John, was treated by Dr. Matthew J. Allen in 1832 in Calvert County (p. 24)

Parsons, Abner, near Little Falls Quaker Meeting House, was treated by Dr. John Archer in 1796 and 1797 (Ledger I, which is missing, was abstracted by Dr. George W. Archer circa 1890; his notes are in the Archives of the Historical Society of Harford County folder "Archer, G. W. Coll. – Ledgers and Day Books")

Paterson, John, see Isaac Tolson, q.v.

Patrick, Hugh, was treated by Dr. John Archer in Jan, Feb and Mar 1778 (Ledger C, p. 100, noted his bill included "ferriage" and payment was finally made "by John Patrick's bond" on 5 Jun 1785)

Patrick, John [1735-1805] (esquire), was visited by Dr. John Archer who treated him in Jan 1777, Jan 1779, Mar 1780 and Jul 1781, a child in Jul 1782, him in Sep 1782, inoculated 13 of his family and Negro Paul's children in 1782, and treated him [John] in Jun 1783 (Ledger C, p. 36, noted on 31 Mar 1780 the doctor was paid "by a iron kettle in full which is but about half so much for depreciation" and then noted "debt forgiven by order of testator;" Ledger D, p. 58, noted "debt forgiven as before") [John Patrick was a Revolutionary War veteran and a signer of the Bush Declaration on March 22. 1775.]; see Hugh Patrick, q.v.

Patten, James, at Buckingham's, was treated by Dr. Matthew J. Allen in Dec 1847 (p. 70)

Patten, John, was mentioned by Dr. Robert H. Archer in a non-medical matter that "paid him in full" in May 1827 (p. 229)

Patten, John, Mrs. (widow), was treated by Dr. John Archer, Jr. in Dec 1819 (p. 15)

Patten, Thomas, see James Evans, of James, q.v.

Patterson, Avarilla (widow), was visited by Dr. John Archer who treated her and her family [no names were given] in 1787 and her and daughters Sally and Polly in 1790 (Ledger F, pp. 174, 212) [account continued in Ledger G, which is missing]

Patterson, Callendar, was treated by Dr. John Archer, Jr. in Aug 1817 and also mentioned John Burrough; was treated by Dr. Robert H. Archer in Sep 1821 (Dr. John Archer, Jr., p. 47; Dr. Robert H. Archer, Ledger F, p. 15)

Patterson, Elizabeth (negro), was treated by Dr. Robert H. Archer in Baltimore before 1822 [no dates or details were given] (Dr. Archer's "Alphabet to Ledger H" is his booklet [filed in the Archives of the Historical Society of Harford County] that contains his index to Ledger H [which is missing] for his patients in Baltimore before 1822 and in Harford County after 1822, according to a notation by Dr. George W. Archer.)

Patterson, Enoch, see Jane Patterson, q.v.

Patterson, Jane, was visited by Dr. John Archer, Jr. who treated her son Enoch in May 1818 and a daughter in Aug 1821 and a grandchild in Sep 1821 (p. 33)

Patterson, George [1748-1808] (schoolmaster), was treated by Dr. John Archer in 1786 and 1789 (Ledger F, pp. 25, 161) [account continued in Ledger G, which is missing] [George Patterson was a Revolutionary War veteran and a signer of the Bush Declaration on March 22, 1775.]

Patterson, John, was visited by Dr. John Archer who treated Miss Bathia in 1786 and him in 1787 (Ledger F, p. 161) [John Patterson was a Revolutionary War veteran.]

Patterson, Orville, was treated by Dr. Matthew J. Allen in Sep 1848 (p. 93)

Patterson, Polly, see Avarilla Patterson, q.v.

Patterson, Sally, see Avarilla Patterson, q.v.

Patterson, William P. [1788-1865], was visited by Dr. Matthew J. Allen who treated his wife in Sep and Oct 1844 (p. 40) [His full name was William Presbury Patterson.]

Patton, Thomas, was treated by Dr. John Archer, Jr. in Mar 1816 (p. 46); see James Evans, q.v.

Paxton, ---- [blank], at John James', was treated by Dr. John Archer in 1778 [exact date not given] (Ledger C, p. 100)

Paxton, Thomas, was treated by Dr. Robert H. Archer in Baltimore before 1822 [no dates or details were given] (Dr. Archer's "Alphabet to Ledger H" is his booklet [filed in the Archives of the Historical Society of

Harford County] that contains his index to Ledger H [which is missing] for his patients in Baltimore before 1822 and Harford County after 1822, according to a notation by Dr. George W. Archer.)

Peacock, G., tavernkeeper(?), was treated by Dr. John Archer, Jr. in June 1821 (p. 38)

Peacock, John, was visited by Dr. John Archer who treated him in Apr 1778, a negro girl in Aug 1779, him in Sep 1780 and Mar and Jul 1781, his brother in Oct 1781 (dressed an ulcer), him [John] in Nov and Dec 1781, his wife in Apr 1782, him in May 1782, and his wife and daughter Molly in Jan 1790 (Ledger C, p. 77; Ledger D, p. 80 [account continued in Ledger E, which is missing]; Ledger F, p. 57); see Negro Margaret, q.v.

Peacock, Molly, see John Peacock, q.v.

Pearl, Nelly, see Andrew Harriott and Nelly Peril, q.v.

Pearce, ---- [blank], at B. Bond's Mill, was treated by Dr. John Archer in 1799 (Ledger I, which is missing, was abstracted by Dr. George W. Archer circa 1890; his notes are in the Archives of the Historical Society of Harford County folder "Archer, G. W. Coll. – Ledgers and Day Books")

Peerson, Thomas, "at the Crossroads," was treated by Dr. John Archer in Sep 1788 (Ledger F, p. 244)

Pemberton, Mrs., was visited by Dr. John Archer who treated daughters Sally, Polly and Nancy in 1796 (Ledger I, which is missing, was abstracted by Dr. George W. Archer circa 1890; his notes are in the Archives of the Historical Society of Harford County folder "Archer, G. W. Coll. – Ledgers and Day Books")

Pennington, H., was prescribed medicine by Dr. Robert H. Archer on 4 Sep 1802 (Rx Book, 1802-1804, p. 19)

Pennington, Isaac, was visited by Dr. James Archer who treated his wife in Apr 1806 and in Nov-Dec 1806, son Luke in Oct 1806 and Negro Cloe in Nov-Dec 1806, all treated for typhus fever (p. 23)

Pennington, Josias, was prescribed medicine by Dr. Robert H. Archer on 12 Mar 1803 (Rx Book, 1802-1804, p. 35)

Pennington, Luke, see Isaac Pennington, q.v.

Peril, Nelly, at P. Quinlan's, now James Hughes' wife in Bellair, [Bel Air] was treated by Dr. John Archer on 3 Oct 1788 (Ledger F, p. 322); Nelly Pearl *(sic)* was treated by Dr. John Archer in Dec 1782 and charged it to Andrew Harriott's account (Ledger C, p. 25); see Andrew Harriott, q.v.

Perine, James, near Charles Baker's, was treated by Dr. John Archer in Aug 1786 (Ledger F, p. 371)

Perkins, John, was treated by Dr. John Archer in Jan 1774 (Ledger B, p. 93) [John Perkins was a Revolutionary War veteran.]

Perkins, Samuel (tanner), at Bald Friar [a landing on Susquehanna River], was treated by Dr. John Archer in 1793 (Ledger F, p. 156, spelled his name Perkens)

Perkins, William, was treated by Dr. John Archer in Dec 1780 (Ledger D, p. 110, noted "debt forgiven as before") [William Perkins was a Revolutionary War veteran.]

Perryman, see James Cunningham, q.v.

Pervail, Elizabeth, see Gideon Pervail, q.v.

Pervail, Gideon [1747-1797] (carpenter), was visited by Dr. John Archer who treated him and his wife, sons John and Samuel and daughter Elizabeth in 1795 and at various times between 1795 and 1797 (Ledger F, p. 42) [continued in Ledger I, which is missing, but it was abstracted by Dr. George W. Archer circa 1890; his notes are in the Archives of the Historical Society of Harford County file "Archer, G. W. Coll. – Ledgers and Day Books" and he spelled the name Prevail]

Pervail, John, see Gideon Pervail, q.v.

Pervail, Mrs. (widow), was visited by Dr. John Archer who treated her and daughter Peggy at various times between 1797 and 1803 (Ledger I, which is missing, was abstracted by Dr. George W. Archer circa 1890; his notes are in Archives of the Historical Society of Harford County file "Archer, G. W. Coll. - Ledgers and Day Books" and he spelled the name Prevail)

Pervail, Peggy, see Mrs. Pervail and Sarah Thomas, q.v.

Pervail, Rachael, see John Stump, q.v.

Pervail, Samuel, see Gideon Pervail, q.v.

Peten, John, see George Benjamin, q.v.

Peters, Thomas, was prescribed various medicines by Dr. Robert H. Archer on 19 Oct 1802 and 24 Dec 1802 and 21 Mar 1803 (Rx Book, 1802-1804, pp. 22, 23, 27, 37)

Phenix, Jacob, near James Pritchet's, was visited by Dr. John Archer who treated his wife in Oct, Nov ("dressing ulcer") and Dec 1785 (Ledger D, p. 9, spelled his name Pheenix and noted "debt forgiven as before")

Phenix, Mrs., was prescribed various medicines for a negro on 16 Aug 1802 by Dr. Robert H. Archer and medicine for herself on 7 Oct 1802 (Rx Book, 1802-1804, pp. 6, 13)

Phillips, see Peter Dixon, q.v.

Phillips, Cordil, see James Phillips, q.v.

Phillips, Jacob, see James Phillips, q.v.

Phillips, James, was treated by Dr. John Archer at times between Jan 1774 and May 1775 and who also treated his child, a son and a negro in Jan 1774, Sally Phrisby in Jan 1775, Jacob in Feb 1775, a child and Negro Phillis in May 1775, Negro Sam in Nov 1775, an infant in Dec 1775, a son in Feb 1776, him [James] 17 times between 7 Feb and 23 Apr 1781, Polly Phrisby in Aug 1784 ("ordered by Aquila Paca") and Sep 1784, his wife and Negro Sall in Jul 1785, his wife in Aug 1785 and him, his sons Cordil, Jacob and William Phillips and Miss Polly Smith in 1787 (Ledger B, p 94; Ledger C, p. 13; Ledger D, p. 118 [account continued in Ledger E, which is missing]; Ledger F, p. 352) [James Phillips was a Revolutionary War veteran.]

Phillips, James (esquire), was treated by Dr. John Archer in Jan 1789 (Ledger F, p. 160) [account continued in Ledger G, which is missing] [James Phillips was a Revolutionary War veteran.]

Phillips, Mrs., was prescribed medicine by Dr. Robert H. Archer for his wife on 16 Aug 1796 (Rx Book, 1796-1801, p. 7)

Phillips, Susan, Miss, was treated by Dr. John Archer in Sep 1787 (Ledger F, p. 24)

Phillips, William, see James Phillips, q.v.

Phrisby, Polly, see James Phillips, q.v.

Phrisby, Sally, see James Phillips, q.v.

Phrisby, William, see Aquila Paca, q.v.

Pinkney, William [1764-1822] (esquire), was treated by Dr. John Archer in Jan 1789 (Ledger F, p. 230) [account continued in Ledger G, which is missing] [William Pinkney was a War of 1812 veteran, U. S. Congressman and Attorney General of Maryland, among other accomplishments.]

Pitt, Francis, was treated by Dr. John Archer in Sep 1788 and Dec 1792 (Ledger D, p. 14, noted "debt forgiven as before;" Ledger F, p. 194)

Points, Mr., was prescribed medicine for his child by Dr. Robert H. Archer on 8 Aug, 9 Aug, 16 Aug and 18 Aug 1802 (Rx Book, 1802-1804, pp. 10, 11, 14)

Points, Mrs., was prescribed medicine for her child by Dr. Robert H. Archer on 7 Aug 1802 (Rx Book, 1802-1804, p. 9)

Poke, Master, see Reuben H. Davis, q.v.

Pollock, Elias, was prescribed medicine for his wife by Dr. Robert H. Archer on 24 Jun 1803 (Rx Book, 1802-1804, p. 45, spelled his name Polock); Elias Pollock was treated by Dr. Archer in Baltimore before 1822 [no dates or details were given] (Dr. Archer's "Alphabet to Ledger H" is his booklet [filed in the Archives of the Historical Society of Harford County] that contains his index to Ledger H [now missing] for his patients in Baltimore before 1822 and Harford County after 1822, according to a notation by Dr. George W. Archer.)

Pooder (Pouder?), Joshua, near Long Calm, was treated by Dr. John Archer in 1795 (Ledger I, which is missing, was abstracted by Dr. George W. Archer circa 1890; his notes are in Archives of the Historical Society of Harford County folder "Archer, G. W. Coll. – Ledgers and Day Books")

Pool, John, was visited by Dr. Matthew J. Allen who treated him and an infant in Jul 1847 (p. 58)

Pool, Mrs., was treated by Dr. Robert H. Archer in Nov 1822 (Ledger F, p. 122)

Pool, Richard, on Mr. Gover's place. treated by Dr. John Archer in Nov 1788 (Ledger F, p. 256)

Poole, Mrs., near Stephen T. Cooper's, was treated by Dr. Robert H. Archer in Nov 1822 (p. 37)

Poor, Master, see Reuben H. Davis, q.v.

Porter, James, was treated by Dr. John Archer in Sep 1774 and Jun 1775 (Ledger B, p. 22)

Porter, John, was treated by Dr. John Archer in Oct 1781 and noted that his security was Thomas Bowles (Ledger D, p. 84, noted "debt forgiven as before")

Porter, John (tailor), Havre de Grace, was treated by Dr. John Archer in 1795 [no dates were given] (Ledger I, which is missing, was abstracted by Dr. George W. Archer circa 1890; his notes are in the Archives of the Historical Society of Harford County folder "Archer, G. W. Coll. – Ledgers and Day Books")

Porter, Moses (mason), was treated by Dr. Robert H. Archer in Apr 1822 (Ledger F, p. 42)

Potee, Peter, was treated by Dr. John Archer in Sep 1779 and Oct 1780 (Ledger D, p. 22, spelled his name Petee and noted "debt forgiven as before") [Peter Potee was a Revolutionary War veteran.]

Poteet, Thomas, was treated by Dr. John Archer in 1780 (Ledger D, p. 43, listed his name as Petete) [Thomas Poteet was a Revolutionary War veteran.]

158

Pouder (Pooder?), Joshua, near Long Calm, was treated by Dr. John Archer in 1795 (Ledger I, which is missing, was abstracted by Dr. George W. Archer circa 1890; his notes are in Archives of the Historical Society of Harford County folder "Archer, G. W. Coll. – Ledgers and Day Books")

Powell, John, was prescribed medicine for his wife by Dr. Robert H. Archer on 24 Feb 1801 (Rx Book, 1796-1801, p. 35)

Power, Nicholas, was visited by Dr. John Archer who treated him in Aug 1772, Sep 1775, Dec 1776, Aug 1779 and Aug 1781 and his son Samuel in Aug 1781 (Ledger B, p. 61; Ledger C, p. 70, noted "debt forgiven by order of testator;" Ledger D, p. 65, noted "debt forgiven as before" and also noted "Dead," but the doctor did not indicate the date of death.]

Power, Samuel, see Nicholas Power, q.v.

Powley, Daniel, was prescribed medicine for his wife and child by Dr. Robert H. Archer in Oct 1804 (Rx Book, 1802-1804, pp. 59, 60)

Prall, Edward & Archer, also Edward & Company (sic) [probably one and the same], was visited by Dr. John Archer in 1795 who inoculated a negro woman and two children and boarded them while inoculated 4 weeks each; also treated Edward for "colic" on 14 Feb 1803 [not 1808 as abstracted since Edward Prall died in 1803] (Ledger I, which is missing, was abstracted by Dr. George W. Archer circa 1890; his notes are in the Archives of the Historical Society of Harford County folder "Archer, G. W. Coll. – Ledgers and Day Books"); see Capt. Edward Prall, q.v.

Prall, Edward, Capt. [c1739-1803] (esquire), was treated by Dr. John Archer in Feb 1803 [and later died; see entry above] (Ledger F, p. 208) [Edward Prall was a Revolutionary War veteran and a signer of the Bush Declaration on March 22, 1775.]; see Thomas Harris, q.v.

Presberry, Rodger (a black man), was treated by Dr. Alonzo Preston several times between 7 Feb and 13 Feb 1826 (p. 65); "Roger Presbury" appeared twice on a list of debts dated 26 Dec 1822 and titled "A List of Allen's Claims" that were due and payable to Dr. Richard N. Allen for services rendered [no dates were given] by him to the said Presbury [or Presberry] (Document filed in the Archives of the Historical Society of Harford County folder "R. N. Allen")

Presbury, Bethia, Miss, was treated by Dr. John Archer in 1787 (Ledger F, p. 283)

Presbury, George, was visited by Dr. John Archer who treated him and child in 1788 (Ledger F, p. 7)

Presbury, Mary, widow of Joseph Presbury, was treated by Dr. John Archer in Nov 1785 and Apr 1788 (Ledger D, p. 15, listed her name as "Mrs. Presbery widow of Joseph" and noted "debt forgiven as before;" Ledger F, p. 232, listed her name as "Mary, of Jos. Presberry")

Presbury, George G., was visited by Dr. Alonzo Preston who treated his wife in Aug 1827 (p. 95)

Presbury, Joseph, see Mary Presbury, q.v.

Presbury, Roger, see Rodger Presberry, q.v.

Presbury, Sophia [1767-1853], was treated by Dr. John Archer in May 1787 (Ledger F, p. 273, noted she "married to William Hall, of Aquila," but he gave no date) [They married on 15 May 1788.]

Presbury, Walter, was treated by Dr. John Archer in Apr 1786 (Ledger F, p. 217)

Preston, Alonzo [1796-1829] (doctor), made oaths before Daniel Wann, a Justice of the Peace, on 7 Dec 1824 and 7 May 1827 and 11 Jun 1828 that the information in his medical book was just and true as stated. [Alonzo Preston was a War of 1812 veteran.]

Preston, Aquila (negro), was murdered in 1814: "Maryland, Harford County, to wit: An Inquisition taken at the late dwelling of Negro Aquila Preston in the County and State aforesaid on the 18th day of January 1814 before Samuel Bradford, one of the Coroners of the said State for the County aforesaid, upon the view of the body of the aforesaid Negro Aquila Preston then and there lying dead upon the oaths of … good and lawful men of the County aforesaid who being sworn upon the holy evangely of almighty God, and affirmed as aforesaid, and charged to enquire when, where, how and after what manner the said Negro Aquila came to his death, do say upon their oaths and affirmation that they are of opinion that the said Negro Aquila was shot by John England whether intentionally or accidentally they are not prepared to say from the Testimony before them. In witness whereof as well the aforesaid coroner as the jurors aforesaid have to this inquisition put their hands and seals on the day and year aforesaid and at the place aforesaid. Samuel Bradford, Coroner." ("Slavery Inquisitions" file in the Archives Department of the Historical Society of Harford County)

Preston, Barnard [1754-1831], son of James [also called Barnard Preston, Jr., of James], was visited by Dr. John Archer who treated him in May, Sep and Nov 1779, Jun 1781, a negro in Feb 1782, him in Jun and Jul 1782 and Aug, Sep, Oct and Nov 1785, him and his wife in Jan 1786, him in May 1786 and sons Ralph and Harry in Sep 1793 (Ledger C, p. 72; Ledger D, p. 55, and p. 119 spelled his name Bernard; Ledger F, pp. 31, 155, 197, spelled it Barnard); see Negro Jack, q.v.

Preston, Barnet, was visited by Dr. John Archer who treated a negro wench in Jun 1774 and him in Jul 1774 and Jun 1775 (Ledger B, p. 30) [Barnet Preston was a Revolutionary War veteran.]

Preston, Barnet, Jr., son of James, was treated by Dr. John Archer in Oct 1794 (Ledger F, p. 128) [account continued in Ledger I, which is missing]; see Barnard Preston, son of James, q.v.

Preston, Benjamin, was treated by Dr. John Archer in Oct 1797 (Ledger F, p. 26) [Benjamin Preston was a Revolutionary War veteran.]

Preston, Betsy, see George Preston, q.v.

Preston, Charlotte, was visited by Dr. Matthew J. Allen who rendered obstetrical services to Negro Jane on 14 Sep 1848 (p. 93)

Preston, Daniel, see James Preston, q.v.

Preston, Darby (a black man), was treated by Dr. Alonzo Preston at various times between 1823 and 1824 (p. 3)

Preston, Dr., see John O'Daniel, John Johnson, James Magraw, Nathaniel W. S. Hays, Mrs. McGaw, William Johns, George Bevard, John Moores, Parker Moores, Samuel Prichard and William Richardson, q.v.

Preston, Edward, was visited by Dr. William Sappington who treated and prescribed medicine for a child in Jan, Mar, Jul and Sep 1833, an infant in Jan 1834 and a child in Jan 1835 (Document filed in Historical Society of Harford County Archives folder "Sappington, Dr. William" and it noted "Mr. Isaac Hoopman is not expected to pay any part of the above to me. W. Sappington")

Preston, George (colored), was visited by Dr. Matthew J. Allen who treated his children [names not given] in Feb 1848, a young child [name not given] and Louisa, Betsy and George in Mar 1848 and George in Apr 1848 (pp. 54, 74, 76, and noted "paid to W. H. Dallam")

Preston, Grafton, was treated by Dr. John Archer in Jun 1775 (Ledger B, p. 83) [Grafton Preston was a Revolutionary War veteran.]

Preston, Harry, see Barnard Preston, q.v.

Preston, Henry, see Luther A. Norris, q.v.

Preston, Henry (Bull?) (sic), was treated by Dr. Robert H. Archer after 1822 [no dates or details were given] (Dr. Archer's "Alphabet to Ledger H" is his booklet [filed in the Archives of the Historical Society of Harford County] that contains his index to Ledger H [which is missing] for his patients in Baltimore before 1822 and Harford County after 1822, according to a notation by Dr. George W. Archer.)

Preston, Jacob A., Dr., see Benedict Hall, Edward Hall, Henry Smith, James Morsel, William W. Hall, Ruthen Garrettson and Cyrus Osborn, q.v.

Preston, James, was treated by Dr. John Archer in July 1786 (Ledger F, p. 218) [account continued in Ledger H which is missing]; see Barnet Preston, Jr. and Bernard Preston, q.v.

Preston, James, appeared on a list of debts dated 26 Dec 1822 and titled "A List of Allen's Claims" that were due and payable to Dr. Richard N. Allen for services rendered [no dates] by him to said Preston (Document filed in Historical Society of Harford County Archives folder "R. N. Allen"); James was later visited by Dr. Alonzo Preston who treated his daughter Sally in Sep 1828 (p. 103, noted "Dead & insolvent" [James Preston, of James, was a War of 1812 veteran.]

Preston, James, of Daniel, was visited by Dr. John Archer who treated his wife in Apr 1780 and him in May 1782 and Mar 1783 (Ledger D, p. 57, noted "debt forgiven as before") and was visited by Dr. John Archer who treated him and his family at various times between 1796 and 1799 (Ledger I, which is missing, was abstracted by Dr. George W. Archer circa 1890; his notes are in the Archives of the Historical Society of Harford County folder "Archer, G. W. Coll. – Ledgers and Day Books") [James Preston, of Daniel, was a Revolutionary War veteran.]

Preston, James B. [1787-1835] [miller], was visited by Dr. Alonzo Preston who treated him, his wife and family and Elizabeth in 1825 (p. 23) [James Bond Preston was a War of 1812 veteran.]

Preston, Louisa, see George Preston, q.v.

Preston, Martin [c1755-c1805], was visited by Dr. John Archer who treated him in Feb, May and Jun 1775 and him and his wife in 1786 (Ledger B, p. 75; Ledger F, p. 141) [Martin Preston was a Revolutionary War veteran.]

Preston, Moses [c1798-1853], was visited by Dr. Matthew J. Allen who treated his son and daughter in Feb 1844 and his son in Jul 1845 (p. 32); Moses Preston signed this note on 27 May 1852: "On demand I promise to pay Matthew J. Allen or order Seven dollars and thirty eight cents for value received." That note, indicating Preston lived in the "neighbourhood of Churchville" and the following statement, written on a separate piece of paper dated 24 Nov 1853, were inserted in the back of Dr. Allen's ledger. This 1853 letter, addressed to Major Bond, was signed by I. Day and stated "I have just returned after 3 days ride to look up the Drs. [probably an abbreviation for debtors] of Dr. Allen and the following is the result." It mentioned several patients, including: "Moses Preston is dead & has left no property."] Moses had died in Jan 1853: "State of Maryland, Harford County, to wit: An inquisition taken near the Union in the county & State aforesaid on the 21st day of January 1853 before me Thomas Cord, one of the Justices of the Peace for said county acting as coronor, upon the view of the body of Moses Preston then & there lying dead … [listed the names of the men who assisted Mr. Cord] … good and lawful men of said county who being sworn on the Holy Evangelly of Allmighty God & charged to enquire where, when, how & in what manner the said Moses Preston cam to his death do say upon their oaths that the said Moses Preston came to his death by intemperance and exposure." (Inquisition document filed in the Archives of the Historical Society of Harford County and Dr. Matthew J. Allen's medical ledger is filed in the Court Records Department of that society.)

Preston, Mrs., see Henry Dorsey and Samuel Dorsey, q.v.

Preston, Ralph, see Barnard Preston, q.v.

Preston, Sally, see James Preston, q.v.

Preston, Samuel (negro), was treated by Dr. Robert H. Archer in Aug 1822 and May 1823 (Ledger F, p. 64)

Preston, Samuel and Harriet (negroes), were visited by Dr. Matthew J. Allen who rendered obstetrical services to Harriet on 25 Jun 1848 and treated her four times in Jul 1848 (p. 87)

Preston, Scott, was treated by Dr. Matthew J. Allen in Aug 1847 (p. 62)

Preston, Thomas, was visited by Dr. Matthew J. Allen who treated a child in Dec 1844, him and a child in Jan 1845 and him in Mar 1845 (p. 41) [The following statement was written on a separate page dated 24 Nov 1853 that was inserted in the back of Dr. Allen's ledger. The letter, addressed to Major Bond, was signed by I. Day and stated "I have just returned after 3 days ride to look up the Drs. of Dr. Allen and the following is the result." It mentioned several patients, including: "I missed Thos. Preston as I passed thro his neighbourhood but have written to him what to do.]

Preston, William, was treated by Dr. Matthew J. Allen in Jan 1845 (p. 42) [The following statement was written on a separate page dated 24 Nov 1853 that was inserted in the back of Dr. Allen's ledger. The letter, addressed to Major Bond and signed by I. Day, stated "I have just returned after 3 days ride to look up the Drs. of Dr. Allen and the following is the result." It mentioned several patients, including this one: "Wm. Preston at Rock Spring Church says he's not the man, that Wm. Preston who lives somewhere near Balto. is the man & so he told the Dr."]

Prevail, see Pervail, q.v.

Price, Charles, was visited by Dr. Matthew J. Allen who treated his wife in Apr and May 1844 (p. 34, noted "good for nothing")

Price, Edward, at Edward Thompson's, was visited by Dr. John Archer who treated him and wife in Feb 1791 (Ledger F, p. 44)

Price, Henry, was prescribed medicine for his wife by Dr. Robert H. Archer on 17 Aug 1802 and medicine for him on 28 Dec 1802 and 15 Jan 1803 (Rx Book, 1802-1804, pp. 14, 28, 32)

Price, Hezekiah, was treated by Dr. Robert H. Archer in Baltimore before 1822 [no dates or details were given] (Dr. Archer's "Alphabet to Ledger H" is his booklet [filed in the Archives of the Historical Society of Harford County] that contains his index to Ledger H [which is missing] for his patients in Baltimore before 1822 and Harford County after 1822, according to a notation by Dr. George W. Archer.)

Price, John, was prescribed medicine for his child by Dr. Robert H. Archer on 7 Aug 1802 (Rx Book, 1802-1804, p. 9)

Price(?), Miss, in Darlington, was prescribed medicine by Dr. Robert H. Archer in 1841 (Rx Book, 1825-1851, p. 115)

Price, Mr., was treated by Dr. Robert H. Archer in Baltimore before 1822 [no dates or details were given] (Dr. Archer's "Alphabet to Ledger H" is his booklet [filed in the Archives of the Historical Society of Harford County] that contains his index to Ledger H [which is missing] for his patients in Baltimore before 1822 and Harford County after 1822, according to a notation by Dr. George W. Archer.)

Price, Rachel, see John Stump, q.v.

Price, Richard, was prescribed medicine for his wife by Dr. Robert H. Archer on 10 Aug 1802 (Rx Book, 1802-1804, p. 11)

Price, Robert, was treated by Dr. John Archer in January 1786 (Ledger F, p. 9)

Price, Warrick, was treated by Dr. Robert H. Archer in Baltimore before 1822 [no dates or details were given] (Dr. Archer's "Alphabet to Ledger H" is his booklet [filed in the Archives of the Historical Society of Harford County] that contains his index to Ledger H [which is missing] for his patients in Baltimore before 1822 and Harford County after 1822, according to a notation by Dr. George W. Archer.)

Price, William, was treated by Dr. John Archer in July 1791 (Ledger F, p. 217) [account continued in Ledger H, which is missing] [William Price was a Revolutionary War veteran.]

Price, William (carpenter), was treated by Dr. Robert H. Archer in Baltimore before 1822 [no dates or details were given] (Dr. Archer's "Alphabet to Ledger H" is his booklet [filed in the Archives of the Historical Society of Harford County] that contains his index to Ledger H [which is missing] for his patients in Baltimore before 1822 and Harford County after 1822, according to a notation by Dr. George W. Archer.)

Prigg, Carvill H., was visited by Dr. Matthew J. Allen who treated his son William in Jul 1843 in consultation with Dr. Johnson and him [Carvill] from Aug to Nov 1843 and in Jan 1844 (p. 27) [His full name was Carvill Hall Prigg.]

Prigg, Christiana, Mrs. [wife of Carvill H. Prigg], was visited by Dr. Matthew J. Allen who treated her son in Sep 1847 (p. 66)

Prigg, Edward, was visited by Dr. John Archer who inoculated him in Feb 1776 and treated him in Aug, Sep and Nov 1779 (Ledger C, p. 29; Ledger D, p. 11) [account continued in Ledger G, which is missing] [Edward Prigg was a Revolutionary War veteran.]

Prigg, Jacob, see William Prigg, Sr., q.v.

Prigg, Polly, see William Prigg, Sr., q.v.

Prigg, William, see Carvill H. Prigg, q.v.

Prigg, William, Jr. [c1753-1833], was visited by Dr. John Archer who inoculated William Wells in Feb 1776 and treated him [William Prigg, Jr.] in Apr 1780, Jun 1781 and Apr 1782, his wife in Mar 1783, and him and a woman in Oct 1783 (Ledger C, p. 31, noted that he was "insolvent" and "debt forgiven by order of testator") [account continued in Ledger E, which is missing] [William Prigg was a Revolutionary War veteran.]

Prigg, William, Sr., was visited by Dr. John Archer who treated him in June 1773 and Sep 1774, son Jacob in June 1773, daughter Polly in Feb 1776 and him [William] in Aug 1780 and Oct 1782 (Ledger B, p. 65; Ledger C, p. 30)

Pringle, Mark [1761-1819], "for Mat. Ridley," was treated by Dr. John Archer in Feb 1786 (Ledger F, p. 108) [Mark Pringle, a prominent Baltimorean and Harford Countian, was a Revolutionary War veteran who owned the estate called Bloomsbury in Havre de Grace]; see Paca Smith, q.v.

Pritchard, Harmon, was visited by Dr. John Archer who treated and inoculated him in Oct 1782 and treated him in Aug 1789 (Ledger D, p. 12, spelled his name Harmin Prichard and noted that Micajah Mitchell had paid £1 for the inoculation; Ledger F, p. 232) [Harmon Pritchard was a Revolutionary War veteran.]

Pritchard, James, was visited by Dr. John Archer who treated his son in Mar 1781, him in May 1784 and his wife in Sep 1784 (Ledger D, p. 125) [account continued in Ledger E, which is missing] [James Pritchard was a Revolutionary War veteran.]

Pritchard, John, was treated by Dr. John Archer in Jan 1787 (Ledger F, p. 213, spelled it Pritchart)

Pritchard, Samuel, near John Kirk's, was visited by Dr. Robert H. Archer who treated his wife in Jan 1828 in consultation with Dr. Preston (p. 261, spelled his name Prichard) [Samuel Pritchard was a War of 1812 veteran.]

Pritchard, Stephen, was inoculated by Dr. John Archer in 1782 (Ledger D, p. 15, spelled his name Pritchet and noted that Micajah Mitchell paid the £1 fee for his inoculation)

Pringle, Mark, see Paca Smith, q.v.

Prisby, William, see Aquila Paca, q.v.

Pue, Caleb, was visited by Dr. Alonzo Preston who treated him in 1824 and his wife and a child and Rebecca in 1826 and 1827 (p. 4)

Pue, Rebecca, see Caleb Pue, q.v.

Pugh, Michael, was treated by Dr. Matthew J. Allen in Aug 1847 (p. 63)

Pyle, Ralph, was visited by Dr. John Archer who treated his wife and child in Sep 1777 and him in Jun 1783 (Ledger C, p. 2) [Ralph Pyle was a Revolutionary War veteran.]

Quarles, John [1777-1846], was visited by Dr. Robert H. Archer who treated his wife in July 1824 in consultation with Dr. Worthington (pp. 112, 113, 114; Ledger F, p. 19)

Quinlan, James [1752-1830], was treated by Dr. John Archer in Dec 1774, Oct 1779 and Jun 1785 (Ledger B, p. 65; Ledger D, p. 33, noted "by transfer from Ledger C, fol. 56," which account was in the name of Philip Quinlan) [continued in Ledger E, which is missing]; James, son of Philip, was treated by Dr. John Archer in Sep 1788 (Ledger F, p. 193); James was treated by Dr. Robert H. Archer in Jul 1823 (pp. 84, 85, Ledger F, p. 69); see Augustus J. Greme and Mr. Baxter, q.v.

Quinlan, James, was visited by Dr. Matthew J. Allen who treated his child for a fractured clavicle [collarbone] on 25 May 1847 and treated him in Jun and Jul 1847 and Jul 1848 (p. 52 listed him as Lee James Quinland and continued the account to p. 57 which listed him as James Quinlan)

Quinlan, James, Jr., see Philip Quinlan, q.v.

Quinlan, Philip, was visited by Dr. John Archer who treated him in Jun 1773, May 1775 and Sep 1777, his son in Sep 1777, him in Apr, Jul and Oct 1778 and Aug 1780, and inoculated his family; also mentioned Nat. Kennedy in Mar 1779 and the daughter of Philip's brother James Quinlan, Jr. circa 1784 and treated Philip in Jul 1792 (Ledger B, p. 66; Ledger C, p. 56; Ledger F, pp. 136, 155); see James Quinlan, Dennis Cain, Henry Neil, Nelly Peril and Jane Jones, q.v.

Quinlan, Philip, appeared on a list of debts dated 26 Dec 1822 and titled "A List of Allen's Claims" that were due and payable to Dr. Richard N. Allen for services rendered [no dates were given] by him to the said Quinlan (Document filed in Historical Society of Harford County Archives folder "R. N. Allen" noted that "Philip Quinlain's acct. on which no balance no balance (sic) is struck")

Rach, Joseph, was prescribed medicine for a child by Dr. Robert H. Archer on 25 Jul 1803 (Rx Book, 1802-1804, p. 51)

Rafferty, Dr. (president), and the Trustees of St. John's College, were mentioned in a non-medical matter regarding tuition expenses for Robert Archer's son Thomas in 1825 (Ledger F, p. 122); see Mrs. Hurst, and St. John's College, q.v.

Ralston, Andrew, was treated by Dr. John Archer in Jun 1778 (Ledger C, p. 114, noted "debt forgiven by order of testator")

Ralston, William, was treated by Dr. John Archer in Jun and Jul 1779 (Ledger C, p. 114, noted "debt forgiven by order of testator")

Ramsay, Charlotte, see Nathaniel Ramsay, q.v.

Ramsay, Col., see Charlotte Hall, q.v.

Ramsay, Cunningham, see James Ramsay, q.v.

Ramsay, Eliza, see James Ramsay, q.v.

Ramsay, James [1742-1806], at Slate Ridge, was visited by Dr. John Archer who treated him, his wife, son Cunningham and daughter Eliza in 1796 (Ledger F, p. 17) [account continued in Ledger K, which is missing]

Ramsay, Nathaniel [1741-1817] (colonel), was visited by Dr. John Archer, Jr. who treated his daughter Charlotte in Mar 1816 and mentioned Mr. Gregg in July 1827 (p. 49); he was treated by Dr. Robert H. Archer in Baltimore before 1817 [no dates or details were given] and listed as Col. Nathan Ramsy (Dr. Archer's "Alphabet to Ledger H" is his booklet [in Historical Society of Harford County Archives] that contains his index to Ledger H [which is missing] for his patients in Baltimore before 1822 and Harford County after 1822, according to Dr. George W. Archer.) [Nathaniel Ramsay was a Revolutionary War veteran.]

Ramsay, William, was treated by Dr. John Archer in Mar 1791 (Ledger F, p. 182) [account continued in Ledger H, which is missing]

Ramsey, James, see Mr. Fraizer, q.v.

Ramsey, Mr., see William Smith (Bayside), q.v.

Ramsey, Mrs. (widow), in the Barrens [area in northwest part of Harford County near Pennsylvania], was visited by Dr. John Archer who treated her and a child in 1787 (Ledger F, p. 345)

Randall, Thomas, was treated by Dr. Robert H. Archer in Baltimore before 1822 [no dates or details were given] (Dr. Archer's "Alphabet to Ledger H" is his booklet [filed in the Archives of the Historical Society of Harford County] that contains his index to Ledger H [which is missing] for his patients in Baltimore before 1822 and Harford County after 1822, according to a notation by Dr. George W. Archer.)

Rankin, John, cooper, at Stump & Co., was visited by Dr. John Archer who treated him, his wife and a child in 1789 (Ledger F, p. 143)

Rankin, Mr., was prescribed medicine by Dr. Robert H. Archer on 13 Nov 1828 (Rx Book, 1825-1851, p. 93)

Rankin, Samuel (cooper), at Stafford Mills, was treated by Dr. John Archer in Dec 1792 (Ledger F, p. 239)

Ratican, James (weaver), at Durham's, was treated by Dr. John Archer in Nov 1781 and Apr 1787 (Ledger D, p. 97, spelled his name Ratigan and noted part of bill was paid by "spinning, raking and binding" in Jul 1786; Ledger F, p. 71) [James Ratican was a Revolutionary War veteran.]

Rawlins, George, at Widow Bull's, was treated by Dr. John Archer in Sep 1788 (Ledger F, p. 215)

Reardon, Dr., see Alonzo Hollis and William W. Hall, q.v.

Reardon, Eleanor, see John Reardon, q.v.

Reardon, James, see Samuel Sutton and John Reardon, q.v.

Reardon, John, was visited by Dr. John Archer who treated him and a child in Sep 1789 (Ledger F, p. 2, spelled his name Rearden). This account was continued in Ledger I, which is missing, but it was abstracted by Dr. George W. Archer circa 1890 as follows: "Jno. Reardon, Bel Air Dpy. Clk, 94-01 [meaning 1794-1801] … To inoculating 4 of yr. family, '95 [1795]: viz., Jno. & Eleanor Reardon, Jno. Riely & Negro – had son James." (Dr. George W. Archer's notes are in the Archives of the Historical Society of Harford County folder "Archer, G. W. Coll. – Ledgers and Day Books") [John Reardon was a Revolutionary War veteran.]

Reardon, Josias, on Bush River Neck, was treated by Dr. John Archer in Sep 1790 (Ledger F, p. 193) [account continued in Ledger G, which is missing]

Redding, Andrew, was visited by Dr. Matthew J. Allen who treated him and "boy Jn." in Aug 1844 and him [Andrew] in Sep 1844 (p. 38) [The following statement was written on a separate page dated 24 Nov 1853 that was inserted in the back of Dr. Allen's ledger. The letter, addressed to Major Bond, was signed by I. Day and stated "I have just returned after 3 days ride to look up the Drs. of Dr. Allen and the following is the result." It mentioned several patients, including: "Andrew Redding says he does not nor never did owe the D. nor will he pay anything." A copy of Allen's bill to Redding for $8 in 1844 noted "beyond Churchville."]; see Thomas Kelly, q.v.

Redman, Mr., was prescribed medicine for a child by Dr. Robert H. Archer circa 1804 (Rx Book, 1802-1804, p. 67)

Reed & Vanbibber, had an account with Dr. Robert H. Archer who treated the following in 1836: Negro Antony in Jan, Sep and Oct, Negro Horace in Jan, Mar and Jul, Negro Scott in Jan, Feb and May, Negro Ophelia in Jan, Apr ("dressing wound'), May, Jul and Aug, Negro Betty on 14 Jan "obstetricand" [in childbirth] and in Apr, May, Jul and Aug, Negro Caroline in Jan, Feb, Jun, Jul, Aug, Sep and Oct, Negro Sharlotte in Jan, Feb and Jul, Negro Eveline in Jan, Apr, Aug and Sep, Negro Jim in Feb, Apr ("dressing wound") and Jul, Negro Tom in Feb, May and Jun, Negro Joe in Feb, Mar, Jul, Aug, Sep and Oct, Negro Bob in Mar and May ("dressing wound"), Negro Martha in Mar and Jul, Negro Louis in Apr, Jul and Aug, Negro Mary in May. Jun, Jul and Aug, Negro Captain in May, Negro Little Mary in Jun, Negro Minerva in Jun and Jul, Negro Harrison in Jun and Jul ("venereal disease"), Negro Joe Watkins in Jul, Negro Susan in Jul and Sep, Negro Mary's child in Jul and Aug, Negro Betty's child in Jul, Negro Sharlotte's child in Jul, negro Mary Watkins in Sep and Oct, negro Antony Watkins in Sep, and Negro Robert in consultation with Dr. Annon in Oct 1836; Negro Martin was treated in Mar 1837 (Document filed in the Archives of the Historical Society of Harford County folder "Archer, Robert H., 1775-1857 – Receipts" and noted the total medical bill from 9 Jan 1836 to 14 Mar 1837 amounted to $839.00)

Reed, ---- [blank] (schoolmaster), in Havre de Grace, was visited by Dr. John Archer who treated him and his wife in 1787 (Ledger F, p. 18)

Reed, David, was treated by Dr. John Archer in Apr 1772 (Ledger B, p. 65)

Reed, Jane (negro), was treated by Dr. Robert H. Archer in Baltimore before 1822 [no dates or details were given] (Dr. Archer's "Alphabet to Ledger H" is his booklet [filed in the Archives of the Historical Society of Harford County] that contains his index to Ledger H [which is missing] for his patients in Baltimore before 1822 and Harford County after 1822, according to a notation by Dr. George W. Archer.)

Reed, John, was visited by Dr. Alonzo Preston who treated his wife in 1827 (p. 89)

Reese, Jean, was treated by Dr. John Archer in Sep 1773 (Ledger B, p. 77)

Reese, John, was visited by Dr. Robert H. Archer who treated him and a child in Aug 1822, a child in Oct 1823 and his wife in Jan 1823 (Ledger F, p. 61)

Reese, John (millwright), was visited by Dr. Robert H. Archer who treated his wife "in partu" [in childbirth] in the night of 29 Aug 1822, a child in Oct 1822, and his wife in Jan 1823 in consultation with Dr. Worthington (pp. 15, 29, 47, 48)

Reese, John, at Tyson's, was treated by Dr. John Archer in Aug 1787 (Ledger F, p. 379)

Reese, John, son of John, now at Col. Norris', was visited by Dr. John Archer who treated him and his wife in Jan1794 (Ledger F, p. 349)

Reese, Joseph, near White Hall, was visited by Dr. John Archer who treated him and his family in 1796 and 1797 (Ledger I, which is missing, was abstracted by Dr. George W. Archer circa 1890; his notes are in the Archives of the Historical Society of Harford County folder "Archer, G. W. Coll. – Ledgers and Day Books"); see William Lee, q.v.

Reese, Joseph, was treated by Dr. John Archer in Jan 1786 (Ledger F, p. 50) [account continued in Ledger H, which is missing]

Reese, Joseph, was prescribed medicine for his wife by Dr. Robert H. Archer on 8 Jul 1803 (Rx Book, 1802-1804, p. 49)

Reese, Mary, see Harford County for Pensioners, q.v.

Reese, Mr., was prescribed medicine by Dr. Robert H. Archer on 19 Aug 1803 (Rx Book, 1802-1804, p. 53)

Reese, Mr., was visited by Dr. Robert H. Archer who treated his wife in Jul 1822 (p. 12)

Reese, Peggy, near Mrs. Gover's, was treated by Dr. John Archer in Jan-Feb 1777 (Ledger C, p. 83)

Reese, Solomon, was treated by Dr. John Archer in 1788 and the bill was charged to Harford County (Ledger F, p. 160, spelled his name Reece) [account continued in Ledger G, which is missing] [Solomon Reese was a Revolutionary War veteran.]; see Harford County for Pensioners, q.v.

Reese, Thomas, see Harford County for Pensioners, q.v.

Reeves, Josias, was treated by Dr. John Archer in Dec 1774 and Jan 1775 (Ledger B, p. 22)

Renshaw, James, see Robert Renshaw, q.v.

Renshaw, Robert, was visited by Dr. John Archer who treated his brother James in Sep 1777 and him in May and Aug 1781 (Ledger C, p. 94, noted "debt forgiven by order of testator;" Ledger D, p. 60, noted "debt forgiven as before") [Robert Renshaw was a Revolutionary War veteran.]

Renshaw, Thomas, was visited by Dr. John Archer who treated his wife in Oct 1773, him in Feb and Aug 1782, and him and a child in Sep 1782 (Ledger B, p. 35; Ledger D, p. 121) [account continued in Ledger E, which is missing]

Renshaw, Widow, was visited by Dr. John Archer who treated a daughter in Nov and Dec 1775, her [widow] and son and a negro in Jan 1776 and inoculated 2 of her family in 1777, and treated her in Oct 1779 (Ledger C, p. 19, noted "debt forgiven by order of testator")

Resin, James, at George Drew's, was treated by Dr. John Archer in Mar 1786 (Ledger F, p. 136)

Reynolds, Ann, Mrs. was visited by Dr. Matthew J. Allen who treated Fanny in Jan 1848 (p. 72)

Reynolds, E. & J., had an account with Dr. John Archer, Jr. in Jan 1817 that mentioned Elisha Reynolds in Oct 1820 (p. 30); see Joel Reynolds and James Fulton, q.v.

Reynolds, Edward, was visited by Dr. Matthew J. Allen who treated his wife in May and Jun 1848 (p. 84, noted the bill was paid "by order to Jas. Fulton" on 30 Aug 1848)

Reynolds, Elisha, was visited by Dr. Robert H. Archer who treated a child in Feb 1823 (p. 54); see E. & J. Reynolds, q.v.

Reynolds, Fanny, see Ann Reynolds, q.v.

Reynolds, J., see Joel Reynolds and E. & J. Reynolds, q.v.

Reynolds, J. W., see Matthew Johnson, James Fulton and A. J. Greme, q.v.

Reynolds, Joel, had an account in the ledger of Dr. Robert H. Archer in Oct 1821 that also mentioned E. & J. Reynolds in Oct 1820 (Ledger F, p. 12)

Reynolds, Joseph, see Mary Reynolds, q.v.

Reynolds, L., see Matthew Johnson and Augustus J. Greme, q.v.

Reynolds, Mary, widow of Joseph, was treated in 1818 by Dr. John Archer, Jr. and the account also mentioned Mr. Magraw in 1820 (p. 46)

Reynolds, Patrick, at James Barnet's, was treated by Dr. John Archer in Mar 1788 (Ledger F, p. 128)

Reynolds, Reuben, West Nottingham Meeting, was treated by Dr. John Archer, Jr. in Mar 1817 and Mar 1820 (pp. 27, 71)

Reynolds, Stephen, was treated by Dr. John Archer, Jr. in Apr 1816 (p. 42)

Rice, James, at Otter Point, was treated by Dr. John Archer who treated him in Sep 1781 and his wife in Oct 1781 (Ledger D, p. 2, noted "debt forgiven as before")

Richard, Thomas, see Joseph Brownley, q.v.

Richards, ----, Jr., see Reuben H. Davis, q.v.

Richards, John, was treated by Dr. Robert H. Archer in Baltimore before 1822 [no dates or details were given] (Dr. Archer's "Alphabet to Ledger H" is his booklet [filed in the Archives of the Historical Society of Harford County] that contains his index to Ledger H [which is missing] for his patients in Baltimore before 1822 and Harford County after 1822, according to a notation by Dr. George W. Archer.)

Richards, L., was prescribed medicine for his wife by Dr. Robert H. Archer circa Dec 1804 (Rx Book, 1802-1804, p. 73); see Reuben H. Davis, q.v.

Richards, Rev., was prescribed medicine for his wife by Dr. Robert H. Archer circa Dec 1804 (Rx Book, 1802-1804, p. 69)

Richardson, Arnold, was treated by Dr. Robert H. Archer in Baltimore before 1822 [no dates or details were given] (Dr. Archer's "Alphabet to Ledger H" is his booklet [filed in the Archives of the Historical Society of Harford County] that contains his index to Ledger H [which is missing] for his patients in Baltimore before 1822 and Harford County after 1822, according to a notation by Dr. George W. Archer.)

Richardson, Benjamin, was visited by Dr. John Archer who treated him in Dec 1780 and Sep 1781, his wife in Dec 1781 and him in Mar 1782 and Apr 1783 (Ledger D, p. 108) [account continued in Ledger K, which is missing]

Richardson, Daniel, was visited by Dr. John Archer who treated a negro in Dec 1781, him [Daniel] in Jan 1782, a negro in Mar 1782, Negro Harry in Jul, Aug and Sep 1782 and him [Daniel] in Oct and Nov 1782 and Apr 1787 (Ledger D, p. 110 [account continued in Ledger E, which is missing]; Ledger F, p. 295) [Daniel Richardson was a Revolutionary War veteran.]

Richardson, James, of Abingdon, was visited by Dr. John Archer who treated him and son James in 1797 and 1798 (Ledger I, which is missing, was abstracted by Dr. George W. Archer circa 1890; his notes are in the Archives of the Historical Society of Harford County folder "Archer, G. W. Coll. – Ledgers and Day Books") [James Richardson was a Revolutionary War veteran.]

Richardson, Margaret, see William Richardson, q.v.

Richardson, Martha, was treated by Dr. Robert H. Archer in Baltimore before 1822 [no dates or details were given] (Dr. Archer's "Alphabet to Ledger H" is his booklet [filed in the Archives of the Historical Society of Harford County] that contains his index to Ledger H [which is missing] for his patients in Baltimore before 1822 and Harford County after 1822, according to a notation by Dr. George W. Archer.)

Richardson, Mrs., see Negro Harry, q.v.

Richardson, Nanny (negro), was prescribed medicine by Dr. Robert H. Archer on 10 Aug 1802 (Rx Book, 1802-1804, p. 11)

Richardson, Robert [c1795-1833], was visited by Dr. Alonzo Preston who treated his wife in Jan 1825 and him nine times between 22 Sep 1827 and 14 Dec 1827 (pp. 12, 99) [Robert Richardson was a War of 1812 veteran.]

Richardson, Sally, was treated by Dr. John Archer in Nov 1782 (Ledger D, p. 53, noted the "debt forgiven as before")

Richardson, Samuel, was visited by Dr. John Archer who treated him, daughter and son in Dec 1780, his daughter and son in Jan 1781 and his wife and an infant in Aug 1782 (Ledger D, p. 107, noted "debt forgiven as before") [Samuel Richardson was a Revolutionary War veteran.]; see William Richardson, q.v.

Richardson, Vincent, was murdered in 1779: "Harford County & State of Maryland – November ye 29th 1779 – Whereas a certain Vincent Richardson has been found dead in the house of Mrs. Elizabeth Finegan and a certain William Eddy (sic) charged with violence offered to said man this sheweth that a jury of twelve free men and theirs have been duly and legally impaneled to examine and enquire into the cause of said Richardson's death who after being duly sworn and have heard the evidences of the witnesses are of opinion and do make a return to the Court of Harford County that the said Vincent Richardson recd. his death by a blow from said Edy (sic) under the right breast; therefore the said …do make this return wherein we are of opinion that the sd. Edey (sic) is guilty of manslaughter. Given under our hands and seals the day and year above written." (File 4.09.26A in the Court Records Department of the Historical Society of Harford County); "William Ady convicted of the murder of Vincent Richardson. Letter [in 1781] from William Ady states he was returning home after an election for sheriff of Harford County on Monday, 29th day of November 1779, accompanied by Vincent Richardson. They stopped at a Public House (operated by Mrs. Elizabeth Finagan) on the road leading toward home. Both under the influence of liquor, there arose an altercation between Ady and Richardson. Ady with his second blow killed Vincent Richardson. Convicted of manslaughter and sent to prison. In his petition Ady stated he and Richardson lived within one mile of each other for 22 years and had never had any malice toward each other. William Ady is married with four children." A petition for his pardon was signed and sent to the Governor of Maryland by a number of citizens. (Pardon Papers, Folder 64, Maryland State Archives, abstracted by F. Edward Wright and published in *Maryland Genealogical Society Bulletin* 32:4 (Fall, 1991), pp. 477-478)

Richardson, William [1752-c1820s], was treated by Dr. John Archer in Aug 1786 (Ledger F, p. 4) [account continued in Ledger H, which is missing]; William Richardson, Sr. was visited by Dr. John Archer who treated him and son Samuel at various times between 1794 and 1798 (Ledger I, which is missing, was abstracted by Dr. George W. Archer circa 1890; his notes are in the Archives of the Historical Society of Harford County folder "Archer, G. W. Coll. – Ledgers and Day Books") [William Richardson was a Revolutionary War veteran.]

Richardson, William [1788-1834], was treated between 1822 and 1824 [no details were given] and in 1828 by Dr. Alonzo Preston who also treated his wife many times in 1825, 1826 and 1827 ("from 24th up to the 9th Dec, visit every other day"), and Course(?) in 1826 and 1827, an unnamed child in 1826, and Margaret in 1827 and 1828 (p. 57, and p. 98, noting "This acct. settled by acct. in bar for $115.93¼ - $105.25, [balance of] $10.68¼ [and] paid 1/3 [or] $3.56"); Maj. William Richardson was visited by Dr. Robert H. Archer who treated his wife in Oct 1827 in consultation with Dr. Preston (p. 251) [William Richardson was a War of 1812 veteran who owned Richardson's Tavern, also known as Eagle Hotel, later the Country Club Inn, in Bel Air.]

Rickets, ---- [blank] (Dublin cooper), was visited by Dr. Robert H. Archer who treated his son in Aug 1824 (pp. 117, 118; Ledger F, p. 104, noted he was "insolvent")

Rickets, Mr., was visited by Dr. Robert H. Archer who treated his wife in Dec 1826 (p. 211, noted "went to western country")

Ricketts, Nathan or Nathaniel [1786-1867], appeared on a list of debts dated 26 Dec 1822 and titled "A List of Allen's Claims" that were due and payable to Dr. Richard N. Allen for services rendered [no dates given] to said Ricketts (Document filed in Historical Society of Harford County Archives folder "R. N. Allen")

Riddle, ---- [blank] (carpenter), was treated by Dr. Robert H. Archer in Baltimore before 1822 [no dates or details were given] (Dr. Archer's "Alphabet to Ledger H" is his booklet [filed in the Archives of the Historical Society of Harford County] that contains his index to Ledger H [which is missing] for his patients in Baltimore before 1822 and Harford County after 1822, according to a notation by Dr. George W. Archer.)

Riddle, John [1784-1850], was treated by Dr. Robert H. Archer in Baltimore before 1822 [no dates or details were given] (Dr. Archer's "Alphabet to Ledger H" is his booklet [filed in the Archives of the Historical Society of Harford County] that contains his index to Ledger H [which missing] for his patients in Baltimore before 1822 and Harford County after 1822, according to a notation by Dr. George W. Archer.)

Ridley, Matthew (esquire), was visited by Dr. John Archer who treated him and his wife and a child named Essex in 1789 (Ledger F, p. 353); see Mark Pringle, q.v.

Riely, George (mulatto), at Samuel Forwood's, was treated by Dr. John Archer in July 1788 (Ledger F, p. 199, listed him as Geor. Riely)

Riely, Jean, Mrs. (widow), was treated by Dr. John Archer in Dec 1786 (Ledger F, p. 64)

Riely, John, see John Reardon, q.v.

Rigbie, James, Jr., was treated by Dr. John Archer in Feb 1791 (Ledger F, p. 245) [account continued in Ledger H, which is missing]

Rigbie, James, Sr. [1721-1791], was visited by Dr. John Archer who treated him in Mar 1782, his wife in Mar 1784 in consultation with Dr. Hall, daughter Nancy in Mar 1784, him in Nov 1784, him and Miss Nancy and Miss Massey [Mercy?] in Jul 1785, May 1787 and Sep 1788 (Ledger D, p. 125, spelled his name Rigby [account continued in Ledger E, which is missing]; Ledger F, pp. 148, 339) [account continued in Ledger G, which is missing] [James Rigbie, at Berkley, near Darlington, hosted Gen. Lafayette and his troops on 13 Apr 1781 on their march to Yorktown.]

Rigbie, James, see Negro Pompey and Thomas Ammons, q.v.

Rigbie, Massey (Mercy?), see James Rigbie, Sr., q.v.

Rigbie, Nancy, see James Rigbie, Sr., q.v.

Rigbie, Robert, was treated by Dr. Robert H. Archer in Baltimore before 1822 [no dates or details were given] (Dr. Archer's "Alphabet to Ledger H" is his booklet [filed in the Archives of the Historical Society of Harford County] that contains his index to Ledger H [which is missing] for his patients in Baltimore before 1822 and Harford County after 1822, according to a notation by Dr. George W. Archer.)

Rigdon, see Ann Johnson and Mr. Nevill, q.v.

Rigdon, Alexander [1742-1820], was visited by Dr. John Archer who treated him in Dec 1781 and Mar 1782, a negro in Apr 1782, him in May, Jun, Sep 1782 and Aug 1783, his wife in Aug 1783 and him in Feb 1790 (Ledger D, p. 106 [account continued in Ledger E, which is missing]; Ledger F, p. 340) [Alexander Rigdon was a Revolutionary War veteran and a signer of the Bush Declaration on March 22, 1775.]; see John Hays, q.v.

Rigdon, Baker, was treated by Dr. John Archer in May 1778 (Ledger C, p. 106, noted "debt forgiven by order of testator") [Baker Rigdon was a Revolutionary War veteran.]

Rigdon, Baker, appeared on a list of debts dated 26 Dec 1822 and titled "A List of Allen's Claims" that were due and payable to Dr. Richard N. Allen for services rendered [no dates] by him to said Rigdon (Document filed in Historical Society of Harford County Archives folder "R. N. Allen")

Rigdon, Martin, was treated by Dr. Matthew J. Allen, at the request of Dr. Bond, ten times between 27 Jul and 7 Aug 1848 (p. 90, noted later that the bill was "settled in part by J. Brown" and part "from Martin Rigdon who is working at B. & O. R.R. Depot")

Rigdon, Stephen, was treated by Dr. John Archer in Sep 1781 (Ledger D, p. 71) [account continued in Ledger G, which is missing] [Stephen Rigdon was a Revolutionary War veteran.]

Riggs, Mr. (merchant) was treated by Dr. Robert H. Archer after 1822 [no dates or details were given] (Dr. Archer's "Alphabet to Ledger H" is his booklet [filed in the Archives of the Historical Society of Harford County] that contains his index to Ledger H [which is missing] for his patients in Baltimore before 1822 and Harford County after 1822, according to a notation by Dr. George W. Archer.); see Mr. Davis, q.v.

Riley, John, see Thomas Huggins & Co., q.v.

Riley, Patrick, was treated by Dr. John Archer in Oct 1788 (Ledger F, p. 145)

Ringgold, Mr., was prescribed medicine by Dr. Robert H. Archer on 28 Jan 1803 (Rx Book, 1802-1804, p. 31)

Ringgold, Thomas, was prescribed medicine by Dr. Robert H. Archer on 11 Mar 1801 (Rx Book, 1796-1801, p. 44)

Riston, Thomas, was treated by Dr. Robert H. Archer in Baltimore before 1822 [no dates or details were given] (Dr. Archer's "Alphabet to Ledger H" is his booklet [filed in the Archives of the Historical Society of Harford County] that contains his index to Ledger H [which is missing] for his patients in Baltimore before 1822 and Harford County after 1822, according to a notation by Dr. George W. Archer.)

Roales, Joseph, "near Stone House," was visited by Dr. John Archer who treated him and his wife in 1788 (Ledger F, p. 329)

Robardet, James, was treated by Dr. Robert H. Archer in Baltimore before 1822 [no dates or details were given] (Dr. Archer's "Alphabet to Ledger H" is his booklet [filed in the Archives of the Historical Society of Harford County] that contains his index to Ledger H [which is missing] for his patients in Baltimore before 1822 and Harford County after 1822, according to a notation by Dr. George W. Archer.)

Roberts, Elizabeth, see James Murray, q.v.

Roberts, James H., was visited by Dr. William T. Munnikhuysen who treated his wife and a Mr. Humphrey in Jan 1842 and on 31 Mar 1845 the doctor filed a complaint that Roberts owed him $12 and "he is credibly informed and verily believes that the said James H. Roberts is actually fled and run away and removed from his place of abode with intention to defraud his creditors." (Court Records Department File 124.05.3A in the Historical Society of Harford County)

Robinson, Charles [1756-1834], was visited by Dr. John Archer who treated him in Nov 1781 and Mar 1782, his wife in Oct 1782 and a negro in Jan 1783 (Ledger D, p. 100, spelled his name Robison and noted "debt forgiven as before") [account continued in Ledger E, which is missing]; see William Robinson, q.v.

Robinson, Edward, was treated by Dr. John Archer in Jan 1786 (Ledger F, p. 45)

Robinson, Daniel, was visited by Dr. John Archer who treated him in Sep 1779 and Oct, Nov and Dec 1780, him and a child in Sep 1783 and him, his wife and a child in 1787 (Ledger D, p. 27, noted "debt forgiven as before;" Ledger F, p. 31, spelled his name Robison)

Robinson, George, was visited by Dr. Alonzo Preston who treated a child in Aug 1827 (p. 96)

Robinson, Grafton, appeared on a list of debts dated 26 Dec 1822 and titled "A List of Allen's Claims" that were due and payable to Dr. Richard N. Allen for services rendered [no dates were given] by him to said Robinson (Document filed in Historical Society of Harford County Archives folder "R. N. Allen"); Grafton was visited by Dr. Robert H. Archer who dressed his wound on 25 Jul and 7 Aug 1825 and treated his wife in Sep 1827 and a child in Aug 1828 (pp. 149, 150, 151, 244, 290; Ledger F, p. 143); also see Grafton Baker, q.v.

Robinson, Isaac, was prescribed medicine by Dr. Robert H. Archer on 21 Apr 1803 (Rx Book, 1802-1804, p. 40)

Robinson, James, see Joseph Robinson, q.v.

Robinson, John, was visited by Dr. Alonzo Preston who treated him in May 1827 and treated "Pater" in Mar 1832(?) [illegible] (p. 28)

Robinson, Joseph [1762-1839], in Bel Air, was visited by Dr. John Archer who treated him and son James at various times between 1796 and 1802 (Ledger I, which is missing, was abstracted by Dr. George W. Archer circa 1890; his notes are in Archives of the Historical Society of Harford County folder "Archer, G. W. Coll. – Ledgers and Day Books")

Robinson, William, was treated by Dr. John Archer in April 1782 (Ledger D, p. 8, noted the "debt forgiven as before" and "Charles Security" was written beneath William's name [i. e., someone named Charles, probably Charles Robinson, was his security] [Two men named William Robinson were Revolutionary War veterans.]; see John Marford, q.v.

Robison, Elenor, at Kent Michel's [most likely referring to Kent Mitchell], was treated by Dr. John Archer in Nov 1785 (Ledger D, p. 57, noted "debt forgiven as before")

Robison, Eliza, see Temperance Robison, q.v.

Robison, Margaret (widow), was treated by Dr. John Archer in Jun 1793 (Ledger F, p. 36) [account continued in Ledger H, which is missing]

Robison, Richard, son of William, was treated by Dr. John Archer in May 1788 (Ledger D, p. 22, noted "debt forgiven as before")

Robison, Temperance, was visited by Dr. John Archer who treated her in Oct 1778 and May and Dec 1785, and her and daughter Eliza in Feb 1786 (Ledger C, p. 30; Ledger D, p. 46, noted "debt forgiven as before;" Ledger F, p. 55)

Robison, William, see Richard Robison, q.v.

Roche, ---- [blank] (carpenter), was treated by Dr. Robert H. Archer in Baltimore before 1822 [no dates or details given] (Dr. Archer's "Alphabet to Ledger H" is his booklet [filed in the Archives of the Historical Society of Harford County] that contains his index to Ledger H [which is missing] for his patients in Baltimore City before 1822 and in Harford County after 1822, according to a notation by Dr. George W. Archer.)

Rockhold, John was treated by Dr. John Archer at various times between 1795 and 1799 and also inoculated him, his wife and Nancy, Ruthy, James and Harriet in 1795 (Ledger I, which is missing, was abstracted by Dr. George W. Archer circa 1890; his notes are in the Archives of the Historical Society of Harford County folder "Archer, G. W. Coll. – Ledgers and Day Books")

Roddam, William, was visited by Dr. Matthew J. Allen who rendered obstetrical services to his wife on 12 May 1848 in consultation with Dr. Bond (p. 81, noted bill was paid in full on 28 Jul 1848)

Rodes, Benjamin, near Salt Box, was treated by Dr. John Archer in 1796 (Ledger I, which is missing, was abstracted by Dr. George W. Archer circa 1890; his notes are in the Archives of the Historical Society of Harford County folder "Archer, G. W. Coll. – Ledgers and Day Books")

Rodes, Mary, Mrs., near Salt Box, was visited by Dr. John Archer who treated her and her family in 1796 (Ledger I, which is missing, was abstracted by Dr. George W. Archer circa 1890; his notes are in the Archives of the Historical Society of Harford County folder "Archer, G. W. Coll. – Ledgers and Day Books")

Rodgers, Betsey, was treated by Dr. John Archer in May 1774 (Ledger B, p. 23)

Rodgers, Elizabeth, was treated by Dr. John Archer in July 1779 (Ledger C, p. 29, noted the "debt forgiven by order of testator")

Rodgers, Joseph, was visited by Dr. John Archer who treated him and his wife and a child in 1804 (Ledger F, p. 11); see William Rodgers, q.v.

Rodgers, Lilburn, was visited by Dr. Alonzo Preston who treated his wife in 1827 and "in partu" [in childbirth] on 2 Oct 1828, charging $5.00 for his obstetrical services (p. 61)

Rodgers, Mrs., widow of Col. John Rodgers, was treated by Dr. John Archer between 1794 and 1801 (Ledger I, which is missing, was abstracted by Dr. George W. Archer circa 1890; his notes are in the Archives of the Historical Society of Harford County folder "Archer, G. W. Coll. – Ledgers and Day Books")

Rodgers, Roland [1775-1848], was visited by Dr. Alonzo Preston who treated his wife in Nov 1825, later noting "acct. in bar passed by the Court" and a second note "Settled by acct. in bar Feb 23rd, 1830" made and initialed by W.B.B. [referring to Dr. William B. Bond] (p. 62) [Rowland Rogers was a War of 1812 veteran.]; see Thomas Rodgers, q.v.

Rodgers, Samuel, son-in-law of William Coale, was visited by Dr. John Archer who treated an infant and a child in Jan 1776 (Ledger C, p. 99)

Rodgers, Thomas, was treated by Dr. John Archer in Nov 1790 (Ledger F, p. 171) [account continued in Ledger G, which is missing]; Thomas Rodgers, of Rowland, was treated by Dr. John Archer in 1797 (Ledger I, which is missing, was abstracted by Dr. George W. Archer circa 1890; his notes are in the Archives of the Historical Society of Harford County folder "Archer, G. W. Coll. – Ledgers and Day Books"); see Thomas Rogers, q.v.

Rodgers, William, son of Joseph, dec'd., was treated by Dr. John Archer in 1787 (Ledger F, p. 240)

Rogers, Benjamin, was prescribed medicine by Dr. Robert H. Archer on 19 Feb 1801 (Rx Book, 1796-1801, p. 34)

Rogers, John, appeared on a list of debts dated 26 Dec 1822 and titled "A List of Allen's Claims" that were due and payable to Dr. Richard N. Allen for services rendered [no dates] by him to said Rogers (Document filed in Historical Society of Harford County Archives folder "R. N. Allen")

Rogers, Joseph, was visited by Dr. John Archer who treated him and his sister in Jan 1781 and him in Jun 1786 [for "hamorrhoid"] (Ledger D, p. 116)

Rogers, Mrs., was prescribed medicine by Dr. Robert H. Archer on 4 Jul 1803 (Rx Book, 1802-1804, p. 47)

Rogers, Roland, was visited by Dr. John Archer who treated him in Sep 1779, Jan 1780, Aug 1781, May 1782, inoculated 3 of his family in 1783 and treated him in Jun 1788 (Ledger D, p. 14, misspelled his name "Rolling Rogers" and noted he paid part of his bill by making 21 pairs of shoes); see Roland Rodgers and Thomas Rodgers, q.v.

Rogers, Samuel, was visited by Dr. John Archer who treated a child in Apr 1780 and May 1781, him in Jun and Aug 1781, his wife in Jul 1782, him in Jul and Aug 1783, his wife in Dec 1783 and him in Apr 1788 (Ledger D, p. 55; Ledger F, p. 254) [continued in Ledger G, which is missing]

Rogers, Thomas, was visited by Dr. John Archer who treated an infant in Dec 1781, him in Jan 1782, inoculated 3 of his family in 1782, treated his wife in Dec 1783 and him in Sep 1784 (Ledger D, p. 103, indicated "to a transfer to Ledger F, fol. 171," where his name was spelled Rodgers)

Rollins, Isaac, was treated by Dr. John Archer in Aug 1772 (Ledger B, p. 3)

Root, Daniel [1750-1808], was visited by Dr. John Archer who treated his daughter in Feb 1777, his son in Oct 1777 and him in Apr 1778 (Ledger C, p. 83) [Daniel Root was a Revolutionary War soldier who served in Harford County and subsequently moved to Frederick County, Maryland.]

Rose, Joseph, was treated by Dr. John Archer in June 1789 (Ledger F, p. 53) [Joseph Rose was a Revolutionary War veteran.]

Ross, ----, near Mr. Bradford's, was visited by Dr. John Archer who treated him in Aug and Oct 1777 and Mary Ross in May 1779 (Ledger C, p. 91, noted "debt forgiven by order of testator")

Ross, Mary, see ---- Ross, q.v.

Roundtree, Thomas (schoolmaster), was treated by Dr. John Archer in Oct and Nov 1772 (Ledger B, p. 54) [Thomas Roundtree or Rowntree was a Revolutionary War veteran.]

Roy, John, was treated by Dr. Robert H. Archer in Sep 1815 (Ledger F, p. 1)

Ruff, Daniel, was visited by Dr. John Archer who treated him in Aug 1781, him and his wife in Sep 1781, him in Mar and Aug 1782, an infant in Feb 1783, a child in Mar 1783, a child in May 1783 and him [Daniel] in Apr 1787 (Ledger D, p. 69 [account continued in Ledger E, which is missing]; Ledger F, p. 197)

Ruff, H., see George Lochary, q.v.

Ruff, Han, see Henry Ruff, Sr., q.v.

Ruff, Harriot, see James Ruff, q.v.

Ruff, Henry, see Mrs. Ruff and James Ruff, q.v.

Ruff, Henry (tanner), was visited by Dr. John Archer who treated him in Aug 1781, his wife "ad partum" [childbirth] on 25 Jan 1781, him in Jun 1781 and Apr, Sep and Oct 1782, him and a child in Sep 1783 and him in Nov 1789 (Ledger D, p. 62 [account continued in Ledger E, which is missing]; Ledger F, p. 294) [account continued in Ledger G, which is missing]

Ruff, Henry, Sr. (farmer), was visited by Dr. John Archer who treated him many times between Feb 1773 and Mar 1775, his wife in May and Aug 1773, a negro in June and July 1774, Samuel and a negro in Aug 1774, an old Negro and a negro boy in Aug 1774, his [Henry's] wife in Aug 1774 and Mar 1775, his son in Nov 1774, an infant in Jan 1775, him, his wife and a child in Jan 1775, a child in Mar and Apr 1778, him in Aug 1778, his wife in May 1779, him in Jun and Sep 1779, a child in Oct 1779 and Jan 1780 him in Mar 1780, son James in Jul and Aug 1780 and Feb and Apr 1781, son Henry in Apr 1781, his mother in Sep 1781, a negro in Mar 1782, son Henry in May 1782, him in Aug 1782, son Jacob in Sep 1782, him [Henry] in Feb 1783, him and sons Henry, Richard and Han *(sic)* in 1791 and him in 1793 (Ledger B, pp. 36, 44; Ledger C, p. 12 [account continued in Ledger E, which is missing]; Ledger D, p. 86 [account continued in Ledger E, which is missing]; Ledger F, pp. 237, 238); see Mrs. Ruff and Henry Touchstone, q.v.

Ruff, Henry [1760-1845], appeared on a list of debts dated 26 Dec 1822 and titled "A List of Allen's Claims" that were due and payable to Dr. Richard N. Allen for services rendered [no dates were given] by him to the said Ruff (Document filed in Historical Society of Harford County Archives folder "R. N. Allen"); he was visited by Dr. Robert H. Archer who treated his wife in Sep 1825, Negro Louisa and Negro George in 1828; he was also treated by Dr. Alonzo Preston at various times between 12 Apr 1826 and 29 Dec 1826 (Archer, p. 154, Ledger F, p. 146; Preston, p. 72) [Henry Ruff, Jr. was a Revolutionary War veteran.]; see James Ruff and John Lochary, q.v.

Ruff, James, of Henry, was treated by Dr. John Archer in March 1793 (Ledger F, p. 288)

Ruff, James [1791-1875], was visited by Dr. Alonzo Preston who treated him at various times between 1824 and 1826 [no dates or details were given], Harriot and Priscilla in 1825 and Henry in 1827; his medical bills were paid in cash in June 1826 and Dec 1829 (p. 9) [James Ruff was a War of 1812 veteran.]

Ruff, John, was treated by Dr. John Archer nine times between 17 Jan and 26 Jan 1777 (Ledger C, p. 59, noted that Richard Ruff paid the medical bill on 21 Jan 1778)

Ruff, John, was treated by Dr. John Archer in July 1787 (Ledger F, pp. 346, 361) [John Ruff was a Revolutionary War veteran.]; see Thomas Jones, q.v.

Ruff, John, was treated by Dr. Robert H. Archer after 1822 [no dates or details were given] (Dr. Archer's "Alphabet to Ledger H" is his booklet [filed in the Archives of the Historical Society of Harford County] that contains his index to Ledger H [which is missing] for his patients in Baltimore City before 1822 and in Harford County after 1822, according to a notation by Dr. George W. Archer.)

Ruff, Mrs., widow of Henry (tanner), was visited by Dr. John Archer who treated her and son Henry at various times between 1795 and 1799 (Ledger I, which is missing, was abstracted by Dr. George W. Archer circa 1890; his notes are in the Archives of the Historical Society of Harford County file "Archer, G. W. Coll. – Ledgers and Day Books")

Ruff, Priscilla, see James Ruff, q.v.

Ruff, Richard, was treated by Dr. John Archer in Feb and Mar 1778, Dec 1780, and Jan and Nov 1781 (Ledger C, p. 104) [account continued in Ledger E, which is missing] [Richard Ruff was a Revolutionary War veteran.]; see John Ruff, q.v.

Ruff, Richard [1791-1822], near Ranger's Lodge, was treated by Dr. Robert H. Archer on 10 Dec 1822 [wrote his will on 17 Dec 1822] and when seen on 19 Dec 1822 the doctor noted he was "moritund" [i. e., near death] (pp. 42, 43; Harford Co. Will Book SR 1, p. 269; Ledger F, p. 127, noted he "died insolvent") [Richard Ruff was a War of 1812 veteran.]; see Henry Ruff, Sr., q.v.

Ruff, Samuel, see John Bull, q.v.

Ruffcord, Simon, was treated by Dr. John Archer in Jul 1781 (Ledger D, p. 47, noted "debt forgiven as before")

Rumsey, see Thomas Garrett, q.v.

Rumsey, Benjamin [1743-1808] (esquire), was visited by Dr. John Archer who treated him and daughter Hannah in 1787 (Ledger F, p. 367) [account continued in Ledger K, which is missing] [Benjamin Rumsey was a Revolutionary War veteran and a prominent attorney in Joppa.]

Rumsey, Hannah, see Benjamin Rumsey, q.v.

Rumsey, John (esquire), was visited by Dr. John Archer who treated a negro in Aug 1780, him [John] in Nov 1780, his wife in Dec 1780, him in Feb 1781, a child in Mar 1781, a negro in Aug 1783, his [John's] wife in Sep 1783, his wife and daughter in 1789 and him in Jan 1792 (Ledger D, p. 92 [account continued in Ledger E, which is missing]; Ledger F, p. 123) [account continued in Ledger H, which is missing]

Rumsey, Mr., see Patrick Sloane, q.v.

Rush, Arnold, son-in-law to Robert Conn, was treated by Dr. John Archer in 1796 (Ledger I, which is missing, was abstracted by Dr. George W. Archer circa 1890; his notes are in the Archives of the Historical Society of Harford County folder "Archer, G. W. Coll. – Ledgers and Day Books")

Rush, Hanna, see William Amoss, q.v.

Russell, William, "at Bal. Town" [Baltimore], was treated by Dr. John Archer in Jul 1787 (Ledger F, p. 324, spelled his name Russel)

Ruth, Joseph (saddler), was treated by Dr. John Archer in Aug 1772, Sep 1775, May 1782 and Feb 1783 (Ledger B, p. 41; Ledger D, p. 10, noted "debt forgiven as before") [Joseph Ruth was a Revolutionary War veteran.]

Ruth, Moses, Jr., was visited by Dr. John Archer who treated a negro woman in Mar 1775, a negro infant in June 1775, him in July 1775, Sep 1778 and Aug 1780, and him and a negro in Sep 1780 (Ledger B, p. 51; Ledger C, p. 123, noted that his account was transferred to his father's account) [Moses Ruth, Jr. was a Revolutionary War veteran.]

Ruth, Moses, Sr., was visited by Dr. John Archer who treated him in Oct 1778, him and his wife in Aug 1779, him in Feb, May and Dec 1780 and Negro Rute in Oct 1781 (Ledger C, p. 101, and p. 111 stated "Moses Ruth Sr., from p. 101, to son's account;" Ledger D, p. 68); see Lawrence Conway, q.v.

Rutter, Charles, was visited by Dr. John Archer, Jr. who treated a child in Jul 1818, a child in Apr 1820, and his wife in Mar 1821; also mentioned "sundries to Chesapeake Academy" in Mar 1821 (p. 62); see Bob Howard, q.v.

Ryan, Betsy, see William Gorrell, q.v.

Ryan, James &ca (sic), was treated by Dr. Robert H. Archer in Baltimore before 1822 [no dates or details were given] (Dr. Archer's "Alphabet to Ledger H" is his booklet [filed in the Archives of the Historical Society of Harford County] that contains his index to Ledger H [which is missing] for his patients in Baltimore before 1822 and Harford County after 1822, according to a notation by Dr. George W. Archer.)

Ryan, John N., was visited by Dr. Robert H. Archer who treated him in Sep 1821 and his account mentioned Joseph Ryan (Ledger F, p. 8)

Ryan, Joseph, see John N. Ryan, q.v.

Ryland, Joseph P., was treated by Dr. Robert H. Archer in Oct 1821 and also mentioned Dr. Miller (Ledger F, p. 17); see Capt. Travis, q.v.

Ryland, Phil., was visited by Dr. John Archer, Jr. who treated his wife in May 1817 and him in Oct 1821 (p. 79)

Sample, Cunningham (esquire), was visited by Dr. John Archer who treated him and his wife in 1791 and Cunningham in 1798 (Ledger F, pp. 16, 61)

Sample, John, at Slate Ridge, was treated by Dr. John Archer in 1792 (Ledger F, p. 131) [account continued in Ledger H, which is missing]

Sampson. Ann, was treated by Dr. Matthew J. Allen in Jun 1847 (p. 57)

Samuels, Eleanor, was prescribed medicine by Dr. Robert H. Archer on 11 Mar 1801 (Rx Book, 1796-1801, p. 44)

Sanders (Saunders), Robert, allegedly murdered in 1838: "Maryland, Harford County. An inquisition taken at the house of Mrs. Hester Waltham in the County of Harford and State of Maryland aforesaid on the 6th day of March 1838 before me John C. Norris one of the Justice of the Peace in and for said county upon the view of the body of Robert Saunders then and there laying dead upon the oaths of … good and lawful men of the county aforesaid who being sworn upon the Holy Evangely of Almighty God and charged to inquire where, when and in what manner the said Robert Sanders came to his death do say upon their oaths that the said Robbert (sic) Sanders (sic) came to his deth (sic) by blows inflicted upon his head by a certain Thomas Dorsey and a certain Dennis Lowrey on Thursday, the 1st day of March inst., in Gunpowder Neck in said county. I witness whereof as well the aforesaid coroner or Justice of the Peace on the Jurors aforesaid have to this inquisition put their hands and seals this 6th day of March 1838. John C. Norris, Justice of the Peace. Inquisition – Robt. Sanders – Received & Recorded the ninth day of March Eighteen Hundred and Thirty Eight in Liber H. D. No. 20, folio 229, one of the Land Record Books of Harford County Court." (Document filed in the Archives Department of the Historical Society of Harford County)

Sanders (Saunders), Velinda, alias Lenney Sanders, sister to Jacob Wheeler, was treated by Dr. John Archer in Mar 1787 and Oct 1790 (Ledger F, pp. 32, 125)

Sankey, George, at Underhill's Mill, was treated by Dr. John Archer in 1795 (Ledger I, which is missing, was abstracted by Dr. George W. Archer circa 1890; his notes are in the Archives of the Historical Society of Harford County file "Archer, G. W. Coll. – Ledgers and Day Books") [Thomas Underhill either owned or operated a grist mill in the northwestern part of the county.]

Sappington, John K., see John Forwood, of Jacob, q.v.

Sappington, Richard [1753-1828] (doctor), was consulted by Dr. John Archer in 1787 and 1801 and he was also treated by Dr. Archer in Nov 1798 (Ledger F, pp. 240, 314) [Richard Sappington was a surgeon's assistant during the Revolutionary War.]

Saunders, ----, son-in-law to Mrs. Armstrong, was visited by Dr. John Archer who treated him and his family in 1797 (Ledger I, which is missing, was abstracted by Dr. George W. Archer circa 1890; his notes are in the Archives of the Historical Society of Harford County folder "Archer, G. W. Coll. – Ledgers and Day Books")

Saunders, Betsey, Mrs., was mentioned in Dr. Robert H. Archer's ledger in a non-medical matter in April 1823 and also mentioned wood cutting by son Wentworth in Dec 1822 and cash paid by Sarah Botts (Ledger F, p. 149)

Saunders, Edward, was visited by Dr. Matthew J. Allen who treated his son in Mar and Apr 1844 and Jan 1845 and rendered obstetrical services to his wife on 25 Jun 1845 (p. 33, noted he paid part of the bill in Sep 1847)

Saunders, Elizabeth, was treated by Dr. John Archer in Apr 1786 (Ledger F, p. 247)

Saunders, Isaac, was treated by Dr. Robert H. Archer in Jul 1824 (Ledger F, p. 101)

Saunders, Sarah, was treated by Dr. John Archer in Feb 1786 (Ledger F, p. 139)

Saunders, Velinda, see Velinda Sanders, q.v.

Saunders, Wentworth, see Betsey Saunders, q.v.

Saunders, William, was treated by Dr. John Archer in Aug 1782 (Ledger D, p. 47, noted the "debt forgiven as before") [William Saunders was a Revolutionary War veteran.]

Savin, Thomas L., was visited by Dr. John Archer, Jr. who treated a child in Dec 1819 (p. 5)

Sayre, John (captain), "Harford County" *(sic)*, was visited by Dr. John Archer who treated him and his wife in July 1787; Elenor ---- [no last name was given] was treated at Capt. Sayre's in Aug 1786 (Ledger F, pp. 16, 17) [John Sayre was most likely John Sear.]; see Negro Abigail, q.v.

Scantlin, John, was treated by Dr. John Archer in Nov 1779 and May 1781 (Ledger D, p. 36, noted "debt forgiven as before")

Scantlin, Mrs. (widow), was treated by Dr. John Archer in Jul 1786 (Ledger F, p. 353)

Scarborough, E., appeared on a list of debts dated 26 Dec 1822 and titled "A List of Allen's Claims" that were due and payable to Dr. Richard N. Allen for services rendered [no dates] to the said Scarborough (Document filed in Historical Society of Harford County Archives folder "R. N. Allen") [Euclidus Scarborough was a Revolutionary War veteran.]

Scarborough, Francis, was treated by Dr. Matthew J. Allen in Jun 1844 (p. 36)

Scarborough, John, Sr., was treated by Dr. Robert H. Archer in Oct 1822 (p. 26; Ledger F, p. 93) John Scarborough also appeared on a list of debts dated 26 Dec 1822 [no dates given] and titled "A List of Allen's Claims" that were due and payable to Dr. Richard N. Allen for services rendered [no dates] by him to the said Scarborough (Document filed in Historical Society of Harford County Archives folder "R. N. Allen")

Scarborough, Joseph, appeared on a list of debts dated 26 Dec 1822 and titled "A List of Allen's Claims" that were due and payable to Dr. Richard N. Allen for services rendered [no dates given] by him to the said Scarborough (Document filed in Historical Society of Harford County Archives folder "R. N. Allen") [Joseph Scarborough was a Revolutionary War veteran.]

Scarborough, Josiah, was treated by Dr. Matthew J. Allen in Aug 1844 (p. 40)

Scarborough, Samuel, appeared on a list of debts dated 26 Dec 1822 and titled "A List of Allen's Claims" that were due and payable to Dr. Richard N. Allen for services rendered [no dates given] by him to the said Scarborough (Document filed in Historical Society of Harford County Archives folder "R. N. Allen") [Two men by this name served in the War of 1812.]

Scarborough, Thomas, appeared on a list of debts dated 26 Dec 1822 and titled "A List of Allen's Claims" that were due and payable to Dr. Richard N. Allen for services rendered [no dates given] by him to the said Scarborough (Document filed in Historical Society of Harford County Archives folder "R. N. Allen"); see William Scarborough, q.v.

Scarborough, William, was visited by Dr. John Archer in 1787 and he treated him and his wife and also treated them and son Thomas in 1799 (Ledger F, p. 360) [account continued in Ledger K, which is missing] [William Scarborough was a Revolutionary War veteran.]

Scarff, Edmund, see John Scarff, q.v.

Scarff, John, near Upper Crossroads, son-in-law to John Talbot, was visited by Dr. John Archer who treated him and his sons Edmund and John in 1792 (Ledger F, p. 262) [John Scarff was a Revolutionary War veteran.]; see Negro Will, q.v.

Schofield, John, was treated by Dr. John Archer in Sep 1789 (Ledger F, p. 306, spelled his name Scophil) [account continued in Ledger H, which is missing]

Schreve, Joseph, was treated by Dr. Robert H. Archer in Baltimore before 1822 [no dates given] (Dr. Archer's "Alphabet to Ledger H" is his booklet [filed in Historical Society of Harford County Archives] that contains his index to Ledger H [which is missing] for his patients in Baltimore before 1822 and Harford County after 1822, according to a notation by Dr. George W. Archer.)

Scott, Abraham, see Joseph Scott, q.v.

Scott, Alexander, see Aquila Scott, of James, q.v.

Scott, Ann, Miss, see Aquila Scott, of James, q.v.

Scott, Ann, Mrs., was visited by Dr. John Archer who treated her and a negro in Apr 1775 (Ledger B, p. 20); widow Ann Scott was visited by Dr. Archer who treated her daughter Patty in June 1779, her [Ann] in Feb, Apr and Jun 1780, May and Dec 1781 and Dec 1782, and negroes Jim and Dermest (or Dermett?) in 1783 (Ledger D, p. 40, noted "This account settled by Aquila Scott.")

Scott, Aquila, of James, was visited by Dr. John Archer who treated him in Jan and Feb 1775, his wife in Nov 1782 and him, his wife, son Benjamin and daughter Ann in Oct 1788; Aquila Scott, at Oldfields, was treated by Dr. Archer in Jul 1781 and in Jun, Jul and Sep 1783 (Ledger B, p. 16; Ledger D, p. 32, and p. 92 noted "debt forgiven as before" [account continued in Ledger E, which is missing]; Ledger F, p. 24); Aquila Scott, near Bel Air, was visited by Dr. John Archer who treated him and his son Alexander in 1798 (Ledger I, which is missing, was abstracted by Dr. George W. Archer circa 1890; his notes are in the Archives of the Historical Society of Harford County folder "Archer, G. W. Coll. – Ledgers and Day Books") [Aquila Scott, of James, was a Revolutionary War veteran and founded Scott's Old Fields, now Bel Air, in 1780.]; see Ann Scott and Benjamin Scott, q.v.

Scott, Aquila [1790-1856], appeared on a list of debts dated 26 Dec 1822 and titled "A List of Allen's Claims" that were due and payable to Dr. Richard N. Allen for services rendered [no dates were given] by him to said Scott (Document filed in Historical Society of Harford County Archives folder "R. N. Allen"); Aquilla Scott was visited by Dr. Alonzo Preston who treated him in Aug 1827 and his wife "in partu" [in childbirth] on 6 Dec 1827 (p. 95) [Aquila "Quiller" Scott was a War of 1812 veteran.]

Scott, Benjamin, see Aquila Scott, q.v.

Scott, Benjamin (captain), was treated by Dr. John Archer eight times between Nov 1774 and Jun 1775, and in Oct and Dec 1780 and Jan 1781 (Ledger B, p. 98; Ledger D, p. 103, noted the bill was settled by Aquila Scott in his account) [Benjamin Scott was a Revolutionary War veteran.]

Scott, Elizabeth, see Joseph Scott, q.v.

Scott, James, see Joseph Scott, q.v.

Scott, James, was visited by Dr. John Archer who treated him in Feb and Mar 1781, a child in Apr 1781, him in Jun and Oct 1781, a negro in May and Jun 1782 and him [James] in Aug and Sep 1782, Aug and Sep 1783 and him and his family in 1786 (Ledger D, p. 123, noted "debt forgiven as before;" Ledger F, p. 105) [James Scott was a Revolutionary War veteran.]

Scott, Jean, see Joseph Scott, q.v.

Scott, Joseph, Jr., was treated by Dr. Robert H. Archer in Baltimore before 1822 [no dates or details were given] (Dr. Archer's "Alphabet to Ledger H" is his booklet [filed in the Archives of the Historical Society of Harford County] that contains his index to Ledger H [which is missing] for his patients in Baltimore before 1822 and Harford County after 1822, according to a notation by Dr. George W. Archer.)

Scott, Joseph, Sr., was prescribed medicine by Dr. Robert H. Archer on 20 Jun 1798 and 22 May 1799 (Rx Book, 1796-1801, pp. 11, 16) and was treated by Dr. Archer in Baltimore, but no dates or details were given in his "Alphabet to Ledger H" which is Dr. Archer's booklet [filed in the Archives of the Historical Society of Harford County] that contains his index to Ledger H [which is missing] for his patients in Baltimore before 1822 and Harford County after 1822, according to a notation by Dr. George W. Archer.)

Scott, Joseph (esquire), York Co., was visited by Dr. John Archer who treated William, Samuel, Abraham, Mary, Jean, James and Elizabeth and "oldest daughter" in June 1775 and him [Joseph] in July 1775 (Ledger B, p. 83)

Scott, Mary, see Joseph Scott, q.v.

Scott, Michael, near S. Osborn's on Gunpowder Neck, was treated by Dr. John Archer circa 1787 (Ledger F, p. 220, and later written in a different handwriting were the words "Great Scott!")

Scott, Mr., was prescribed medicine for his child by Dr. Robert H. Archer on 5 May 1799 (Rx Book, 1796-1801, p. 15)

Scott, Mrs., daughter of Mr. Giles, was visited by Dr. John Archer who treated her in Mar 1781 and an "African domestic" named Tim in Apr 1783 (Ledger D, p. 124) [account continued in Ledger E, which is missing]

Scott, Nathaniel, in Colegate's Old Fields, was treated by Dr. John Archer in 1786 (Ledger F, p. 345)

Scott, Otho [1797-1864], was visited by Dr. Robert H. Archer who treated his wife "parturiend" [in childbirth] on 12 Jun 1825 in consultation with Dr. Forwood (p. 134; Ledger F, p. 84) [Otho Scott was a War of 1812 veteran and a prominent attorney in Bel Air.]

Scott, Patrick, at Slate Ridge, was treated by Dr. John Archer in Apr 1779 (ledger C, p. 4); see Thomas Smith and ---- Bryarly, q.v.

Scott, Samuel, see Joseph Scott, q.v.

Scott, Susanna, Mrs., was treated by Dr. John Archer in Aug 1794 (Ledger F, pp. 316, 324) [account continued in Ledger I, which is missing]; Susanna Scott (widow) was treated by Dr. John Archer in 1797 (Ledger I, which is missing, was abstracted by Dr. George W. Archer circa 1890; his notes are in the Archives of the Historical Society of Harford County folder "Archer, G. W. Coll. – Ledgers and Day Books")

Scott, William, see Negro Sarah and Joseph Scott, q.v.

Scott, William, was treated by Dr. Robert H. Archer in Baltimore before 1822 [no dates or details were given] (Dr. Archer's "Alphabet to Ledger H" is his booklet [filed in the Archives of the Historical Society of Harford County] that contains his index to Ledger H [which is missing] for his patients in Baltimore before 1822 and Harford County after 1822, according to a notation by Dr. George W. Archer.)

Scotten, Martha, Miss, at Ring Factory [on Winters Run, west of Bel Air], was treated by Dr. Matthew J. Allen in Jun, Jul, Aug, Sep and Oct 1848 (p. 87)

Scotton, William, at William Morgan's place on B. R. Neck [Bush River Neck], was visited by Dr. John Archer who treated him and his wife in 1790 (Ledger F, p. 18)

Seales, H., see ---- Ferril, q.v.

Sear, John (captain), see Negro Abigail, James Bond and John Sayre, q.v.

Sears, James (postmaster), Havre de Grace, was treated by Dr. John Archer, Jr. in Jun 1815 (p. 15)

Sears, John [1752-1802], was prescribed medicine by Dr. Robert H. Archer on 19 Jun 1801 (Rx Book, 1796-1801, p. 53) and he was treated by Dr. Archer in Baltimore before 1822 [no dates or details were given] (Dr. Archer's "Alphabet to Ledger H" is his booklet [filed in the Archives of the Historical Society of Harford County] that contains his index to Ledger H [which is missing] for his patients in Baltimore before 1822 and Harford County after 1822, according to a notation by Dr. George W. Archer.)

Sears, Mrs., was prescribed medicine by Dr. Robert H. Archer on 25 Jul 1799 and 24 Oct 1799 and 25 Dec 1799 (Rx Book, 1796-1801, pp. 18, 23, 26)

Sears, Simon, see Thomas Huggins & Co., q.v.

Sedgwick, Benjamin, was treated by Dr. John Archer in Apr 1781 and Apr 1786 (Ledger D, p. 9, noted "debt forgiven as before" and misspelled his name Seduwick; Ledger F, p. 235)

Senate, Thomas (shoemaker), "X Roads," was visited by Dr. John Archer who rendered treatment "by inoculating yr. family Martha & Geo. Senate & Saml. Hathorn" in 1795 (Ledger I, which is missing, was abstracted by Dr. George W. Archer circa 1890; his notes are in Archives of the Historical Society of Harford County file "Archer, G. W. Coll. – Ledgers and Day Books")

Sewell, Bill, see Charles S. Sewell, q.v.

Sewell, Charles (reverend), was visited by Dr. John Archer who treated a negro in Jul 1779 and him [Charles] in Aug 1779 (Ledger C, p. 105, noted that the doctor had forgiven the bill, stating "by a donation of the acct. to him as a clergyman")

Sewell, Charles S. [1779-1848] (esquire), was visited by Dr. Robert T. Allen who treated a girl in Jan 1825, Harry in Mar 1825, his [Charles'] wife in Jun 1825, Harry in Sep 1825, Bill in Nov 1825, him [Charles] in Jan and Apr 1826, Miss Morea [Maria?] in Apr 1826, Benjamin Shelden and Harry in Jun 1826, him [Charles] in Jan 1827, W. Wright in Feb 1827 and a negro female (tooth extraction) in Mar 1827; also noted William Allen [in behalf of Dr. Allen] received full payment in Jul 1828 (Document filed in Historical Society of Harford County Archives file "R. N. Allen" misspelled his name Sewall) [Charles Smith Sewell, of Abingdon, was a War of 1812 veteran.]

Sewell, Harry, see Charles S. Sewell, q.v.

Sewell, Morea or Maria, see Charles S. Sewell, q.v.

Sewell, Thomas, was treated by Dr. Robert H. Archer in Baltimore before 1822 [no dates or details were given] (Dr. Archer's "Alphabet to Ledger H" is his booklet [filed in the Archives of the Historical Society of

Harford County] that contains his index to Ledger H [which is missing] for his patients in Baltimore before 1822 and Harford County after 1822, according to a notation by Dr. George W. Archer.)

Shanley, Dr., was consulted by Dr. John Archer in 1788 (Ledger F, p. 291)

Shannon, George (blacksmith), was visited by Dr. John Archer who inoculated two of his family in 1782 and treated him in Nov 1788 (Ledger D, p. 40, noted "debt forgiven as before;" Ledger F, p. 317) [account continued in Ledger G, which is missing]

Sharewood, William, see William Sherewood, q.v.

Shaw, Araminta (widow), was visited by Dr. John Archer who treated her in May 1773, a child in Nov 1774 and her [Araminta] in May-June 1775 (Ledger B, p. 98, listed her as Aramyta Shaw)

Shaw, John, was visited by Dr. John Archer, Jr. who treated his daughter in June 1816 (p. 54)

Shaw, Samuel, was treated by Dr. John Archer before 1772 and his child, his wife and maid in Sep 1772 and him [Samuel] in May 1773 (Ledger B, p. 18)

Shelden, Benjamin, see Charles S. Sewell, q.v.

Shepherd, William, was treated by Dr. John Archer in Jul 1780, Mar 1782, Aug and Oct 1783 and Aug 1786 (Ledger D, p. 78, noted "debt forgiven as before;" Ledger F, p. 5)

Sherewood, William, was visited by Dr. John Archer who treated his wife in June 1775, him in Jun 1780, Jan and Apr 1781, him and his wife in Feb 1785 and Mar 1788, and him, his wife and child in Apr 1788 (Ledger B, p. 26, spelled his name Sharwood; Ledger D, p. 71, spelled his name Sheerwood; Ledger F, p. 64, spelled his name Sharewood, and p. 69 spelled it Sherewood) [account continued in Ledger G, which is missing]; William Sherwood (sic) was visited by Dr. John Archer who treated him and his family in 1797 (Ledger I, which is missing, was abstracted by Dr. George W. Archer circa 1890; his notes are in the Archives of the Historical Society of Harford County folder "Archer, G. W. Coll. – Ledgers and Day Books")

Sheridan (Sheredine), James, was visited by Dr. John Archer who treated him in Nov 1774, a child in Dec 1777, him in Jul 1779, Sep 1780 and Jun 1783, son Thomas in 1787 and him [James] in Aug 1790; Dr. James Archer treated him [James] in Feb 1806 for "nervous fever" (Ledger B, p. 100, spelled his name Sheredine; Ledger C, p. 98, spelled his name Sheridine and noted "debt forgiven by order of testator;" Ledger D, p. 98, spelled his name Sheridon and noted "debt forgiven as before;" Dr. John Archer, Ledger F, p. 154, spelled his name Sheridin) [account continued in Ledger G, which is missing]; Dr. James Archer, p. 24, spelled his name Sheridane) [James Sheredine was a Revolutionary War veteran.]

Sheridan, James, Jr. [1773-1838], was visited by Dr. John Archer who treated him and his family at various times between 1796 and 1803 (Ledger I, which is missing, was abstracted by Dr. George W. Archer circa 1890; his notes are in Archives of the Historical Society of Harford County folder "Archer, G. W. Coll. – Ledgers and Day Books")

Sheridan, Mr. (cooper), was mentioned in Dr. Robert H. Archer's ledger in a non-medical matter in Oct 1827 (p. 251)

Sheridan, Thomas, was treated by Dr. Robert H. Archer in Baltimore before 1822 [no dates or details were given] (Dr. Archer's "Alphabet to Ledger H" is his booklet [filed in the Archives of the Historical Society of Harford County] that contains his index to Ledger H [which is missing] for his patients in Baltimore before 1822 and Harford County after 1822, according to a notation by Dr. George W. Archer.); see James Sheridan (Sheredine), q.v.

Sherwood, William, see William Sherewood, q.v.

Shewel, Benjamin, was treated by Dr. Alonzo Preston in 1824 and 1825 who noted that Benjamin had "removed out of the state," but the doctor did not indicate the date or where he went (p. 54)

Shields, Jacob (negro), was treated by Dr. Robert H. Archer in Apr 1826 (p. 186)

Shields, Paul, near Isaac Webster's, was visited by Dr. John Archer who treated his wife in Jan 1776, him in Nov 1776 and a daughter in Dec 1777 (Ledger C, p. 21, noted "debt forgiven by order of testator")

Shields, Rosannah, near Samuel Forwood, was treated by Dr. John Archer in 1791 (Ledger F, p. 271)

Shineflu, Conrad, was prescribed medicine by Dr. Robert H. Archer on 17 Mar 1801 and on 2 Sep and 18 Oct and 13 Nov 1802 (Rx Book, 1796-1801, p. 49; Rx Book, 1802-1804, pp. 17, 22, 25); Conrad was treated by Dr. Archer in Baltimore before 1822 [no dates or details were given] (Dr. Archer's "Alphabet to Ledger H" is his booklet [filed in the Archives of the Historical Society of Harford County] that contains his index to Ledger H [which is missing] for his patients in Baltimore City before 1822 and in Harford County after 1822, according to a notation by Dr. George W. Archer.)

Short, Cotty, see Catherine Boardsman, q.v.

Short, Edward, was visited by Dr. John Archer who treated a child in Aug 1772 and him in Jul 1773 and Apr 1775 (Ledger B, p. 19) [Edward Short was a Revolutionary War veteran.]

Short, Polly, Miss, was treated by Dr. Robert H. Archer in Baltimore before 1822 [no dates or details were given] (Dr. Archer's "Alphabet to Ledger H" is his booklet [filed in the Archives of the Historical Society of Harford County] that contains his index to Ledger H [which is missing] for his patients in Baltimore before 1822 and Harford County after 1822, according to a notation by Dr. George W. Archer.)

Shriard, Francis, near William Luckie's, was treated by Dr. John Archer in 1787 (Ledger F, p. 301)

Silver, B., see William Aiken, q.v.

Silver, Benjamin, was visited by Dr. John Archer who treated his daughter in Mar 1775, him and Sally and a grandchild in Apr 1775, a young man and Benjamin's brother William in Feb 1777, his [Benjamin's] wife and Sally Smith in Apr 1783, and his sister Sarah and brother John in June 1783 (Ledger B, p. 20, and Ledger C, p. 9, both spelled his name Silvers); see Mary King, q.v.

Silver, Benjamin [1753-1818], was visited by Dr. John Archer who treated him and his wife in 1796 (Ledger F, p. 39, spelled his name Silvers) [account continued in Ledger K, which is missing] [Benjamin Silver, near Darlington, was a Revolutionary War veteran.]; see Millicent Silver, q.v.

Silver, David, was visited by Dr. John Archer who treated "Malisson Silvers" [Millicent Silver] in 1795 (Ledger I, which is missing, was abstracted by Dr. George W. Archer circa 1890; his notes are in the Archives of the Historical Society of Harford County folder "Archer, G. W. Coll. – Ledgers and Day Books; spelled his name Silvers); see William Silver, q.v.

Silver, Gershom, was treated by Dr. John Archer in March and April 1775 and who also treated 5 children in Mar 1775, his wife and 2 children in Apr 1775 at which time he mentioned Billy and Peggy (Ledger B, p. 52, spelled his name Silvers)

Silver, John, was treated by Dr. Robert H. Archer after 1822 [no dates or details were given] (Dr. Archer's "Alphabet to Ledger H" is his booklet [filed in the Archives of the Historical Society of Harford County] that contains his index to Ledger H [which is missing] for his patients in Baltimore City before 1822 and in Harford County after 1822, according to a notation by Dr. George W. Archer); see Benjamin Silver, q.v.

Silver, Joseph, see William Silver, q.v.

Silver, Mary, see William Silver, q.v.

Silver, Millicent (widow), was treated by Dr. John Archer in 1801 and he also mentioned Benjamin Silver (Ledger I, which is missing, was abstracted by Dr. George W. Archer circa 1890 and her name was listed as Mrs. Mellison Silvers; George's notes are in the Archives of the Historical Society of Harford County folder "Archer, G. W. Coll. – Ledgers and Day Books")

Silver, Mrs., was visited by Dr. John Archer who treated her son William in Mar 1777 and her in Jun 1783 (Ledger C, p. 44, spelled her name Silvers)

Silver, Sally, see Benjamin Silver, q.v.

Silver, Silas, was treated by Dr. Robert H. Archer in July 1828 (p. 2856)

Silver, William [1778-1838], was visited by Dr. Robert H. Archer who treated a child in July 1823, him and son David in Aug 1823, wife in Aug and Sep 1824, son Joseph and Negro Rachel in Mar 1826, daughter Mary in Mar 1827, a child in July 1827 and son David in Oct 1827 (pp. 85, 86, 120, 175, 177, 219, 239, 251; Ledger F, p. 46) [William Silver was a War of 1812 veteran.]

Silver, William, see Benjamin Silver, q.v.

Simco, William, see Christopher Little, q.v.

Simmons, James, see Thomas Huggins & Co., q.v.

Simmons, Thomas, had an account in Dr. John Archer, Jr.'s ledger that mentioned his son Nimrod or Winstod (?) [name illegible] in Oct 1841 (sic) (p. 41)

Simpers, D., see Thomas Huggins & Co., q.v.

Sims, George, was treated by Dr. John Archer in Nov 1779(?) [the year was not entered in the ledger and "McCallis" was written in smaller letters after his name] (Ledger D, p. 17, noted "debt forgiven as before")

Sims, Mary, see John Lynch, q.v.

Sinclair, William, was treated by Dr. John Archer in Mar 1786 (Ledger F, p. 188) [William Sinclare or Sinclair was a Revolutionary War veteran.]

Sinnet, Nicholas, see Francis Maybury, q.v.

Slack, Heny or Henry, see John Slack, q.v.

Slack, Jacob, was visited by Dr. John Archer who treated him in Sep 1781, his wife "obstetriend" [pregnant and probably in childbirth] on 2 Mar 1782, a child in Apr 1784, his wife in Aug 1784 and him in Dec 1790 and Sep 1793 (Ledger D, p. 70; Ledger F, pp. 112, 122) [Jacob Slack was a Revolutionary War veteran.]

Slack, John, was visited by Dr. John Archer who treated him in July 1773 and Feb 1774, his wife in Aug 1773, an infant in Oct 1774, a child in 1776, him [John] in Sep and Oct 1779, his sister and her child in Jul 1781, him in Nov 1782, a child in Mar 1783, him in Jul and Oct 1783, Aug 1784 and Jan 1785, a child in Sep and Oct 1785, a child named Heny or Henry [unclear] in 1786 and him [John] in Jan 1792 (Ledger B, 69; Ledger C, p. 61; Ledger D, pp. 51, 123, noted "debt forgiven as before;" Ledger F, pp. 112, 122, 302)

Slack, Mrs. (widow), was treated by Dr. John Archer in Mar 1781 (Ledger D, p. 126, noted "debt forgiven as before")

Slade, William, near Cooptown, was treated by Dr. John Archer in March 1787 (Ledger F, p. 235)

Slade, William (tavern keeper), at Manor Chapel, was treated by Dr. John Archer in consultation with Dr. Bradford circa 1794 [date not given] (Ledger I, which is missing, was abstracted by Dr. George W. Archer circa 1890; his notes are in the Archives of the Historical Society of Harford County folder "Archer, G. W. Coll. – Ledgers and Day Books")

Slater, William, was prescribed medicine by Dr. Robert H. Archer for his wife on 14 Feb 1803 and 24 Apr 1803, for his child on 14 Apr 1803 and for him on 18 May 1803 (Rx Book, 1802-1804, pp. 32, 39, 41, 43)

Slee, John, was visited by Dr. Robert H. Archer who treated his wife in Mar 1823 and him in Oct 1823, daughter Eliza and a negro in May 1824,Timothy and Hannah and John Johnson and a child in Aug 1824, him [John] in Jun 1825, a child Fra.(?) in July 1825 and a child in Aug 1827; John was also treated in 1824 by Dr. Alonzo Preston and was prescribed medicine for a child by Dr. Robert H. Archer on 6 May 1825 and 26 Sep 1830 (Dr. Archer, pp. 57, 90, 107, 145, 146, 243, Ledger F, pp. 129, 140; Rx Book, 1825-1851, pp. 77, 102; Dr. Preston, p. 3)

Slemmons, John (reverend), was visited by Dr. John Archer who inoculated 6 of his family in 1782 and treated him, his wife and an infant in Oct 1788 and him and his wife in Apr 1792 (Ledger D, p. 7, noted "debt forgiven as before;" Ledger F, pp. 25, 136)

Slemmons, Mr., see Mr. Cunningham," q.v.

Sloane, Patrick, on Mr. Rumsey's place, was treated by Dr. John Archer in July 1787 (Ledger F, p. 288) [account continued in Ledger I, which is missing]

Small, Robert, was visited by Dr. John Archer who treated his brother [no name was given] in June 1776, a child in July 1777 and his brother [no name was given] in May 1778 (Ledger C, p. 50) [Robert Small was a Revolutionary War veteran.]

Smith & Giles, had an account with Dr. John Archer who treated Negro Andrew in Mar 1780 and others [not named] in Apr 1780 and Jul 1781 (Ledger D, p. 53, noted "debt forgiven as before")

Smith, Alex, see Buchanan Smith, q.v.

Smith, Alizanna, was treated by Dr. John Archer in July 1789 (Ledger F, p. 361) [account continued in Ledger K, which is missing]

Smith, Ally, Miss, was treated by Dr. John Archer in Nov 1782 and Jan and Feb 1783 (Ledger D, p. 4, noted "debt forgiven as before")

Smith, Basil, at Otter Point, was visited by Dr. John Archer who treated him in Dec 1774 and "Bazil Smith, at the Point," in Mar 1787 (Ledger B, p. 85; Ledger F, p. 251) [account continued in Ledger H, which is missing] [Basil Smith was a Revolutionary War veteran.]

Smith, Benjamin, was visited by Dr. John Archer who inoculated 3 of his family in 1777 and treated him in Oct 1782 and Mar 1788 (Ledger C, p. 73, noted "debt forgiven by order of testator" in 1782, but no note in 1788; Ledger F, p. 85) [Benjamin Smith was a Revolutionary War veteran.]

Smith, Buchanan, was visited by Dr. John Archer who treated him at times between Jan 1773 and Jul 1775, an infant in Jan 1773, his wife in Jun 1773 and Jan 1775, a child in Sep 1773 and Jul 1774, and son Alex in Jul 1775 (Ledger B, p. 73)

Smith, Cal, was prescribed medicine for his wife by Dr. Robert H. Archer on 20 May 1830 (Rx Book, 1825-1851, p. 100)

Smith, Caroline, see Mary Ann Smith, q.v.

Smith, Catherine, daughter of Widow Smith, at Freeborn Brown's, was treated by Dr. John Archer in Jun 1792 (Ledger F, p. 171)

Smith, Cathy, see Martha Smith, q.v.

Smith, David, see Samuel Smith (blacksmith), q.v.

Smith, David (pedagogue), was treated by Dr. John Archer in Dec 1788 (Ledger F, p. 349) [account continued in Ledger I, which is missing, but was abstracted by Dr. George W. Archer circa 1890: David Smith (pedagogue) was treated in 1794.] (Archives of the Historical Society of Harford County folder "Archer, G. W. Coll. – Ledgers and Day Books")

Smith, Davixter, was treated by Dr. John Archer in Apr 1788 and the medical bill was charged to Harford County (Ledger F, p. 160)

Smith, Delia, see Mary Ann Smith, q.v.

Smith, Dr., was consulted by Dr. John Archer in 1792 (Ledger F, p. 233)

Smith, Elenor, was treated by Dr. John Archer in Aug 1781 and Feb 1788 (Ledger D, p. 67, noted "debt forgiven as before;" Ledger F, p. 194)

Smith, Elizabeth, widow of Nathaniel Smith, was visited by Dr. John Archer who treated a negro boy in Jul 1780 and her in Oct 1780, Feb 1781 and Apr 1791; account was paid by Miss Polly Smith in 1792 (Ledger D, p. 77; Ledger F, p. 303)

Smith, Fanny, see William Smith (bayside), q.v.

Smith, Francis, Sr., in Baltimore, was visited by Dr. John Archer who treated his son John in Sep 1781, Hugh Jeffrey in May 1782 and him [Francis] in Sep 1782 and Aug 1788 (Ledger D, p. 74, noted "debt forgiven as before;" Ledger F, p. 226); see Paca Smith, q.v.

Smith, George, "for mother," was treated by Dr. John Archer in Sep 1780 (Ledger D, p. 99, noted "debt forgiven as before")

Smith, George, was treated by Dr. Robert H. Archer in Mar 1825 and Aug 1827 (Ledger F, p. 125); see George Lochary, q.v.

Smith, George [1773-1835] (blacksmith), was paid by Dr. Robert H. Archer for sundry smith work in Apr 1827, and treated him in Aug 1828 and son Samuel in Sep 1828 (pp. 221, 293, 296, 297) [George Smith was a War of 1812 veteran.]

Smith, George, Mrs. (widow), was treated by Dr. Robert H. Archer after 1822 [no dates or details were given] (Dr. Archer's "Alphabet to Ledger H" is his booklet [filed in the Archives of the Historical Society of Harford County] that contains his index to Ledger H [which is missing] for his patients in Baltimore before 1822 and Harford County after 1822, according to a notation by Dr. George W. Archer.) [Her name listed as "Smith, Mrs., widow of Geo., see Smith, Samuel."]

Smith, Hannah &ca (sic), was treated by Dr. Robert H. Archer in Baltimore before 1822 [no dates or details were given] (Dr. Archer's "Alphabet to Ledger H" is his booklet [filed in the Archives of the Historical Society of Harford County] that contains his index to Ledger H [which is missing] for his patients in Baltimore before 1822 and Harford County after 1822, according to a notation by Dr. George W. Archer.)

Smith, Henry (colored), was visited by Dr. Matthew J. Allen who treated him in Apr and May 1844 and his wife 16 times in Jun, Jul and Aug 1847 and once in Sep and Nov 1847 (pp. 33, 56, and p. 60 later noted "Dead," but did not give a date of death or indicate who had died, him or his wife)

Smith, Henry, was treated by Dr. Jacob A. Preston 18 times between 7 Dec 1821 and 15 Feb 1822; he was also treated by Dr. Robert H. Archer in Feb 1827 in consultation with Dr. Norris (Document filed in Historical Society of Harford County Archives folder "Preston, Jacob A.;" Dr. Archer's ledger, pp. 214, 215) [Henry Smith was a War of 1812 veteran.]; see Joseph Husband, q.v.

Smith, Hugh, son of Thomas, was treated by Dr. John Archer in May 1787 (Ledger F, p. 298)

Smith, Hugh, Jr. [c1785-1836], was treated by Dr. Robert H. Archer in Oct 1827 in consultation with Dr. John Archer, Jr. (p. 249)

Smith, Isabel, was treated by Dr. John Archer in Sep 1786 (Ledger F, p. 2); see Isabel Finagan, q.v.

Smith, Jabish, see John Smith, q.v.

Smith, James, see George Morrison, q.v.

Smith, James, was treated by Dr. Matthew J. Allen in 1823 in Calvert County (p. 8b)

Smith, James (blacksmith), was visited by Dr. Robert H. Archer who treated his son James in June 1825, himself in July 1825 and his wife in Aug 1825 and Apr 1826 (pp. 138, 143, 150, 180; Ledger F, p. 135)

Smith, James (tailor) was treated by Dr. John Archer in Mar 1778 (Ledger C, p. 92, noted "debt forgiven by order of testator")

Smith, James, was visited by Dr. Matthew J. Allen who rendered obstetrical services to his wife [in childbirth] on 14 Feb 1844 and also noted $5 paid to Dr. Johnson (p. 31)

Smith, James, son of Thomas, at G. Ferry [Gunpowder Ferry], was treated by Dr. John Archer in Sep 1799 (Ledger F, p. 232)

Smith, Job (blacksmith), was treated by Dr. Robert H. Archer in Baltimore before 1822 [no dates or details were given] (Dr. Archer's "Alphabet to Ledger H" is his booklet [filed in the Archives of the Historical Society of Harford County] that contains his index to Ledger H [which is missing] for his patients in Baltimore before 1822 and Harford County after 1822, according to a notation by Dr. George W. Archer.)

Smith, John, see Francis Smith, Capt. Samuel Smith and Thomas Harris, q.v.

Smith, John [1747-1832] (captain), was treated by Dr. John Archer in Sep 1781, Feb, Mar and Aug 1783 and May and Jun 1784 (Ledger D, p. 78) [account continued in Ledger E, which is missing] [Capt. John Smith was a Revolutionary War veteran.]

Smith, John (carpenter), was treated by Dr. John Archer at times between 1786 and 1795 (Ledger F, pp. 101, 271, 292)

Smith, John (fuller), was visited by Dr. John Archer who treated him in Jul 1781, a child in Aug 1781, his wife in Sep 1781, a daughter in Mar 1782, a daughter in Feb 1783 and his wife in Aug 1783 (Ledger D, p. 27) [account continued in Ledger E, which is missing]

Smith, John (lieutenant), was treated by Dr. John Archer in Dec 1776 and May 1778 (Ledger C, p. 74) [Lieut. John Smith was a Revolutionary War veteran.]

Smith, John, son of Jabish (sic), was visited by Dr. John Archer who treated him in Oct 1779, Bowman (sic) and George Swarts in Mar 1783, and him in Oct 1783 and Jun 1785 (Ledger D, p. 30, noted "debt forgiven as before")

Smith, John, son of Robert, near Ignatius Wheeler's, was treated by Dr. John Archer in Nov 1787 (Ledger F, p. 202)

Smith, John, Green Street, in Baltimore, was treated by Dr. Robert H. Archer before 1822 [no dates or details were given] (Dr. Archer's "Alphabet to Ledger H" is his booklet [filed in the Archives of the Historical Society of Harford County] that contains his index to Ledger H [which is missing] for his patients in Baltimore before 1822 and Harford County after 1822, according to a notation by Dr. George W. Archer.)

Smith, Jonathan, was treated by Dr. John Archer at various times between 1788 and 1798 and his wife in 1795 (Ledger F, pp. 179, 185, 200, 240); see Samuel Smith (blacksmith), q.v.

Smith, Joseph, was treated by Dr. John Archer twice in Jan 1773 (Ledger B, p. 69) [Joseph Smith was a Revolutionary War veteran.]

Smith, Joseph, was prescribed medicine for his wife on 22 Mar 1803 by Dr. Robert H. Archer (Rx Book, 1802-1804, p. 37) [Joseph Smith was a Revolutionary War veteran.]

Smith, Joseph (reverend), was treated by Dr. John Archer in Aug 1779 (Ledger D, p. 9, noted "debt forgiven as before")

Smith, Martha, was visited by Dr. John Archer who treated her daughter in Feb 1781, her [Martha] in May 1782, a child in Sep 1781, her [Martha] in Sep 1782 and Mar 1783, Miss Cathy in Mar 1783 and a negro in Aug 1783 (Ledger D, p. 122) [continued in Ledger E, which is missing]

Smith, Martha (widow), was visited by Dr. John Archer who treated her and son Ralph in 1789 and also mentioned Daniel Harris (Ledger F, pp. 293, 306, 307); see John Van Cleave, q.v.

Smith, Mary Ann, Mrs., was visited by Dr. Matthew J. Allen who treated Caroline in Apr 1844, her [Mary Ann] and Delia in Sep 1844, her [Mary Ann] in Jan and Feb 1845, a child in Jan 1845 and also mentioned Mary Ann was the guardian for Miss M. Herbert in 1845; he also treated Delia (tooth extraction) in Jan 1848 and in Mar 1848 (pp. 34, 43, 72)

Smith, Molly, see John Barney, q.v.

Smith, Mr., son-in-law of Mrs. Greme, was visited by Dr. Robert H. Archer who treated his wife in Aug 1825 (p. 147; Ledger F, p. 118)

Smith, Mrs., was prescribed medicine by Dr. Robert H. Archer on 1 Aug 1825 (Rx Book, 1825-1851, p. 82); see George Kidd and Thomas Lilley, q.v.

Smith, Nancy, see William Smith (blacksmith), q.v.

Smith, Nathan, son of William, was treated by Dr. John Archer in 1795 (Ledger F, p. 150) [Nathan or Nathaniel Smith was a Revolutionary War veteran.]

Smith, Nathaniel, see Elizabeth Smith, q.v.

Smith, Paca [1779-1830], was visited by Dr. John Archer, Jr. who treated Francis Smith and Negro Sam in May 1816 and also mentioned Mark Pringle, dec'd., in 1815 (p. 7); "Paca Smith on his death bed addressing himself to his wife & me, said, indistinctly, that he had lent cousin Betsy Archer some money between 150 & 200 dollars which he wished to be given her – and at the time appeared to be well in his senses. Wm. M. Dallam, August 21st 1831." (Document filed in Historical Society of Harford County Archives folder "Medical Bills – Dr. William M. Dallam") [Paca Smith was a War of 1812 veteran.]; see William Smith, q.v.

Smith, Patty, Miss, was treated by Dr. John Archer in July 1791 (Ledger F, p. 308)

Smith, Polly, Miss, was treated by Dr. John Archer in Oct 1789 (Ledger F, p. 368); see Elizabeth Smith and James Phillips, q.v.

Smith, Ralph, was treated by Dr. John Archer in Sep 1790 (Ledger F, pp. 175, 308) [Ralph Smith was a Revolutionary War veteran.]; see Martha Smith, q.v.

Smith, Ralph, son of Thomas, was treated by Dr. John Archer in Dec 1778, Nov 1779 and Oct 1782 (Ledger C, p. 37)

Smith, Richard, was treated by Dr. Robert H. Archer after 1822 [no dates or details were given] (Dr. Archer's "Alphabet to Ledger H" is his booklet [filed in the Archives of the Historical Society of Harford County] that contains his index to Ledger H [which is missing] for his patients in Baltimore City before 1822 and in Harford County after 1822, according to a notation by Dr. George W. Archer.)

Smith, Robert (storekeeper), at Susquehanna [i. e., Smith's Ferry, now Lapidum, on the Susquehanna River], was visited by Dr. John Archer who treated his brother in Aug 1772 and him [Robert] in Sep 1773, and Mar and Apr 1776 (Ledger B, p. 17; Ledger C, p. 45, noted that Robert lived "at R: Mills" which was most likely referring to Rock Run Mill nearby on the Susquehanna River)

Smith, Robert, was treated by Dr. John Archer five times in Dec 1783 and in Jan 1786 (Ledger D, p. 94; Ledger F, p. 10) [Robert Smith was a Revolutionary War veteran.]; see Thomas Hall, q.v.

Smith, Robert, appeared on a list of debts dated 26 Dec 1822 and titled "A List of Allen's Claims" that were due and payable to Dr. Richard N. Allen for services rendered [no dates given] to said Smith (Document filed in Historical Society of Harford County Archives folder "R. N. Allen")

Smith, Ruth (widow), was visited by Dr. John Archer many times between Dec 1772 and May 1774 and treated her child [or children?] in Dec 1772 and Feb 1773 (Ledger B, pp. 80, 84)

Smith, Sally, see William Smith (blacksmith), q.v.

Smith, Samuel (blacksmith), was visited by Dr. John Archer who treated him six times between May 1773 and May 1775, his child in Apr 1775, Jonathan in 1776 [no date or relationship given, probably his son], son David in Dec 1776, Sep 1777, Dec 1778 and Jan 1779, him [Samuel] in Jul 1777 and Sep 1778, his wife in Dec 1778, son Samuel in Dec 1778 and Jan 1779, wife in Mar 1779 and him [Samuel] and his wife in Jun 1780 (Ledger B, p. 67; Ledger C, p. 68)

Smith, Samuel (captain), was visited by Dr. John Archer who treated him nine times in Jul 1780, him and son John in Dec 1780, an infant in Feb 1782 and William Wills in Jul 1782 (Ledger D, p. 74) [continued in Ledger E, which is missing] [Samuel Smith was a Revolutionary War veteran.]

Smith, Samuel (cooper), was visited by Dr. John Archer who treated him in Aug 1780, his wife in Jun 1781, him in Feb 1783, his wife in Mar 1783, his children in Apr 1785, a child in May 1785, him in Dec 1785, and him and a child in Nov 1789 (Ledger D, p. 93, noted "debt forgiven as before;" Ledger F, p. 337)

Smith, Samuel, was treated by Dr. Robert H. Archer after 1822 [no dates or details were given] (Dr. Archer's "Alphabet to Ledger H" is his booklet [filed in the Archives of the Historical Society of Harford County] that contains his index to Ledger H [which is missing] for his patients in Baltimore before 1822 and Harford County after 1822, according to a notation by Dr. George W. Archer); see George Smith and Mrs. George Smith, q.v.

Smith, Samuel, was visited by Dr. Alonzo Preston who treated his wife in Mar 1825 (p. 22)

Smith, Samuel, was treated by Dr. Matthew J. Allen who dressed a hand wound in Jun 1848 (p. 86)

Smith, Samuel E., see George Morrison, q.v.

Smith, Sarah, Mrs., was prescribed medicine for a negro by Dr. Robert H. Archer on 6 Aug 1802 (Rx Book, 1802-1804, p. 9)

Smith, Sarah H., was prescribed medicine for a negro on 9 Aug 1802 by Dr. Robert H. Archer (Rx Book, 1802-1804, p. 10)

Smith, Thomas, at Joseph Miller's, was treated by Dr. John Archer in May 1787 (Ledger F, p. 289)

Smith, Thomas, at Slate Ridge, son-in-law to Patrick Scott, was treated by Dr. John Archer in Apr 1787 (Ledger F, p. 244)

Smith, Thomas, at Susquehanna Ferry, was visited by Dr. John Archer who inoculated 10 of his family in Feb 1777 and treated him in Aug 1780 (Ledger C, p. 73, noted "debt forgiven by order of testator") [Thomas Smith, possibly this one, was a Revolutionary War veteran.]

Smith, Thomas son of Thomas, "at Susquehanna, at the ferry" [i. e., Susquehanna River at Smith's Ferry, now Lapidum], was visited by Dr. John Archer who treated him and his wife in 1787 and him and a child in 1791 (Ledger F, pp. 25, 329) [continued in Ledger H, which is missing]

Smith, Thomas (laborer), "X Roads," was treated by Dr. John Archer in 1795 (Ledger I, which is missing, was abstracted by Dr. George W. Archer circa 1890; his notes are in the Archives of the Historical Society of Harford County file "Archer, G. W. Coll. – Ledgers and Day Books")

Smith, Thomas (millwright), was treated by Dr. John Archer at various times between 1797 and 1802 (Ledger I, which is missing, was abstracted by Dr. George W. Archer circa 1890; his notes are in the Archives of the Historical Society of Harford County folder "Archer, G. W. Coll. – Ledgers and Day Books")

Smith, Thomas (saddler), was treated by Dr. John Archer in 1782 [no dates were given] and Sep 1783 (Ledger D, p. 113, noted "debt forgiven as before")

Smith, Thomas, see Capt. McCrackin (McCackin?), Hugh Smith, Ralph Smith and James Smith, q.v.

Smith, Widow, see William Stott, James Walker, Patrick Dimsey and Catherine Smith, q.v.

Smith, William, see Nathan Smith, Negro Orange and Winston Smith, q.v.

Smith, William (Baltimore), see Thomas Harris, q.v.

Smith, William (Bayside), was visited by Dr. John Archer who treated his wife in Oct 1781, son Paca in Nov 1781, a negro in Apr and May 1782, him [William] at Mr. Ramsey's in Nov 1782, him in Dec 1782 and Feb 1783, and him and his children Fanny and Paca Smith in Oct 1789 (Ledger D, p. 84 [account continued in Ledger E, which is missing]; Ledger F, p. 3); see William Hill, q.v.

Smith, William (blacksmith), was visited by Dr. John Archer who treated him in Sep 1774 and him and daughters Sally and Nancy from 1796 to 1799 (Ledger B, p. 103; Ledger I, which is missing, was abstracted by Dr. George W. Archer circa 1890; his notes are in the Archives of the Historical Society of Harford County folder "Archer, G. W. Coll. – Ledgers and Day Books")

Smith, William (captain), was treated by Dr. Matthew J. Allen in 1832 in Calvert County (p. 18)

Smith, William (captain), brother-in-law to A. Hays, was visited by Dr. Robert H. Archer who treated Negro Ben in Apr 1826 in Harford County (p. 181; Ledger F, p. 46)

Smith, William [1770-1835] (colonel), was visited by Dr. Robert H. Archer who treated his wife in Feb 1828, him in Jan, May, June and July 1828, daughter Sally in Jul 1828 and him and a child in Aug 1828 (pp. 258, 259, 263, 275, 279, 285, 287, 290) [William Smith, of Churchville, was a War of 1812 veteran who donated an acre of his land for Smith's Chapel.]; see Mrs. Dever, q.v.

Smith, William (esquire), in Barrens [area in northwest part of county near Pennsylvania], was visited by Dr. John Archer who treated him and his wife in Oct 1786 and him in Apr 1788 (Ledger F, pp. 129, 305, 333) [last page noted "of William," but it was written in a different handwriting.]

Smith, William, overseer for Jos. Lee, was visited by Dr. John Archer who treated him and a child in 1786 (Ledger F, p. 351)

Smith, William, on Samuel Wilson's place, was visited by Dr. John Archer who treated him in 1790 and inoculated five of his family, but no names were given (Ledger F, p. 363)

Smith, William, of William, was visited by Dr. John Archer who treated his wife in Aug and Sep 1781 in consultation with Dr. Sappington, and him, his wife and a negro child in Aug [possibly Oct] 1781 (Ledger D, p. 69) [account continued in Ledger E, which is missing] [William Smith, of William, was a Revolutionary War veteran.]; see William Smith (esquire), q.v.

Smith, William, son of Capt. William, was treated by Dr. John Archer in Sep 1773 (Ledger B, p. 76)

Smith, Winston, of William, was treated by Dr. John Archer in Jan 1786 (Ledger F, p. 38) [Winston Smith was a Revolutionary War veteran.]

Smith, Winston Dallam, was visited by Dr. Robert H. Archer who treated a child in Sep 1825 (p. 160; Ledger F, p. 10)

Smithson, see Caesar Clark, q.v.

Smithson, Archibald [1765-c1825], was visited by Dr. John Archer who treated him and his wife in 1799 (Ledger F, p. 40)

Smithson, Daniel [1743-1798], was visited by Dr. John Archer who treated him in Aug and Sep 1780 and him and his wife in Jan 1782 (Ledger D, p. 88, noted "debt forgiven as before"); State vs. Thomas Durham: "Harford

County, to wit: The Jurors of the State of Maryland for the body of Harford county upon their oaths, present, that Thomas Durham late of Harford county aforesaid, yeoman, on the tenth day of February in the Year of our Lord one thousand seven hundred and ninety eight with force and arms at the county aforesaid, in and upon one Daniel Smithson in the peace of God and our said State, then and there being, did make an assault and him the said Daniel then and there did beat, wound and ill treat, so that his life was greatly despaired of, and other wrongs to the said Daniel then and there did to the great damage of the said Daniel and against the peace, government and dignity of the State of Maryland." [He died on 22 Feb 1798.] (File 22.10.3A in the Court Records Department of the Historical Society of Harford County)

Smithson, Maria, see William Smithson, q.v.

Smithson, Mariam, see Thomas Smithson, q.v.

Smithson, Nat., see Thomas Smithson, q.v.

Smithson, Polly, Miss, niece to James Barton's wife, was treated by Dr. John Archer in 1797 (Ledger I, which is missing, was abstracted by Dr. George W. Archer circa 1890; his notes are in the Archives of the Historical Society of Harford County folder "Archer, G. W. Coll. – Ledgers and Day Books")

Smithson, Thomas, was visited by Dr. John Archer who treated his daughter Mariam in 1787 and him in 1790 (Ledger F, p. 259, noted that Nat. Smithson paid the account in full on 24 Mar 1803)

Smithson, William, see Mr. McLaughlin, Vincent Goldsmith and Thomas Thruston, q.v.

Smithson, William [1745-1809] (esquire), was visited by Dr. John Archer who treated him n Apr 1781, a negro in Jan 1785 and him, a child named Maria and his cousin William in 1789 (Ledger D, p. 23; Ledger F, p. 99) [account continued in Ledger G, which is missing] [William Smithson was a Revolutionary War veteran and a signer of the Bush Declaration on March 22, 1775.]

Smithson, William, Jr. [1779-1836], son of Daniel Smithson, was treated by Dr. John Archer in 1798 (Ledger I, which is missing, was abstracted by Dr. George W. Archer circa 1890; his notes are in Archives of the Historical Society of Harford County folder "Archer, G. W. Coll. – Ledgers and Day Books"); William Smithson, Jr. was visited by Dr. James Archer who treated a negro in Jan 1806 ("by bleeding" and medicating) and a negro (tooth extraction) and an infant in Nov 1806 (p. 25); William Smithson was visited by Dr. Robert H. Archer who treated him in Nov 1822, Negro Ned in Mar 1824, him [William] in Nov 1825 (medicated on 23 Nov 1825), his wife and a child in June 1827, and him in Dec 1827 and Jan and Feb 1828 (pp. 35, 100, 101, 169, 170, 234, 258-262; Rx Book, 1825-1852, p. 84) [William Smithson was a War of 1812 veteran.]

Smoot, Mr. &ca (sic), was treated by Dr. Robert H. Archer in Baltimore before 1822 [no dates or details were given] (Dr. Archer's "Alphabet to Ledger H" is his booklet [filed in the Archives of the Historical Society of Harford County] that contains his index to Ledger H [which is missing] for his patients in Baltimore before 1822 and Harford County after 1822, according to a notation by Dr. George W. Archer.)

Snowdy, ---- [blank] (joiner), was treated by Dr. John Archer in 1787 (Ledger F, p. 64) [There was a Matthew Snody who was a Revolutionary War veteran.]

Sommers, Mr., was prescribed medicine by Dr. Robert H. Archer for his child circa Dec 1804 (Rx Book, 1802-1804, p. 71)

Soward, Richard (captain), was visited by Dr. John Archer who inoculated him and his wife and son in Dec 1774 (Ledger B, p. 22)

Speake, Townsend, see Gabriel P. Vanhorn, q.v.

Spence, Henry, was treated by Dr. John Archer in Dec 1777 (Ledger C, p. 98, noted "debt forgiven by order of testator")

Spence, James was treated by Dr. John Archer in Aug 1782 and "on Samuel Gover's place" in Aug 1788 (Ledger D, p. 15, noted "debt forgiven as before"); Ledger F, p. 178) [account continued in Ledger H, which is missing] [James Spence was a Revolutionary War veteran.]

Spence, Richard, near Horner's Stone House, was visited by Dr. John Archer who treated him, his wife and children [no names were given] in 1791 (Ledger F, p. 45) [account continued in Ledger K, which is missing]

Spencer, Enoch, near Little Falls, was visited by Dr. John Archer who treated him and a child in Sep 1790 (Ledger F, p. 320)

Spencer, Roland, was treated by Dr. John Archer in Sep 1787 (Ledger F, p. 273)

Spicer, Abraham [1795-1873], was visited by Dr. Alonzo Preston who treated a child on 13 Jul 1826; Spicer paid the $2.25 bill on 4 Dec 1830 and it was noted in the account by "W. B. B." [referring to Dr. William B. Bond] (p. 80) [Abraham Spicer was a War of 1812 veteran.]

Spicknall, James, see R. N. and M. J. Allen, q.v.

Spicknall, William G., was treated by Dr. Matthew J. Allen in 1832 in Calvert County (p. 23); see William Lawrence, q.v.

Spriard, Francis, near William Luckie's, was treated by Dr. John Archer in 1787 (Ledger F, p. 301)

St. John's College, Trustees of, had an account in Dr. Robert H. Archer's ledger that mentioned Dr. Rafferty (college president) and also tuition for Thomas Archer in 1825-1827 and $10 paid for a diploma (Ledger F)

Stake, Mrs., was treated by Dr. Robert H. Archer forty-eight times between 23 Jan 1823 and 24 Jun 1823 and the medical bill was $73.25 (pp. 49-52, 59, 63-81; Ledger F, pp. 139, 151, 164, gave no date or details, but simply stated "This account has been closed.")

Stallins, James, at Mr. Ballard's, was treated by Dr. Matthew J. Allen in Calvert Co. in 1823 (p. 10b)

Standiford, Aquila, was treated by Dr. John Archer in Oct 1778 and Mar 1780 (Ledger C, p. 39, noted "insolvent")

Stanley, John, was treated by Dr. John Archer in Aug 1787 (Ledger F, p. 344)

Stanley, William, was treated by Dr. John Archer in Oct 1781 (Ledger D, p. 87, noted "debt forgiven as before")

Stansbury, John, was treated by Dr. Robert H. Archer in Baltimore before 1822 [no dates or details were given] (Dr. Archer's "Alphabet to Ledger H" is his booklet [filed in the Archives of the Historical Society of Harford County] that contains his index to Ledger H [which is missing] for his patients in Baltimore before 1822 and Harford County after 1822, according to a notation by Dr. George W. Archer.); see Mr. Stansbury, q.v.

Stansbury, Master, see F. A. Bond, q.v.

Stansbury, Mr., at Tipton's, was prescribed medicine by Dr. Robert H. Archer on 28 Jan 1803 (Rx Book, 1802-1804, p. 30); see John Stansbury, q.v.

Stansbury, Mrs. (widow), was treated by Dr. Robert H. Archer in Baltimore before 1822 [no dates or details were given] (Dr. Archer's "Alphabet to Ledger H" is his booklet [filed in the Archives of the Historical Society of Harford County] that contains his index to Ledger H [which is missing] for his patients in Baltimore before 1822 and Harford County after 1822, according to a notation by Dr. George W. Archer.)

Stansbury, Thomas, was treated by Dr. Robert H. Archer in Baltimore before 1822 [no dates or details were given] (Dr. Archer's "Alphabet to Ledger H" is his booklet [filed in the Archives of the Historical Society of Harford County] that contains his index to Ledger H [which is missing] for his patients in Baltimore before 1822 and Harford County after 1822, according to a notation by Dr. George W. Archer.)

Stapleton, Joshua, in Baltimore, was visited by Dr. John Archer who treated him and his wife in 1801 and was prescribed medicine for himself and his wife by Dr. Robert H. Archer in March 1801 (Ledger F, p. 58; Rx Book, 1796-1801, pp. 41, 45, 48, 49)

Steel, Abraham, was visited by Dr. John Archer who treated his wife in July 1775 (Ledger B, p. 8)

Steel, Abram, at Mr. F. Brown's, was treated by Dr. John Archer in Mar 1777 (Ledger C, p. 31, noted "debt forgiven by order of testator")

Steel, James (captain), was treated by Dr. John Archer in Oct 1787 (Ledger F, p. 11) [James Steel was a Revolutionary War veteran.]

Steel, John, at James Hall's, was treated by Dr. John Archer in Jun 1786 (Ledger F, p. 227) [John Steel was a Revolutionary War veteran.]

Steele, John, at Stafford Mills [occupation illegible], was treated by Dr. John Archer in 1794 [no dates were given] (Ledger I, which is missing, was abstracted by Dr. George W. Archer circa 1890; his notes are in the Archives of the Historical Society of Harford County folder "Archer, G. W. Coll. – Ledgers and Day Books")

Steele, John (general), see Robert Maxwell, q.v.

Steele, Joseph, stage driver at Mr. Barney's, was treated by Dr. John Archer in 1796 (Ledger I, which is missing, was abstracted by Dr. George W. Archer circa 1890; his notes are in Archives of the Historical Society of Harford County folder "Archer, G. W. Coll. – Ledgers and Day Books")

Stephens, George, at Ring Factory [on Winters Run west of Bel Air], was visited by Dr. Matthew J. Allen who treated his wife (neck problem) in Jul 1848 (p. 89)

Stephenson, Ann, see Robert Stephenson, q.v.

Stephenson, Brison, see Robert Stephenson, q.v.

Stephenson, George, Mrs. (widow), was visited by Dr. Robert H. Archer who treated a negro "in partu" [in childbirth] on 2 Nov 1825; consult with Dr. John Archer, Jr. (Ledger F, p. 36)

Stephenson, James, was treated by Dr. Robert H. Archer in Feb 1823, in July 1825 in consultation with Dr. John Archer, and in Oct 1832 (pp. 53, 141; Ledger F, p. 142)

Stephenson, Brison, see Robert Stephenson, q.v.

Stephenson, John, a student at Abingdon [Cokesbury College], was treated by Dr. John Archer in Aug 1789 (Ledger F, p. 30)

Stephenson, Robert, was visited by Dr. John Archer who treated his wife in Oct 1772, him in Jan, Feb and Mar 1773 and son Brison in Sep 1773 (Ledger B, p. 12, noted that part of the bill was paid by Ann Stephenson); see Ann Stevenson, q.v.

Stephenson, William [1793-1870], was treated by Dr. Robert H. Archer in Oct 1822 (p. 27; Ledger F, p. 96) [William Stephenson was a War of 1812 veteran]; see John Lochary, q.v.

Steuart, George, was visited by Dr. John Archer who treated Will in Sep 1772 (tooth extraction), Anny and Boby *(sic)* in Jan 1773, Anny and Tommy in Mar 1773, Negro Tyrone in Oct 1773, and him [George] in Apr, May, Jun, Jul, Oct 1773 and Feb, Mar and Jun 1774 (Ledger B, p. 68)

Steven, Miss, see James White Hall, q.v.

Stevenson, Alex, see Ann Stevenson, q.v.

Stevenson, Andrew (wheelwright), was visited by Dr. John Archer who treated him and his family at various times between 1796 and 1800 (Ledger I, which is missing, was abstracted by Dr. George W. Archer circa 1890; his notes are in the Archives of the Historical Society of Harford County folder "Archer, G. W. Coll. – Ledgers and Day Books"); see Ann Stevenson, q.v.

Stevenson, Ann, was visited by Dr. John Archer who treated her seven times between Apr 1773 and May 1775, her children "Gulielma" [William] and "Alios" [Alex] in July 1773 and "Andream" [Andrew] in June 1774; "Ann Stevenson, widow of Robert," was visited by Dr. John Archer who treated her in Apr 1777, son James in May and Nov 1779, and her in Dec 1779 and Dec 1792 (Ledger B, p. 92; Ledger C, p. 87; Ledger F, p. 205) [account continued in Ledger H, which is missing]; also see Robert Stephenson, q.v.

Stevenson, Edward, was treated by Dr. John Archer in Dec 1781 and Jul 1784 (Ledger D, p. 104, spelled his name Stevinson and noted "debt forgiven as before"); see William Boardsman, q.v.

Stevenson, George, see Mrs. Stevenson, q.v.

Stevenson, James, see Ann Stevenson, q.v.

Stevenson, John, was visited by Dr. John Archer who treated John Finney in Aug 1772, him [John Stevenson] at various times between October 1772 and June 1774 and between Feb 1777 and Oct 1783 (Ledger B, p. 9; Ledger C, p. 20) [John Stevenson was a Revolutionary War veteran.]

Stevenson, John, alias Bond, was visited by Dr. Matthew J. Allen who treated his wife in Nov and Dec 1847 and a child in Apr, Jul and Aug 1848 (p. 68)

Stevenson, Mrs., widow of George, was visited by Dr. Robert H. Archer who treated a negro "in partu" [in childbirth] on 2 Nov 1825; consulted with Dr. J. Archer (p. 166)

Stevenson, Rachel, Mrs. (widow), was treated by Dr. John Archer at avarious between May 1787 and Apr 1794 (Ledger F, p. 189) [account continued in Ledger I, which is missing]; see William Stevenson, q.v.

Stevenson, Robert, see Ann Stevenson, q.v.

Stevenson, Thomas, was treated by Dr. John Archer in Jun 1778 and Aug 1782 (Ledger C, p. 114, and "debt forgiven by order of testator") [Thomas Stevenson was a Revolutionary War veteran.]

Stevenson, William, son of R. R. [Rock Run] Rachel Stevenson, was visited by Dr. John Archer who treated him and his family from 1796 to 1798 (Ledger I, which is missing, was abstracted by Dr. George W. Archer circa 1890; his notes are in the Archives of the Historical Society of Harford County folder "Archer, G. W. Coll. – Ledgers and Day Books"); see Ann Stevenson, q.v.

Stewart, James [c1746-1781], was treated by Dr. John Archer in consultation with Dr. Annon in Aug 1781 (Ledger D, p. 61, noted "debt forgiven as before") [James Stewart was a Revolutionary War veteran.]

Stewart, Mr., at Edward Prigg's, was treated by Dr. John Archer in Sep 1779 (Ledger D, p. 15 note "debt forgiven as before")

Stiles, Eliza (widow), was treated by Dr. John Archer in 1791 (Ledger F, p. 333) [account continued in Ledger H, which is missing]; see Joseph Stiles, q.v.

Stiles, Joseph, was visited by Dr. John Archer who treated a child in Dec 1776, him [Joseph] in Jan 1777 and him and daughter Eliza in 1789 (Ledger C, p. 18; Ledger F, p. 230) [Joseph Stiles was a Revolutionary War veteran.]; see Richard Kroesen, q.v.

Stinson, Widow, see James Nickleston, q.v.

Stockdill, Thomas, at R. Howard's, was visited by Dr. John Archer who treated his wife in Feb 1782 and him in Mar 1782 (Ledger D, p. 122) [Thomas Stocksdale was a Revolutionary War veteran.]

Stokes, Joseph, was visited by Dr. John Archer who treated a child in Jan 1773 and "for boys" in Sep 1779 (Ledger B, p. 71; Ledger D, p. 23) [account continued in Ledger E, which is missing]; see Sarah Harvey, q.v.

Stokes, Mr., was prescribed medicine by Dr. Robert H. Archer on 30 Jan 1801 (Rx Book, 1796-1801, p. 30)

Stokes, Sarah, Mrs., was visited by Dr. Richard Sappington who treated her in May 1785 ("vomiting powder"), on 7 Sep 1785 ("drawing tooth" and treated with fever powder and wine drops, followed by "bleeding" her two days later) and treated her again in Oct 1785; he also charged her for 5 years interest ending in Jan 1791 (Document filed in Historical Society of Harford County Archives folder "Sappington, Dr. Richard – Accounts, 1783-1830")

Stokes, William, "Master, charged in James W. Hall's account," was treated in Jun and Jul 1786 by Dr. Richard Sappington who also dressed a wound to his hand in Nov 1786 (Document filed in Historical Society of Harford County Archives folder "Sappington, Dr. Richard – Accounts, 1783-1830;" on the back of the paper was written "This extravagant and cannot be allowed" and it was signed by C. Brooke); see James White Hall, q.v.

Stokes, William B., was visited by Dr. John Archer, Jr. who treated him and his wife and children in Sep 1815 (p. 13)

Stone, Joseph, was visited by Dr. John Archer who treated him in Jun 1781 and a child in Aug 1782 (Ledger C, p. 65, noted Henry Waters was his security and also "debt forgiven by order of testator"); see Samuel Lee, q.v.

Stots, Hannah, was treated by Dr. John Archer in 1788 (Ledger F, p. 224)

Stott, William, at Widow Smith's Mill, was treated by Dr. John Archer in 1786 (Ledger F, p. 275)

Street, David (blacksmith), was mentioned in Dr. Robert H. Archer's ledger in a non-medical matter in Aug 1828 (p. 289)

Street, Dr., see Thomas Butler, q.v.

Strickland, ---- [blank], Union Mills, was visited by Dr. Matthew J. Allen who rendered obstetrical services to his wife in Jul 1852 [the day was not given] in consultation with Dr. Finney (p. 97)

Strickland, Joshua, was treated by Dr. Matthew J. Allen in Jun 1847 (p. 53, noted the bill was paid by Mr. Hutton)

Strong, Rachel, was prescribed medicine by Dr. Robert H. Archer on 9 Feb 1801 (Rx Book, 1796-1801, p. 33)

Stroud, Thomas, appeared on a list of debts dated 26 Dec 1822 and titled "A List of Allen's Claims" that were due and payable to Dr. Richard N. Allen for services rendered [no dates] by him to said Stroud (Document filed in Historical Society of Harford County Archives folder "R. N. Allen")

Stubbins, George, see William Fisher, q.v.

Stump & Parker, had an account with Dr. Robert H. Archer that mentioned Herman Stump and son Thomas in May 1824 (Ledger F, p. 6)

Stump, Ann, at Havre de Grace, was treated by Dr. John Archer, Jr. in Jun 1815 (p. 17)

Stump, Cassandra, Mrs., was treated by Dr. Robert H. Archer in Oct 1822 (p. 26; Ledger F, p. 94)

Stump, Herman [1798-1881], was treated by Dr. Robert H. Archer reportedly in Baltimore before 1822 [no dates or details given] (Dr. Archer's "Alphabet to Ledger H" is his booklet [filed in the Archives of the Historical Society of Harford County] that contains his index to Ledger H [which is missing] for his patients in Baltimore before 1822 and Harford County after 1822, according to a note by Dr. George W. Archer); Herman Stump, at Stafford [in Harford County], was treated by Dr. Archer in Aug 1822 (p. 14; Ledger F, p. 70); see Stump & Parker and ---- Adams, q.v.

Stump, John [1756-1828], was visited by Dr. Robert H. Archer who treated him in Oct 1815 and Rachel Price in Oct 1822 (p. 30; Ledger F, pp. 17, 106); John Stump was treated by Dr. Robert H. Archer in Baltimore before 1822 [no dates or details were given] (Dr. Archer's "Alphabet to Ledger H" is his booklet [filed in the Archives of the Historical Society of Harford County] that contains his index to Ledger H [which is missing] for his patients in Baltimore before 1822 and Harford County after 1822 [although John Stump was a resident of Harford County before 1822], according to a notation by Dr. George W. Archer); see Mrs. Coulston, q.v.

Stump, John [1752-1816], at Stafford, was treated by Dr. John Archer, Jr. on 19 Nov 1815 and died on 14 Feb 1816 (p. 38) [John Stump was a Revolutionary War veteran.]

Stump, John, Jr., was visited by Dr. John Archer who treated him and his wife and a child in 1792 (Ledger F, p. 101)

Stump, Margaret M., was treated five times by Dr. Robert H. Archer in Feb 1828 (pp. 263-265)

Stump, Margaret, Mrs. [1786-1870], was visited by Dr. Matthew J. Allen who treated Richard and Edward in Jul, Sep and Oct 1844 and Edward in Feb, Mar (by "carterising tonsils") and May 1845 (p. 36); see Mrs. Stump and Peggy Stump, q.v.

Stump, Mrs., was visited by Dr. Alonzo Preston who treated Miss Miller in Feb 1826 (p. 70, noted "This acct. paid by Doctr. R. N. Allen, Mar 1st 1831" and initialed by W. B. B. [referring to Dr. William B. Bond]

Stump, Peggy, Mrs., was visited by Dr. Robert H. Archer who treated her in Sep and Oct 1822, Miss Miller in Sep 1822, Miss A. Miller in Aug 1825, her [Peggy] and Negro Stephen in Apr 1826, Negro Nancy in May 1826, H. Miller in July 1826 and Negro Stephen in Sep 1826 (pp. 24, 149, 180, 193; Ledger F, p. 80); see Mrs. Margaret Stump, q.v.

Stump, Reuben [1765-1841], was visited by Dr. Robert H. Archer who treated Negro Polly and another Negro [not named] in Oct 1822 (pp. 29, 33)

Stump, Thomas, see Stump & Parker, q.v.

Sullivan, John, near Daniel Dunnevan's, was visited by Dr. John Archer who treated him and a child in 1791 (Ledger F, p. 3) [John Sullivan was a Revolutionary War veteran.]

Sullivan, Mrs. (widow), was treated by Dr. Robert H. Archer in Baltimore before 1822 [no dates or details were given] (Dr. Archer's "Alphabet to Ledger H" is his booklet [filed in the Archives of the Historical Society of Harford County] that contains his index to Ledger H [which is missing] for his patients in Baltimore before 1822 and Harford County after 1822, according to a notation by Dr. George W. Archer.)

Sutton, Mary, see Reuben Sutton, q.v.

Sutton, Oswell, was visited by Dr. John Archer who inoculated 9 of his family in 1777 (Ledger C, p. 73, and "debt forgiven by order of testator") [Ozwain Sutton was a Revolutionary War veteran.]

Sutton, Reuben, was visited by Dr. Robert H. Archer who treated him and his son Solomon in Aug and Sep 1825, daughter Mary in Sep 1825, and Solomon promised to pay the bill (pp. 152-154; Ledger F, p. 117, noted on 11 Sep 1825 that Solomon had "moved to Ohio without paying") [Reuben Sutton was a Revolutionary War veteran.]; see Richard Hargrove, q.v.

Sutton, Samuel, in Bush River Neck, was treated by Dr. John Archer in Jun 1779 (Ledger C, p. 87, noted James Reardon was his security)

Stump, S., see John Gregg & Co., q.v.

Sutton, Solomon, see Reuben Sutton, q.v.

Swan, Frederick, was treated by Dr. John Archer in May 1779 (Ledger C, p. 72, noted "debt forgiven by order of testator")

Swan, Mr., at Deer Creek, was treated by Dr. Robert H. Archer between 1800 and 1822 [no dates or details were given] (Dr. Archer's "Alphabet to Ledger H" is his booklet [filed in the Archives of the Historical Society of Harford County] that contains his index to Ledger H [which is missing] for his patients in Baltimore before 1822 and Harford County after 1822 [even though Mr. Swan was treated in Harford County before 1822], according to a notation by Dr. George W. Archer.)

Swan, Samuel, was treated by Dr. Robert H. Archer in Baltimore before 1822 [no dates or details were given] (Dr. Archer's "Alphabet to Ledger H" is his booklet [filed in the Archives of the Historical Society of Harford County] that contains his index to Ledger H [which is missing] for his patients in Baltimore before 1822 and Harford County after 1822, according to a notation by Dr. George W. Archer.)

Swart, Samuel, was treated by Dr. John Archer in Sep 1780 (Ledger D, p. 97, spelled his name Swath and noted "debt forgiven as before") [Samuel Swart (Swarts) was a Revolutionary War veteran.]

Swartz, George, see John Smith, of Jabish, q.v.

Sweeney, David, was treated by Dr. John Archer in 1775 who also treated him and his daughter in 1786 and him in 1789 (Ledger B, p. 82, spelled his name Sweny; Ledger F, pp. 126 and 246 spelled his name Sweney) [David Sweney, Jr. was a Revolutionary War veteran.]

Sweeney, Matthew (schoolmaster), was treated by Dr. John Archer in Jan 1781 and Jul 1792 (Ledger D, p. 113, listed him as "Mr. Swany, schoolmaster" and noted "debt forgiven as before"); Ledger F, p. 331, listed his name as Mathew Sweney) [Matthew Sweeney or Sweny was a Revolutionary War veteran.]; see James Wells, q.v.

Sweeney, Richard, was prescribed medicine by Dr. Robert H. Archer on 9 Feb 1801 and was visited by Dr. James Archer who treated his family three times in Oct 1806 (Rx Book, 1796-1801, p. 33; Dr. James Archer, p. 26)

Swift, James, was visited by Dr. Matthew J. Allen who treated his wife in Dec 1843, rendered obstetrical services to his wife on 1 Nov 1844 and treated her again in Jun 1845 (p. 28)

Swift, Mark, appeared on a list of debts dated 26 Dec 1822 and titled "A List of Allen's Claims" that were due and payable to Dr. Richard N. Allen for services rendered [no dates] to said Swift (Document filed in Historical Society of Harford County Archives folder titled "R. N. Allen")

Tabbs, Mr., was treated by Dr. Robert H. Archer in Baltimore before 1822 [no dates or details given] (Dr. Archer's "Alphabet to Ledger H" is his booklet [filed in the Archives of the Historical Society of Harford County] that contains his index to Ledger H [which is missing] for his patients in Baltimore before 1822 and Harford County after 1822, according to a notation by Dr. George W. Archer.)

Tagart, Jacob, see Samuel Calwell, q.v.

Tagart, James, at Maj. Calwell's, was visited by Dr. John Archer who treated him and a child in 1777 and him and his son William in 1787 (Ledger C, p. 8; Ledger F, p. 60); see Samuel Calwell, q.v.

Tagart, William, see James Tagart and Samuel Calwell, q.v.

Talbot, Anna (colored), was treated by Dr. Matthew J. Allen in Mar, Apr and Jul 1848 (p. 77)

Talbot, John, was prescribed medicine by Dr. Robert H. Archer in 1804 (Rx Book, 1802-1804, p. 67); see John Scarff, q.v.

Talbott, Jos:, was prescribed medicine by Dr. Robert H. Archer on 24 Aug 1802 (Rx Book, 1802-1804, p. 16)

Talbott, Mr., was prescribed medicine for his wife by Dr. Robert H. Archer on 5 Mar 1801 (Rx Book, 1796-1801, p. 39)

Talbott, William, see Negro Hagar, q.v.

Tate, Peggy, see Robert Kerr, q.v.

Taylor, Aquila (millwright), was treated by Dr. John Archer in Jun 1786 (Ledger F, p. 279)

Taylor, Ashberry, of James, was treated by Dr. John Archer in Sep 1789 (Ledger F, p. 321)

Taylor, Eacy, see Matthew McClintock, q.v.

Taylor, Edward, was treated by Dr. J. Archer in Jun 1786 (Ledger F, p. 172); see Elenor Taylor, q.v.

Taylor, Elenor, widow of Edward, was treated by Dr. John Archer in July 1788 (Ledger F, p. 269)

Taylor, Emily, see Lydia Taylor, q.v.

Taylor, George, was treated by Dr. John Archer, Jr. in 1818 and noted that William Taylor paid the bill (Ledger F, p. 42)

Taylor, Hannah, see William Taylor, q.v.

Taylor, James, was treated by Dr. John Archer in Aug 1780 (Ledger D, p. 85, noted "debt forgiven as before")

Taylor, James, in Bel Air, was treated by Dr. John Archer in Aug 1789 (Ledger F, p. 29); see Ashberry Taylor, q.v.

Taylor, James, "Nichs. Sr." *(sic)*, was visited by Dr. John Archer who treated him, his wife and a child in 1787 (Ledger F, p. 137)

Taylor, James J. M., was treated by Dr. Matthew J. Allen in 1832 in Calvert County (p. 19)

Taylor, John, near Slate Ridge, was visited by Dr. John Archer who treated his daughter in May 1778 and him in Jun 1778 (Ledger C, p. 106, noted "debt forgiven by order of testator")

Taylor, John (esquire), was visited by Dr. John Archer who treated him and his wife in 1791 (Ledger F, p. 378) [account continued in Ledger H, which is missing]; Maj. John Taylor and children Betsey, Eliza, Polly and Arnold were treated by Dr. Archer at times between 1794 and 1807 and noted "Cr. by poverty" (Ledger I, which is missing, was abstracted by Dr. George W. Archer circa 1890; his notes are in Archives of the Historical Society of Harford County folder "Archer, G. W. Coll. – Ledgers and Day Books") [John Taylor was a Revolutionary War veteran.]

Taylor, John, was prescribed medicine for his wife by Dr. Robert H. Archer on 17 Aug 1796 and medicine for a negro on 13 Jul 1803 (Rx Book, 1796-1801, p. 8; Rx Book, 1802-1804, p. 50); Maj. John Taylor was treated by Dr. Archer in Baltimore before 1822 [no dates or details given] (Dr. Archer's "Alphabet to Ledger H" is his booklet [filed in the Archives of the Historical Society of Harford County] that contains his index to Ledger H [which is missing] for his patients in Baltimore before 1822 and Harford County after 1822, according to a notation by Dr. George W. Archer.); see Thomas Taylor, q.v.

Taylor, John, Jr., was treated by Dr. John Archer in July 1780 (Ledger D, p. 76, noted "debt forgiven as before")

Taylor, Littleton, see Lydia Taylor, q.v.

Taylor, Lydia, widow of Thomas, was visited by Dr. John Archer, Jr. who treated her in May 1819, grandson Littleton in Jul 1821 and daughter Emily in Aug 1821 (p. 80, noted that the account was paid by Mr. Coudon(?) [unclear] in Mar 1823)

Taylor, Nancy, see William Taylor, q.v.

Taylor, Robert, was visited by Dr. John Archer who treated him and his wife in Sep 1789 (Ledger F, p. 12) [Robert Taylor was a Revolutionary War veteran.]; see Mrs. Wheeler (widow), q.v.

Taylor, Robert, "in the Necks," was treated by Dr. John Archer in Jun 1785 (Ledger D, p. 60, noted "debt forgiven as before") [Robert Taylor was a Revolutionary War veteran.]

Taylor, Sarah (widow), was treated by Dr. John Archer in Apr 1787 (Ledger F, p. 228)

Taylor, Stephen, was treated by Dr. John Archer in Nov 1804 (Ledger F, p. 78) [Stephen Taylor was a Revolutionary War veteran.]

Taylor, Thomas, see Lydia Taylor, q.v.

Taylor, Thomas (deputy sheriff), was visited by Dr. John Archer who treated him and his family at various times between 1796 and 1799 (Ledger I, which is missing, was abstracted by Dr. George W. Archer circa 1890; his notes are in Archives of the Historical Society of Harford County folder "Archer, G. W. Coll. – Ledgers and Day Books")

Taylor, Thomas (ship carpenter), near Old Fields, was visited by Dr. John Archer who treated him, his wife and child in 1791 (Ledger F, p. 372) [account continued in Ledger H, which is missing]

Taylor, Thomas, son of John, was treated by Dr. John Archer in Jul 1791 (Ledger F, p. 348) [account continued in Ledger H, which is missing]

Taylor, Thomas, was treated by Dr. Robert H. Archer in Feb 1822 (Ledger F, p. 33)

Taylor, Walter (weaver), was treated by Dr. John Archer in Sep 1779 and Mar 1783 (Ledger D, p. 16, noted "debt forgiven as before") [Walter Taylor was a Revolutionary War veteran.]; see John Hamilton, q.v.

Taylor, William (sicklemaker and blacksmith), "X Roads," was visited by Dr. John Archer who treated him and his daughters Nancy and Hannah at various times in 1797 and 1798 (Ledger I, which is missing, was abstracted by Dr. George W. Archer circa 1890; his notes are in Archives of Historical Society of Harford County folder "Archer, G. W. Coll. – Ledgers and Day Books")

Taylor, William, was treated by Dr. John Archer, Jr. in July 1815 (p.2 4); see George Taylor and Thomas Huggins & Co., q.v.

Taylor, William, was prescribed medicine by Dr. Robert H. Archer on 18 May 1829 (Rx Book, 1825-1851, p. 93)

Tees, Andrew, was treated by Dr. John Archer in Sep 1778 (Ledger C, p. 123, noted the account was paid in cash in full [nearly 11 years later] on 13 May 1789)

Temple, William, was treated by Dr. Alonzo Preston in Apr 1826 (p. 74)

Terbert, Robert, at Slate Ridge, was visited by Dr. John Archer who treated his wife in Jan 1779, son Robert in Mar 1790 (fractured femur) and him in Apr and May 1790 (Ledger C, p. 27; Ledger D, p. 78, noted the bill was paid in full in cash on 15 Apr 1793)

Thomas, A. J. [1777-1841], was visited by Dr. John Archer, Jr. who treated his wife in Oct 1815 and Aug 1818 and was visited by Dr. Robert H. Archer who treated his wife on 16 Sep and 19 Sep 1826 when the doctor noted "ux moritund" [i. e., wife near death] (Dr. John Archer, Jr., p. 34; Dr. Robert Archer, p. 200); A. Jarrett Thomas was treated by Dr. Robert H. Archer reportedly in Baltimore before 1822 [no dates or details were given] (Dr. Archer's "Alphabet to Ledger H" is his booklet [filed in the Archives of the Historical Society of Harford County] that contains his index to Ledger H [which is missing] for his patients in Baltimore City before 1822 and Harford County after 1822, according to Dr. George W. Archer.) [However, A. J. Thomas, whose full name was Abraham Jarrett Thomas, was a resident of Havre de Grace.]

Thomas, Benjamin, was treated by Dr. John Archer in Aug 1778, Jul 1779 and Aug 1780 (Ledger C, p. 120, noted "debt forgiven by order of testator")

Thomas, Cath., see Philip, Thomas, q.v.

Thomas, Charles, was treated by Dr. John Archer in Mar 1786 (Ledger F, p. 151)

Thomas, Chil:, see Philip Thomas, q.v.

Thomas, Daniel, was treated by Dr. John Archer in Nov 1786 (Ledger F, p. 146) [Daniel Thomas was a Revolutionary War veteran.]

Thomas, David, was treated by Dr. John Archer in Oct 1788 and William Grafton was his security (Ledger F, p. 92) [David Thomas was a Revolutionary War veteran.]

Thomas, George, see Sarah Thomas, q.v.

Thomas, Giles, was treated by Dr. John Archer in Dec 1794 (Ledger F, p. 274) [account continued in Ledger I, which is missing]

Thomas, Henry, near John Forwood's, was visited by Dr. John Archer who treated him in Apr 1775, a child in May 1775, an infant in Apr 1781 and him [Henry] in May 1782 and Apr 1783 (Ledger B, p. 91; Ledger D, p. 19, noted "debt forgiven as before") [Henry Thomas was a Revolutionary War veteran.]

Thomas, Hetty, see Philip, Thomas, q.v.

Thomas, James (millwright), was treated by Dr. John Archer from 1797 to 1799 (Ledger I, which is missing, was abstracted by Dr. George W. Archer circa 1890; his notes are in the Archives of the Historical Society of Harford County folder "Archer, G. W. Coll. – Ledgers and Day Books") [James Thomas was a Revolutionary War veteran.]; see Philip Thomas and Sarah Thomas, q.v.

Thomas, John, was treated by Dr. John Archer in Sep 1777 (Ledger C, p. 91, noted that part was paid "by yr. proportion of the Boston money, 3/6") [John Thomas was a Revolutionary War veteran.]

Thomas, John, was treated by Dr. Robert H. Archer in Baltimore before 1822 [no dates or details were given] (Dr. Archer's "Alphabet to Ledger H" is his booklet [filed in the Archives of the Historical Society of Harford County] that contains his index to Ledger H [which is missing] for his patients in Baltimore before 1822 and Harford County after 1822, according to a notation by Dr. George W. Archer.)

Thomas, John W., was visited by Dr. Robert H. Archer who treated him in Mar 1822, his wife in Feb and Mar 1823 and a child in Mar 1823 and three times in July 1824 (pp. 54, 55, noting "trans fluis" [i. e., "across the water," which meant they lived across the Susquehanna River in Cecil County] (pp. 111-113; Ledger F, p. 50)

Thomas, Jonah, was treated by Dr. Robert H. Archer in Baltimore before 1822 [no dates or details were given] (Dr. Archer's "Alphabet to Ledger H" is his booklet [filed in the Archives of the Historical Society of Harford County] that contains his index to Ledger H [which is missing] for his patients in Baltimore before 1822 and Harford County after 1822, according to a notation by Dr. George W. Archer.)

Thomas, Kitty, see Philip, Thomas, q.v.

Thomas, Ludlow, see Philip Thomas, q.v.

Thomas, Marsha, see Philip Thomas, q.v.

Thomas, Mary, see Sarah Thomas, q.v.

Thomas, Mr., was prescribed medicine by Dr. Robert H. Archer on 5 Mar 1801 (Rx Book, 1796-1801, p. 39)

Thomas, Mrs., see Philip Thomas, q.v.

Thomas, Nancy, Miss, was visited by Dr. Robert H. Archer who treated George Davidson's children James and Sarah in July 1824 (Ledger F, p. 127)

Thomas, P., see ---- Aitken, q.v.

Thomas, Philip, "trans fluis" [i. e., "across the water," which meant he lived across the Susquehanna River in Cecil Co.], was visited by Dr. John Archer who treated him and his wife, son Philip and daughters Hetty and Kitty in 1787, and treated him [Philip] and his wife and children named Chil: (sic) and Cath. (sic) in Sep 1799; also mentioned Eliza Weems and Miss Betsy Weems (Ledger F, pp. 35, 37, 49, 371) [account continued in Ledger G, which is missing]

Thomas, Philip, was visited by Dr. Robert H. Archer who treated him and Sarah Thomas in Aug 1815, his wife "obstetricant placent" [post childbirth] on 29 Aug 1818, daughter Marsha and son Ludlow in Jan 1819, and negroes Isaac, Peg and George between 1816 and 1818; mentioned James Thomas and Mrs. Thomas in Feb 1826 and was paid $20.00 in Jul 1826; the doctor noted "by cash recd. in a letter from his wife at New York last winter if not before credited." (p. 195; Ledger F, p. 26); see Sarah Thomas and Thomas Huggins Co., q.v.

Thomas, R., see George Lisly and Benjamin Horsey, q.v.

Thomas, Richard, was treated by Dr. John Archer in Aug 1794 (Ledger F, p. 206)

Thomas, Samuel, was treated by Dr. John Archer "trans fluis" [i.e., "across the water" which meant that he lived across the Susquehanna River in Cecil Co.] in Apr 1781 (Ledger D, p. 16, noted "debt forgiven as before")

Thomas, Samuel, son of Samuel, was visited by Dr. John Archer who treated him and son William in 1791 (Ledger F, p. 327) [account continued in Ledger H, which is missing]

Thomas, Sarah (widow), was visited by Dr. John Archer, Jr. who treated Philip Thomas in Dec 1815, Miss Nancy, George, James and Mary Thomas and Peggy Prevail in Oct 1819 and Negro Maria in Jul 1821 (p. 32); Mrs. Sarah M. Thomas was treated by Dr. Robert H. Archer in Nov 1821 and mentioned Philip, James and George A. Thomas; treated again in May 1824 (pp. 106, 107; Ledger F, p. 3); see Philip Thomas, q.v.

Thomas, Thomas, was visited by Dr. John Archer who treated his wife in Dec 1781, him and his wife in Jan 1782 and him in Feb 1782 (Ledger D, p. 110, noted "debt forgiven as before") [Thomas Thomas was a Revolutionary War veteran.]

Thomas, William, see Samuel Thomas, q.v.

Thompkins, James, see William W. Lawrence, q.v.

Thompson, Alexander, see Mrs. Grafton and Hugh Anderson, q.v.

Thompson, Andrew, was treated by Dr. Robert H. Archer in Baltimore before 1822 [no dates or details were given] (Dr. Archer's "Alphabet to Ledger H" is his booklet [filed in the Archives of the Historical Society of Harford County] that contains his index to Ledger H [which is missing] for his patients in Baltimore before 1822 and Harford County after 1822, according to a notation by Dr. George W. Archer.) [Andrew Thompson was a Revolutionary War veteran.]

Thompson, Aquila, near Bethel P. Church [Bethel Presbyterian Church at Madonna], was treated by Dr. John Archer in 1789 (Ledger F, p. 292, spelled his name Thomson)

Thompson, Aquila, was treated by Dr. John Archer in Feb 1780 and Jan 1783(?) [date illegible] (Ledger D, p. 48, noted "debt forgiven as before"); see James Thompson, q.v.

Thompson, Charles, son-in-law of James Oliver, was treated by Dr. John Archer in Feb 1786 (Ledger F, p. 125)

Thompson, David, "in the Necks," was treated by Dr. John Archer in Dec 1788 (Ledger F, p. 185) [account continued in Ledger G, which is missing] [David Thompson was a Revolutionary War veteran.]; see Mary Thompson, q.v.

Thompson, Edward, was visited by Dr. John Archer in 1777 and inoculated 6 of his family, treated in Jul 1779 and Jul 1780 and him and his wife in Oct 1788 (Ledger C, p. 126, noted in 1780 the doctor was paid "by cash in Continental rec'd. from Charles Gilbert for the inoculation when it was not more than 1 p. a piece" [account continued in Ledger E, which is missing] [Edward Thompson was a Revolutionary War veteran.]; Ledger F, p. 54); see Edward Price, q.v.

Thompson, Gilbert, at Thomas Gash's, was treated by Dr. John Archer in Jul 1788 (Ledger F, p. 289, spelled his name Thomson)

Thompson, Ingree (captain), at Otter Point, was visited by Dr. John Archer who treated him in 1787, his wife and child in 1790 and his sister-in-law in 1795 (Ledger F, pp. 74, 249, 293)

Thompson, James, was treated by Dr. John Archer in Nov 1781 (Ledger D, p. 92, noted the "debt forgiven as before") [James Thompson was a Revolutionary War veteran.]

Thompson, James (tailor), in Bel Air, brother of Aquila, was visited by Dr. John Archer who treated him and a child in 1788 (Ledger F, p. 62)

Thompson, James, dec'd., appeared on a list of debts dated 26 Dec 1822 and titled "A List of Allen's Claims" that were due and payable to Dr. Richard N. Allen for services rendered [no dates were given] by him to the said James (Document filed in the Archives of Historical Society of Harford County folder "R. N. Allen")

Thompson, John, see Benjamin Howard, q.v.

Thompson, John (ferryman), was treated by Dr. John Archer in Jul 1790 (Ledger F, p. 119)

Thompson, John, son of John, was treated by Dr. John Archer in Mar 1786 (Ledger F, p. 207)

Thompson, John, was treated by Dr. John Archer in Aug 1791 (Ledger F, p. 182) [John Thompson was a Revolutionary War veteran.]

Thompson, Mary, widow of David, was treated by Dr. John Archer at various times from Mar 1787 to Mar 1791 (Ledger F, pp. 216, 327, noted "gone to western country," but did not give the date)

Thompson, Robert, was prescribed medicine by Dr. Robert H. Archer on 5 Sep 1802 (Rx Book, 1802-1804, p. 18)

Thompson, Thomas Alexander, was treated by Dr. John Archer in Jan 1790 (Ledger F, p. 215, noted that payment was made by Mordecai Amoss on 2 Nov 1790)

Thorn, Widow, near Jos. W. Dallam's, was treated by Dr. John Archer in Nov and Dec 1781 (Ledger D, p. 91, noted the £3.16 bill was paid in full by Griffith Jones on 22 Oct 1793)

Thornton, Elizabeth, was treated by Dr. John Archer in Dec 1772 and Jan-Feb 1774 (Ledger B, p. 32)

Thornton, John, was visited by Dr. John Archer who treated him in Oct 1780 and Aug 1782, his wife in Mar 1783 and him in Jul 1783, John Thornton, "freed by Dr. Archer," was visited by Dr. John Archer who treated him in Jul 1786 and him, his wife and child in Aug 1794; "Negro John Thornton" was prescribed medicine by Dr. Robert H. Archer on 31 Oct 1802 (Ledger D, p. 101, noted "debt forgiven as before;" Ledger F, pp. 111, 365 [account continued in Ledger I, which is missing]; Dr. Robert Archer's Rx Book, 1802-1804, p. 23)

Thruston, Thomas, near W. Smithson's, was treated by Dr. John Archer in Oct and Dec 1778 (Ledger C, p. 30, noted "debt forgiven by order of testator") [Thomas Thruston was a Revolutionary War veteran.]

Tilbrook, John (schoolmaster), was treated by Dr. John Archer in Oct 1778 (Ledger C, p. 125, noted "debt forgiven by order of testator")

Tipton, see Mr. Stansbury, q.v.

Tixier, Monsr., at Rev. J. Ireland's, was treated by Dr. John Archer in 1794 (Ledger I, which is missing, was abstracted by Dr. George W. Archer circa 1890; his notes are in Archives of the Historical Society of Harford County file "Archer, G. W. Coll. - Ledgers and Day Books")

Toberdier, Mr., see John Wilson, q.v.

Tolley, James W., was treated by Dr. Alonzo Preston in Feb 1826 (p. 70)

Tollinger, Daniel (hatter), "X Roads," was treated by Dr. John Archer in 1794 [no dates were given] (Ledger I, which is missing, was abstracted by Dr. George W. Archer circa 1890; his notes are in the Archives of the Historical Society of Harford County folder "Archer, G. W. Coll. – Ledgers and Day Books")

Tollinger, George, was visited by Dr. John Archer who treated his wife in Dec 1772, Oct 1773 (or 1774?), and Mar 1774 (or 1775?), him in Jul 1781, his wife in Jul 1785 and him in Aug 1791 (Ledger B, p. 53, spelled his name Tullinger; Ledger D, p. 50, spelled his name Tollenger and noted the "debt forgiven as before;" Ledger F, p. 166) [George Tollinger or Tollenger was a Revolutionary War veteran.]

Tolly, Edward [1753-1790], was treated by Dr. John Archer on 19 Aug 1790 (Ledger F, p. 377) [Edward Carvel Tolley was a Revolutionary War veteran.]

Tolson, Isaac, at John Paterson's, was treated by Dr. John Archer in Apr and May 1780 (Ledger D, p. 59, noted "debt forgiven as before")

Touchstone, Henry (saddler), "at the Roads," was visited by Dr. John Archer who treated him in Mar 1779, a negro in Aug 1779 and inoculated 3 of his family in 1783 (Ledger C, p. 1; Ledger D, p. 77, noted "debt forgiven as before," but part of bill was paid by making a pair of saddle bags and also by Henry Ruff paying 10 shillings); see Thomas Huggins & Co., q.v.

Touchstone, L., see Moses Whitlock, q.v.

Tourk, James, at Mathew Conelton's, was treated by Dr. John Archer in Jun 1788 (Ledger F, p. 151)

Townsley, John, was visited by Dr. John Archer who treated him in May and June 1773 and Sep 1774, a child in Jan 1778, him [John] in Feb 1778, a child in Sep 1781, and inoculated two sons in Feb 1782 (Ledger B, p. 97, spelled his name Townsly; Ledger C, p. 46, noted "debt forgiven by order of testator") [John Townley or Townsley was a Revolutionary War veteran.]

Townsley, Mary, widow of William, was treated by Dr. John Archer at various times in 1797 and 1798 (Ledger I, which is missing, was abstracted by Dr. George W. Archer circa 1890; his notes are in the Archives of the Historical Society of Harford County folder "Archer, G. W. Coll. – Ledgers and Day Books")

Townsley, William, see Mary Townsley, q.v.

Toy, John, was treated by Dr. Matthew J. Allen in Feb 1848 ("by laying open finger in 2 places") and also treated him eight times in Mar 1848 (p. 75)

Toy, Joseph, was treated by Dr. John Archer in Feb 1787 (Ledger F, p. 205)

Trago, John (weaver), brother-in-law to J. Michel (sic), was treated by Dr. John Archer in Sep 1789 (Ledger F, p. 284)

Trago, Thomas, was visited by Dr. John Archer who treated his family in 1796 (Ledger I, which is missing, was abstracted by Dr. George W. Archer circa 1890; his notes are in the Archives of the Historical Society of Harford County folder "Archer, G. W. Coll. – Ledgers and Day Books")

Traplin, James, was treated by Dr. John Archer in Dec 1800 (Ledger F, p. 287)

Traver, Robert, see Robert Travis, q.v.

Travis, Robert, "near Fall Quakers Meeting" [i. e., Little Falls Friends Meeting House in Fallston], was treated by Dr. John Archer in Aug 1786 and "Robert Traver, near Quaker Meeting" in Feb 1788 (Ledger F, pp. 163, 224)

Travis, Captain, was treated by Dr. John Archer, Jr. in Sep 1818 and also mentioned J. P. Ryland, constable, in Oct 1819 (p. 75)

Tredaway, Carvel, was treated by Dr. Robert H. Archer after 1822 [no dates or details were given] (Dr. Archer's "Alphabet to Ledger H" is his booklet [filed in the Archives of the Historical Society of Harford County] that contains his index to Ledger H [which is missing] for his patients in Baltimore City before 1822 and in Harford County after 1822, according to a notation by Dr. George W. Archer.)

Treadway, Carvil, was visited by Dr. Matthew J. Allen who treated his mother in Aug 1847 and Jul and Aug 1848 (p. 60, noted his mother paid part of the bill in Jan 1848 and part was paid "by cash to Wm. Dallam" in May 1850)

Treadway, Thomas, was treated by Dr. Matthew J. Allen in Aug 1847 (p. 61)

Treadway, William, see William Tredway, q.v.

Treadwell, Eliza, see James Treadwell, q.v.

Treadwell, James, was visited by Dr. Alonzo Preston who treated daughter Eliza in Oct 1825 (p. 59)

Treadwell, William, was visited by Dr. Alonzo Preston who treated his wife in Apr 1826 (p. 72)

Tredway, William, appeared on a list of debts dated 26 Dec 1822 and titled "A List of Allen's Claims" that were due and payable to Dr. Richard N. Allen for services rendered [no dates were given] to the said Tredway (Document filed in Historical Society of Harford County Archives folder "R. N. Allen" spelled his name Tredway) [William Tredway was a War of 1812 veteran.]

Tredwell, ---- [blank], was visited by Dr. Alonzo Preston who treated his wife in Jun-Jul 1826 and child in Sep 1826 (p. 78)

Trimble, Isaac, at Ashmead's Mill, was visited in 1789 by Dr. John Archer who treated him and his wife (Ledger F, p. 90, spelled his name Tremble)

Trimble, John, was prescribed medicine for a child by Dr. Robert H. Archer on 5 Dec 1804 (Rx Book, 1802-1804, p. 66)

Trimble, Jos., Mr., was prescribed medicine by Dr. Robert H. Archer for Rachel [daughter?] on 8 Feb 1843 (Rx Book, 1825-1851, p. 118)

Trimble, Joseph, see Negro John, q.v.

Trotter, William, was treated by Dr. John Archer in June 1775 (Ledger B, p. 74)

Troutner, David, near Dublin, was visited by Dr. Robert H. Archer who treated a child on 25 May 1825 and prescribed medicine for the child on 26 May 1825 (Ledger F, p. 132; Rx Book, 1825-1851, pp. 78, 132)

Trustees of the Poor, had an account with Dr. Matthew J. Allen who treated Eliza ---- [last name not given] for a burn in Dec 1847 and an unnamed colored woman for a burn in Jan 1848 (p. 72); see Alms House, q.v.

Turner, Charity, see Samuel Turner, q.v.

Turner, Hannah, see Samuel Turner, q.v.

Turner, Jacob, was visited by Dr. Robert H. Archer who treated his wife in July 1822 (p. 9)

Turner, Samuel (colored), was visited by Dr. Matthew J. Allen who treated a child [daughter?] [name illegible] in Feb and Mar 1848, Charity and Hannah in Mar and Apr 1848 and Samuel, Hannah and Charity in Apr 1848 (pp. 74, 80)

Tyson, see John Reese, q.v.

Underhill, Thomas, see George Sankey, q.v.

Underwood, Elihu, was prescribed medicine by Dr. Robert H. Archer on 4 Aug and 5 Aug 1802 (Rx Book, 1802-1804, pp. 7, 8)

Underwood, Enoch, was prescribed medicine by Dr. Robert H. Archer on 11 Jul 1803 (Rx Book, 1802-1804, p. 52)

Vanbibber, see Reed & Vanbibber, q.v.

Van Cleave, John, was treated by Dr. John Archer in Mar 1773 and July 1774 and Feb and Apr 1780 and also stated Martha Smith was his security in Feb 1780 (Ledger B, p. 94, and continued in Ledger D, p. 41, where his name was spelled Vancleff and also noted "debt forgiven as before")

Vance, David, was visited by Dr. John Archer who treated his wife in Aug 1782, an infant in Jan 1784 and a child in Nov 1785 (Ledger D, p. 93)

Vance, John, was treated by Dr. John Archer in Jun 1782 (Ledger D, p. 65) [John Vance was a Revolutionary War veteran.]

Vanclief, see Elizabeth Lee and also John Van Cleave, q.v.

Vandegrift, George, was visited by Dr. John Archer who treated him in Oct 1773, his wife in labor on 13 Feb 1774, him in Mar, May and Jun 1774, an infant in Feb 1775 and him and a child in Jun 1775 (Ledger B, p. 14 noted "to cash paid you, $1.10" on 13 Feb 1777); visited by Dr. John Archer who treated him, his wife and a child in Sep 1793 (Ledger F, pp. 14, 47) [continued in Ledger I, which is missing, but it was abstracted by Dr. George W. Archer circa 1890 who noted "inoculated 6 of your family, viz., Elizabeth, John, George, Polly and Nancy, and a negro, in 1794" and he also noted "had a child Marcan(?)"] (Archives of the

Historical Society of Harford County folder "Archer, G. W. Coll. – Ledgers and Day Books") [George Vandegrift was a Revolutionary War veteran.]; see Thomas Harris, q.v.

Vanhorn, Ezekiel, was visited by Dr. John Archer who treated his wife in Jan 1777 and his brother in Jan and Feb 1777 (Ledger C, p. 81) [Ezekiel Vanhorn was a Revolutionary War veteran.]

Vanhorn, Gabriel P., was visited by Dr. John Archer who inoculated 4 of his family in 1781, treated his wife and son in Jul 1781, him in Aug and Dec 1781, Feb, Sep and Oct 1782 and Mar 1788, and noted medicine purchased of Townsend Speake in Sep 1782 (Ledger D, p. 41; Ledger F, p. 298) [Gabriel Peterson Vanhorn was a Revolutionary War veteran.]

Vanhorn, Richard (tanner), was visited by Dr. John Archer who treated him and his wife in May 1786 (Ledger F, p. 122)

Vansant, John, was treated by Dr. Thomas Archer at times before Dec 1804 as noted in a complaint filed by the doctor who stated, in part, that "as a physician … [he had] performed and bestowed in and about the visiting of prescribing and furnishing and physic to and for the said John … labouring and languishing under divers diseases, maladies and disorders ..." and he had not been paid for his services. (Court Records File 39.24.4C at the Historical Society of Harford County)

Vansickle, Bennet, was visited by Dr. James Reardon who treated his mother in Sep 1817 and him in Dec 1817; the bill was acknowledged by Thomas S. Bond. Register of Wills, on 21 Aug 1821, who stated "This account will pass when paid." (Document filed in Historical Society of Harford County Archives folder titled "Reardon, James Dr.")

Vansickle, Henry, see Jonathan Fosset, John Nelson and ---- Gale, q.v.

Varney, James, was visited by Dr. John Archer who treated him and his wife and a child in 1793 (Ledger F, p. 63) [account continued in Ledger I, which is missing]

Veachworth, William, was visited by Dr. John Archer who treated him, his wife and daughter Sally in 1795 (Ledger F, p. 134)

Veachworth, Sally, see William Veachworth, q.v.

Veech, James, was visited by Dr. John Archer who treated his wife in Aug 1779 (Ledger D, p. 10, noted "debt forgiven as before"); see Thomas Bowles, q.v.

Vogan, Mr., was treated by Dr. John Archer in Feb, Mar, Jul and Dec 1782 and May 1783 (Ledger D, p. 120, noted "debt forgiven as before")

Vogan, Richard, see Ignatius Wheeler, q.v.

Wadley, Mr., was prescribed medicine by Dr. Robert H. Archer on 26 Nov 1802 (Rx Book, 1802-1804, p. 26)

Waldrom, Sarah, was treated by Dr. John Archer in Mar 1787 (Ledger F, p. 244)

Waldron, Richard, was listed in Dr. John Archer's ledger circa 1773, but no entries were made in his account; subsequently visited by Dr. Archer who treated his grandson in Jun 1778, him [Richard] and a daughter in Sep 1779, and him in Nov 1779 (Ledger B, p. 80; Ledger C, p. 70)

Waldron, Sucky, was visited by Dr. John Archer who treated Nancy's child in Sep 1782 (Ledger D, p. 68, noted £6 bill was transferred to Edward Elliot's account in Ledger G) [which is missing]

Walker, Betsey, Miss, was treated by Dr. Robert H. Archer in July and Aug 1823 and mentioned John Barkley in Nov 1825 (pp. 85a, 86; Ledger F, p. 57)

Walker, Eleanor, widow of James, was visited by Dr. John Archer who treated her and son James at various times between 1796 and 1798 and also noted "Geo. Walker, Exr." (Ledger I, which is missing, was abstracted by Dr. George W. Archer circa 1890; his notes are in the Archives of the Historical Society of Harford County folder "Archer, G. W. Coll. – Ledgers and Day Books")

Walker, George, son-in-law of Joseph Gallion, now at Hughes Works, was treated by Dr. John Archer in Jan, May and Aug 1780 (Ledger D, p. 112, noted "debt forgiven as before"); see James Walker and Eleanor Walker, q.v.

Walker, James, was visited by Dr. John Archer who treated him at times between Nov 1722 and Apr 1774, daughter Kitty in Feb 1773, a child in Apr 1774, children in Apr 1775; account noted "a visit to widow Smith's daughter at the widow Bartley's" in Dec 1772; treated a child and "assumption of Ruth Smith's account" in Apr 1776; treated his son in Aug 1777, him [James] in Feb 1778 and "19 visits, dressing, etc." in Oct 1779, son George in Mar 1780, sister in Mar 1782 and him in Jul 1782, Aug 1783 and Sep 1788 (Ledger B, p. 74; Ledger C, p. 43; Ledger F, p. 246, indicated George Walker was administrator *de bonis non* on 20 Dec 1808) [James Walker was a Revolutionary War veteran.]; see Eleanor Walker and Negro Sam, q.v.

Walker, Kitty, see James Walker, q.v.

Walker, Peggy, see Benedict Edward Hall, q.v.

Wallace, ---- [blank] (deputy clerk), Bel Air, was treated by Dr. John Archer at various times between 1796 and 1800 (Ledger I, which is missing, was abstracted by Dr. George W. Archer circa 1890; his notes are in the Archives of the Historical Society of Harford County folder "Archer, G. W. Coll. – Ledgers and Day Books")

Wallace, Andrew, was treated by Dr. John Archer in Aug 1787 and was treated and medicated by Dr. Robert H. Archer on 11 Jan 1803 (Ledger F, p. 167; Rx Book, 1802-1804, p. 30)

Wallace, John, was visited by Dr. Robert H. Archer who treated a child in Oct 1822, him [John] in Aug 1823, a child in Aug and Sep 1824, and a sister and a negro in Sep 1824 (pp. 26, 86; Ledger F, p. 92)

Wallace, Joseph, was visited by Dr. John Archer who treated him in Oct 1779, his wife in Jun and Aug 1782, a negro in Jun 1783 and him [Joseph] in Oct 1783 (Ledger D, p. 28) [account continued in Ledger E, which is missing]

Wallace, Randal, see Randall Wallis, q.v.

Wallace, Samuel, was visited by Dr. John Archer who treated his son Randel in 1788, him [Samuel] in 1790 and him and son Samuel between 1795 and 1797 (Ledger F, p. 197 [account continued in Ledger H, which is missing]; also listed in Ledger I, which is missing, but it was abstracted by Dr. George W. Archer circa 1890; his notes are in the Archives of the Historical Society of Harford County folder "Archer, G. W. Coll. – Ledgers and Day Books")

Wallace, Samuel, was treated by Dr. Matthew J. Allen in Apr and Sep 1848 (p. 79)

Wallace, Thomas, was visited by Dr. John Archer who treated a child in Sep 1779, him [Thomas] in Aug 1782, a negro in Sep 1783 and him [Thomas] in Dec 1783, Aug 1785 and Jun 1786 (Ledger D, p. 24, noted "debt forgiven as before;" Ledger F, p. 320)

Wallace, William, was prescribed medicine by Dr. Robert H. Archer on 6 Aug 1802 and 26 Dec 1802 (Rx Book, 1802-1804, pp. 9, 27)

Wallace, William, was visited by Dr. Robert H. Archer who treated a child in consultation with Dr. Worthington in July 1823 (p. 83; Ledger F, p. 62)

Wallis, ---- [blank], was treated by Dr. Robert H. Archer in Baltimore before 1822 [no dates or details were given] (Dr. Archer's "Alphabet to Ledger H" is his booklet [filed in the Archives of the Historical Society of Harford County] that contains his index to Ledger H [which is missing] for his patients in Baltimore before 1822 and Harford County after 1822, according to a notation by Dr. George W. Archer.)

Wallis, John, was visited by Dr. Robert H. Archer who treated a child in Nov 1822, him in Apr 1823, a child in Aug 1824 and John's sister's child and a negro in Sep 1824 (pp. 37, 62, 117, 120)

Wallis, Samuel, was visited by Dr. John Archer who treated him and son Samuel in 1788 (Ledger F, p. 204)

Walmsley, William G., see Cecil Furnace, q.v.

Waltham, Hester see Robert Sanders (Saunders), q.v.

Walton, Elijah, was visited by Dr. Robert H. Archer who treated a child in July 1823, rendered obstetrical services to his wife on 23 Jun 1824 and treated his wife in July 1825, a child in Jan 1828, and him in Bel Air in Aug 1828 (pp. 83, 84, 110, 143, 260, 291, 292; Ledger F, p. 93)

Walton, Mr. was visited by Dr. Robert H. Archer who treated his wife in March 1827 and prescribed medicine for his wife on 28 May 1829 (p. 219; Rx Book, 1825-1851, p. 94)

Wand, ---- [blank] (pedlar), was treated by Dr. Robert H. Archer in Baltimore before 1822 [no dates or details were given] (Dr. Archer's "Alphabet to Ledger H" is his booklet [filed in the Archives of the Historical Society of Harford County] that contains his index to Ledger H [which is missing] for his patients in Baltimore before 1822 and in Harford County after 1822, according to a notation by Dr. George W. Archer.)

Wann, also see Whan and Whann, q.v.

Wann, Daniel, was treated by Dr. Alonzo Preston eight times in June 1827 (p. 91, noting "Settled by acct. in bar"); see Alonzo Preston, q.v.

Wann, John, Jr. [1787-1870], appeared on a list of debts dated 26 Dec 1822 and titled "A List of Allen's Claims" that were due and payable to Dr. Richard N. Allen for services rendered [no dates] by him to said Wann (Document filed in Historical Society of Harford County Archives folder "R. N. Allen") [John Wann was a War of 1812 veteran.]

Wann, Thomas, was visited by Dr. Alonzo Preston who treated his wife "in partu" [in childbirth] on 20 Sep 1825 and treated him at times in 1825 and 1827, and his wife again in 1827 (p. 55)

Wann, William [1791-1865], was treated by Dr. Alonzo Preston on 26 Jun 1826 and he paid the $1.50 medical bill in cash on 15 Sep 1826 (p. 79) [William Wann was a War of 1812 veteran.]

Wann, William, Jr., was visited by Dr. Matthew J. Allen who treated a child in Sep 1847, Miss E. Norris in Oct 1847, and children [no names were given] in Oct 1847 (p. 64)

Ward, Benjamin, was treated by Dr. Robert H. Archer in Aug 1822 (Ledger F, p. 71)

Ward, Betsy, see James Ward (tailor), q.v.

Ward, Charles, near Ashmead's Mill, was treated by Dr. John Archer in Dec 1774 (Ledger B, p. 5)

Ward, Charles [1791-1865], was prescribed medicine for his wife by Dr. Robert H. Archer in Jul 1832 (Rx Book, 1825-1851, p. 107) [Charles Ward was a War of 1812 veteran.]

Ward, Harry, see James Ward (tailor), q.v.

Ward, James (mason), was treated by Dr. John Archer in May 1779, Aug 1781, Jan 1782 and Sep 1782 (Ledger C, p. 122, noted "debt forgiven by order of testator") [account was continued in Ledger E, which is missing] [James Ward was a Revolutionary War veteran.]

Ward, James (tailor), was treated by Dr. John Archer from 1794 to 1797 and inoculated Mrs. Ward and Betsy, John and Harry Ward and William Knox (Ledger I, which is missing, was abstracted by Dr. George W. Archer circa 1890; his notes are in the Archives of the Historical Society of Harford County folder "Archer, G. W. Coll. – Ledgers and Day Books")

Ward, John, see Reuben H. Davis and James Ward (tailor), q.v.

Ward, John, was visited by Dr. Matthew J. Allen who treated a child six times in Dec 1847, rendered obstetrical services to his wife on 6 Mar 1848 and treated daughter Mary and son John in Aug 1847 (p. 69, noted part of bill was paid "to cash pd. you for me by W. H. Dallam" in Mar 1851)

Ward, John D., was treated by Dr. Matthew J. Allen in 1832 in Calvert County (p. 20)

Ward, Mary, see John Ward, q.v.

Warfield, Henry, was visited by Dr. John Archer who treated his wife and a negro in Feb 1781 and him [Henry] in Jan 1783 (Ledger D, p. 120) [account continued in Ledger G, which is missing]

Warfield, Jacob, was treated by Dr. Robert H. Archer in Baltimore before 1822 [no dates or details were given] (Dr. Archer's "Alphabet to Ledger H" is his booklet [filed in the Archives of the Historical Society of Harford County] that contains his index to Ledger H [which is missing] for his patients in Baltimore before 1822 and Harford County after 1822, according to a notation by Dr. George W. Archer.)

Warner, Aaron, "Friend," was visited by Dr. James Archer who treated Ellie(?) [illegible] four times in Oct 1807 (p. 27)

Warner, Benjamin, was treated by Dr. John Archer in Feb 1786 (Ledger F, p. 143)

Warner, Brinton, see Jonathan Warner, q.v.

Warner, Cudwith, was visited by Dr. John Archer who treated an infant in Jan 1779 and a child in Aug 1779 (Ledger C, p. 51, noted "debt forgiven by order of testator"); Cuddy Warner was visited by Dr. John Archer who treated him, his wife and an infant in 1799 (Ledger F, p. 68)

Warner, Jonathan [1789-1879], was visited by Dr. Alonzo Preston who treated his son Brinton five times in Sep 1827 (p. 96) [account continued in Ledger K, which is missing]

Warner, Joseph, was visited by Dr. John Archer who treated his son Mordecai in 1786 and him in Oct 1799 (Ledger F, p. 284) [account continued in Ledger K, which is missing]

Warner, Mordecai, see Joseph Warner, q.v.

Warnock, Philip [1753-1813], was treated by Dr. John Archer in Jul 1781, Jun and Sep 1785 and May 1795 (Ledger D, p. 29, spelled his name Warnick; Ledger F, p. 241) [account continued in Ledger L, which is missing] [Philip Warnock was a Revolutionary War veteran.]

Wary, Joseph, was treated by Dr. Robert H. Archer in Baltimore before 1822 [no dates or details were given] (Dr. Archer's "Alphabet to Ledger H" is his booklet [filed in the Archives of the Historical Society of Harford County] that contains his index to Ledger H [which is missing] for his patients in Baltimore before 1822 and Harford County after 1822, according to a notation by Dr. George W. Archer.)

Waskey, Christian, in Abingdon, was visited by Dr. John Archer who treated him and his family in 1795 (Ledger I, which is missing, was abstracted by Dr. George W. Archer circa 1890 and listed his name as Whaskey; his notes are in the Archives of the Historical Society of Harford County file "Archer, G. W. Coll. – Ledgers and Day Books")

Waters, Amos, was treated by Dr. Alonzo Preston from 1824 to 1826 [no details were given] and also between 6 Sep 1827 and 8 Jan 1828, running up $19.00 in medical bills (pp. 21 and 97, noting on 7 Jan 1833, "This acct. settled by acct. in bar & paid $1.00 on his acct. – May 20th 1824 paid also as 1/3 of balance due A.M."); see Benjamin Watters, q.v.

Waters, Charles, see William Kitely, q.v.

Waters, Godfrey, was treated by Dr. John Archer in Apr 1774 (Ledger B, p. 18)

Waters, Godfrey, of Henry, was treated by Dr. John Archer in Aug 1781 and Jul 1791 (Ledger D, p. 58, spelled his name Watters; Ledger F, p. 261) [account continued in Ledger H, which is missing]; see Henry Waters, q.v.

Waters, Henry, was visited by Dr. John Archer who treated his sons in Jan 1773, him in May 1774 and Feb and Mar 1781, a child in Aug 1781, his wife in Dec 1781 and him [Henry] in Oct 1782 (Ledger B, p. 17, spelled his name Waters; Ledger D, p. 121, spelled his name Watters and noted the bill was paid "by 1 half Johan:" on 21 Sep 1783 and "by cash in full" in 18 Mar 1784); see Godfrey Waters and Henry Watters, q.v.

Waters, Henry, Jr., see Frances Bull and John Bull and Richard Bull, q.v.

Waters, Henry, Sr., was visited by Dr. John Archer who treated his son Godfrey in 1786 and him in 1789 (Ledger F, p. 295); see Henry Watters, Sr., Mary Miller and Elisha Daws, q.v.

Waters, Henry G., see Henry G. Watters, q.v.

Waters, Jane, was treated by Dr. Alonzo Preston in 1825 (p. 43)

Waters, Joanna, was treated by Dr. John Archer in Jul 1787 (Ledger F, p. 285)

Waters, John, was visited by Dr. Matthew J. Allen who treated a child in May 1848 (p. 82, noted that W. H. Dallam paid the bill in full in Mar 1850)

Waters, Nicholas, was visited by Dr. John Archer who treated a child (or children) in Mar 1773, May 1775 and a child in Sep 1775 (Ledger B, p. 62; Ledger C, p. 59, noted "assumption of Thomas Barnes' account"); see William Watson, q.v.

Waters, P., Mrs., was prescribed medicine by Dr. Robert H. Archer on 19 Apr 1799 (Rx Book, 1796-1801, p. 14)

Waters, Sally, see Walter Waters, q.v.

Waters, Susan, Miss, was prescribed medicine by Dr. Robert H. Archer on 2 Aug 1841 (Rx Book, 1825-1851, p. 116)

Waters, Thomas, was visited by Dr. John Archer who treated him and a child in 1787 (Ledger F, p. 285)

Waters, Walter, was visited by Dr. John Archer who treated his daughter Sally in 1788 and him in Dec 1792 (Ledger F, p. 162) [account continued in Ledger K, which is missing]

Watkins, Antony (negro), see Reed & Vanbibber, q.v.

Watkins, Joe (negro), see Reed & Vanbibber, q.v.

Watkins, John [1755-1826], was treated by Dr. John Archer in Oct 1781 (Ledger D, p. 93, noted "debt forgiven as before") [John Watkins was a Revolutionary War veteran.]

Watkins, Mary (negro), see Reed & Vanbibber, q.v.

Watson, ---- [blank] (schoolmaster), near Salt Box, was treated by Dr. John Archer at various times between 1796 and 1799 (Ledger I, which is missing, was abstracted by Dr. George W. Archer circa 1890; his notes are in the Archives of the Historical Society of Harford County folder "Archer, G. W. Coll. – Ledgers and Day Books")

Watson, ---- [blank], innkeeper, "X roads," was treated by Dr. Robert H. Archer in Jan 1828 (p. 260)

Watson, Abraham, was visited by Dr. John Archer, Jr. who treated him, his wife and child in 1820 and mentioned Joseph Watson in 1823 (p. 73); see Joseph Watson, Sr., q.v.

Watson, Abram, see Joseph Watson, Sr., q.v.

Watson, Archibald, was visited by Dr. John Archer who treated him in Apr 1781 and inoculated 7 of his family; Archibald's widow had her own account by 1785 when she was visited by Dr. Archer who treated a child in Sep 1785 and a son in Nov 1785 (Ledger D, p. 128, listed the account twice and noted "debt forgiven as before" both times)

Watson, Bromfield, see Joseph Watson, Sr., q.v.

Watson, Cunningham, see Joseph Watson, Sr., q.v.

Watson, James, near Clindennan's, was treated by Dr. John Archer in Nov 1796 (Ledger F, p. 58) [James Watson was a Revolutionary War veteran.]

Watson, Joseph, Sr., was visited by Dr. John Archer, Jr. who treated his son Abraham or Abram in Feb 1816 and Jul 1817 and his wife and sons Cunningham and Bromfield in Oct 1820 (p. 41); see Abraham Watson, q.v.

Watson, Mrs. (widow), was treated by Dr. John Archer in Apr 1786 (Ledger F, p. 226)

Watson, William, at Nicholas Waters', was visited by Dr. John Archer who treated his wife in June 1774 (Ledger B, p. 3)

Watt, John, was visited by Dr. John Archer who treated him in Jan and Feb 1781, his son John in Nov 1781 and him in Oct 1786 (Ledger D, p. 116; Ledger F, p. 83)

Watt, Joseph, was treated by Dr. John Archer in 1786 and 1789 (Ledger F, pp. 6, 357) [account continued in Ledger G, which is missing]

Watters, Benjamin, was treated by Dr. Alonzo Preston four times in 1827, the last time being 30 Jul 1827 (p. 94, spelled his name Waters, but it was later noted the $6.25 medical bill was "pd. 7 Jan 1830 by A. Watters, adm. of Benjn. Watters")

Watters, Daniel R. [1792-1857], appeared on a list of debts dated 26 Dec 1822 and titled "A List of Allen's Claims" that were due and payable to Dr. Richard N. Allen for services rendered [no dates were given] by him to said Watters (Document filed in Historical Society of Harford County Archives folder "R. N. Allen"); Daniel "Dan" Watters was visited by Dr. Robert H. Archer who treated his wife in July 1825 and both of them in Sep 1825, prescribed medicine for him on 13 Aug 1825, treated his wife in Mar 1830 and a child in Sep 1830 and Mar and Apr 1831, and prescribed medicine for his son Henry on 20 May 1832 (pp. 143, 154, 155; Rx Book, 1825-1851, pp. 93, 105; Ledger F, p. 118) [Daniel R. Watters was a War of 1812 veteran.]

Watters, Godfrey, see Henry G. Watters, Godfrey Waters and Henry Waters, Sr., q.v.

Watters, Henry, see Daniel R. Watters and Henry Waters, q.v.

Watters, Henry, Sr., was visited by Dr. James Archer who treated his wife in Feb 1806 and a negro man in Nov 1806 (p. 28); see Joseph Stone, Negro Jacob and Henry Waters, Sr., q.v.

Watters, Henry G. [1790-1865], was visited by Dr. Robert H. Archer who treated a negro in Aug 1822, Henry's sister Margaret several times between May and Aug 1824, S. Bradford and sister F.(?) S. Bradford in July 1824, "Sam, Sally Green's man" in June and July 1825 and July 1826, sister Susan in Sep 1825, wife and child in Oct 1825; also treated Henry's father several times in April and May 1826, an infant in Apr 1826, Henry's son Godfrey in May 1826, a child in May 1827 and Miss Margaret in Nov 1827 and sister Susan in Aug 1828 (pp. 108, 109, 110, 112, 120, 139, 140, 156, 179-181, 183-185, 188, 194, 230, 254, 294; Ledger F, p. 126, spelled his name Waters Wilson); H. G. Watters was treated by Dr. Robert H. Archer after 1822 [no other dates or details were given] as noted in Dr. Archer's "Alphabet to Ledger H" which is his booklet [filed in the Archives of the Historical Society of Harford County] that contains his index to Ledger H [which is missing] for his patients in Baltimore before 1822 and in Harford County after 1822, according to a notation by Dr. George W. Archer.) [His full name was Henry Godfrey Watters and he was a War of 1812 veteran.]; see James Clendenin, q.v.

Watters, Margaret, see Henry G. Watters, q.v.

Watters, Mr., on I. Wheeler's place, was treated by Dr. Robert H. Archer after 1822 [no dates or details were given] (Dr. Archer's "Alphabet to Ledger H" is his booklet [filed in the Archives of the Historical Society of Harford County] that contains his index to Ledger H [which is missing] for his patients in Baltimore before 1822 and Harford County after 1822, according to a notation by Dr. George W. Archer.)

Watters, Susan, see Henry G. Watters, q.v.

Watters, William, of Henry, was treated by Dr. John Archer from 1794 to 1799 (Ledger I, which is missing, was abstracted by Dr. George W. Archer circa 1890; his notes are in the Archives of the Historical Society of Harford County folder "Archer, G. W. Coll. – Ledgers and Day Books")

Watterson, William, was mentioned in Dr. Robert H. Archer's ledger in a non-medical matter in 1828 (p. 293)

Way, James and John, were mentioned in Dr. Robert H. Archer's ledger in non-medical matters between 8 May 1824 and 22 Feb 1833 (p. 222; Ledger F, p. 121)

Webb, George, in the Barrens [an area in the northwest part of the county near Pennsylvania], was visited by Dr. John Archer who treated him and his wife in Oct 1782 (Ledger D, p. 31, noted "debt forgiven as before")

Webb, George, was treated by Dr. Robert H. Archer in Oct 1815 and Dr. John Archer, Jr. treated his wife in 1816 at Havre de Grace and him in Apr 1817 (Dr. Robert H. Archer Ledger F, p. 121; Dr. John Archer, Jr., p. 59)

Webb, Mr., see John Jacob Albert and ---- Halfpenny, q.v.

Webb, Richard, in the Barrens [an area in the northwest part of the county near Pennsylvania], was treated by Dr. John Archer in Nov 1781 and Jul 1787 (Ledger D, p. 98, noted "debt forgiven as before;" Ledger F, p. 342)

Webb, Samuel, Jr. [1746-1813], was visited by Dr. John Archer who treated him and an infant in Jul 1779, him in Feb, Apr, Jun, Jul and Dec 1780 and Jan, Feb, Mar and April 1781, George and a negro in Jun 1781, a child in Aug and Oct 1781, inoculated a daughter in 1782, and treated his wife in Sep 1782 (tooth extraction) him in Oct 1782, an infant in Aug 1783 and him in Sep and Oct 1783 (Ledger C, p. 78; Ledger D, p. 62, noted the account was continued on p. 95, but that account was titled Samuel Webb, Sr. and did not pertain to Samuel Webb, Jr.) [Samuel Webb, Jr. was a Revolutionary War veteran.]

Webb, Samuel, Sr., was visited by Dr. John Archer who treated him eight times between Aug 1778 and Dec 1778 and in Mar, Apr, Jun and Nov 1779, him and a negro in Jan 1781, him in Mar 1781, him and Negro Sampson in Sep 1781, Sally Webb in Nov 1781 (tooth extraction), him [Samuel] in May and July 1782, his wife in Sep 1782 and him in Jan, Apr and May 1783; at various times between 1781 and 1788 this account mentioned Samuel Crockett, William Webb, Robert Amoss and Micajah Mitchell; also treated an infant in 1786, him [Samuel] in 1789, a child in 1800; mentioned Thomas Archer, Elizabeth Archer and John Forwood in 1803 (Ledger C, p. 119, noted "debt forgiven by order of testator;" Ledger D, p. 95 [account continued in Ledger E, which is missing]; Ledger F, pp. 40, 114, 187, 222) [account continued in Ledger G, which is missing]; see Micajah Mitchell, William Webb and Samuel Webb, Jr., q.v.

Webb, William [1732-1778], was visited by Dr. John Archer and treated him at times between Mar 1773 and Jul 1775, a child in Mar 1773, Johanna Logue in Aug 1774, brother Samuel in Jun and Jul 1775, Samuel Crocket in July 1775, him [William] in Nov 1775, and inoculated 19 of his family in Jan 1776; also treated him, his overseer, and "patrem" [father] in Jun 1776, Negro Shelah in Dec 1776, brother Samuel in Apr and May 1777, his [William's] son in May 1777, a negro in May 1777, "Brown" in Sep 1777, Negro George in Feb 1778, and inoculated 5 of his family in Feb 1778 (Ledger B, p. 81; Ledger C, p. 5) [William Webb was a Revolutionary War veteran and a signer of the Bush Declaration on March 22, 1775.]; see Samuel Webb, q.v.

Webb, William (doctor), was treated by Dr. John Archer in May 1788 (Ledger F, p. 169)

Webster, Aliz., see Samuel Webster, q.v.

Webster, Betsy, was treated by Dr. John Archer in Apr 1782 and Mar 1783 (Ledger D, p. 114, noted part of the bill was paid in cash in Nov 1783 and apparently the balance of the "debt forgiven as before"); see Richard Webster, q.v.

Webster, Elizabeth, see Ann Dallam, q.v.

Webster, George, see Isaac Webster and Richard Webster, q.v.

Webster, Grace, see Samuel Webster, Jr., q.v.

Webster, Hannah, Miss, was treated by Dr. John Archer in Oct and Dec 1790 (Ledger F, pp. 220, 296, 350) [account continued in Ledger H, which is missing]; see Michael Webster, q.v.

Webster, Harry [or Henry], was visited by Dr. Robert H. Archer who treated his wife in Oct 1822, "for his father" in Apr 1824, his wife in May 1825, July 1826 and several times in May 1827; Dr. Archer also noted on 13 Feb 1828 that $25.00 was "Recd. of him which (after deducting $6.10 because he said he was a poor man) is in full of all a/cs to this day" (pp. 30, 133, 193, listed him as Harry; pp. 132, 228, 229, 262, listed him as Henry, and Ledger F, p. 104, listed him as Harry)

Webster, Isaac, was visited by Dr. John Archer who treated him in Jan 1781, him and his wife in Apr 1783, a child in Jun 1783 and him in Oct 1783 (Ledger D, p. 115) [account continued in Ledger E, which is missing]; see James Lawrence, Paul Shields, Negro David, Abram Huff and John Lee Webster, q.v.

Webster, Isaac, Jr., was visited by Dr. John Archer who treated him and his wife in Nov 1787 and Aug 1789 (Ledger F, pp. 14, 38) [account continued in Ledger H, which is missing]

Webster, Isaac, Sr., was treated by Dr. John Archer in Aug 1789 (Ledger F, p. 176)

Webster, Isaac (reverend), was visited by Dr. Robert H. Archer who treated his wife in June 1825 and son George in Apr 1828 (pp. 136, 272; Ledger F, p. 116, noted "debt forgiven causa paupertatis & religionis") [Isaac Webster and Isaac P. Webster were both veterans of the War of 1812.]

Webster, J. S. [probably John Skinner Webster, Esq.], was also prescribed medicine by Dr. Robert H. Archer in Baltimore on 8 Nov 1802 (Rx Book, 1802-1804, p. 25)

Webster, James, see Owen McCartey, q.v.

Webster, James (carpenter), was treated by Dr. John Archer in Sep 1788 (Ledger F, p. 200) [account continued in Ledger G, which is missing]

Webster, James, of Samuel, was treated by Dr. John Archer in Jun 1780 and he inoculated "Jon: & Negro" in Jul 1780 (Ledger D, p. 71, noted "debt forgiven as before")

Webster, John Lee [1735-1795], was visited by Dr. John Archer who inoculated 31 negroes in 1777 and treated him in Jul 1779, a child in Aug 1779, him in Oct 1780 and Aug 1781, William Kelsy in Aug 1781, John in Nov 1781, son Isaac in 1787, him [John] in 1788, and inoculated 31 negroes in 1795 (Ledger D, p. 59

[account continued in Ledger E, which is missing]; Ledger F, pp. 198, 221 [account continued in Ledger H, which is missing]; Ledger I, which is missing, was abstracted by Dr. George W. Archer circa 1890; his notes are in the Archives of the Historical Society of Harford County file "Archer, G. W. Coll. – Ledgers and Day Books;"] [John Lee Webster was a Revolutionary War veteran.]; see Samuel Webster, Sr., q.v.

Webster, John Skinner, see J. S. Webster, q.v.

Webster, Jon:, see James Webster, of Samuel, q.v.

Webster, Joseph, was treated by Dr. John Archer in Oct 1778 (Ledger C, p. 30)

Webster, Marian or Mariam, see Samuel Webster, q.v.

Webster, Mary, see Samuel Webster, q.v.

Webster, Michael, was visited by Dr. John Archer who treated him before 1772 [no date or details were given], a child in Aug 1772, him in May 1778, him and a child in Jun 1778, him in Jul and Oct 1779, Oct 1781, Sep 1781 and Jan 1783, him and his daughter Hannah in Mar 1788 and him in Jan 1790 (Ledger B, p. 82; Ledger C, p. 110 [account continued in Ledger E, which is missing]; Ledger F, pp. 180, 184)

Webster, Mrs. "widow senr." *(sic)*, was treated by Dr. John Archer in Feb 1780 (Ledger D, p. 47, noted "debt forgiven as before")

Webster, Peggy, Miss, was treated by Dr. John Archer in July 1787 (Ledger F, p. 163)

Webster, Phebe, see Richard Webster, q.v.

Webster, Richard, was visited by Dr. John Archer who treated him in Aug and Sep 1779, Mar 1781 and Apr 1782 and him and sons William, George and Samuel in 1792 (Ledger D, p. 10, noted "debt forgiven as before" [account continued in Ledger E, which is missing]; Ledger F, p. 16); see John Wiles, q.v.

Webster, Richard, was visited by Dr. Robert H. Archer who treated him in July 1825, daughter Phebe in May and Sep 1825, him, his wife and daughter Betsy in Sep 1825, and daughter Phebe was prescribed medicine ("laxative pills") on 6 May 1825 and daughter Betsy on 6 Sep 1825 (pp. 134, 141, 154, 158; Rx Book, 1825-1851, pp. 79, 83; Ledger F, p. 142)

Webster, Sally, see Samuel Webster (pedagogue), q.v.

Webster, Samuel, see Richard Webster, William Cowin, John Mohon and James Webster, of S., q.v.

Webster, Samuel, was treated by Dr. Thaddeus Jewett before 25 Sep 1775 by which time he was indebted to the doctor for medicines and treatment costs that he thought were not reasonable [final disposition not given]; Samuel was treated by Dr. John Archer in Jan 1776, Nov 1777 and Oct 1778 (Court Records File 3.03.4 in the Historical Society of Harford County; Dr. Archer's Ledger C, p. 20)

Webster, Samuel (pedagogue), of Isaac, was visited by Dr. John Archer who treated him and his daughter Sally at various times between 1797 and 1800 (Ledger I, which is missing, was abstracted by Dr. George W. Archer circa 1890; his notes are in the Archives of the Historical Society of Harford County file "Archer, G. W. Coll. - Ledgers and Day Books")

Webster, Samuel, Jr., was visited by Dr. John Archer who treated him in Aug 1772 and Apr 1774, Indian Mary in Apr 1774; Samuel, son of Samuel, was visited by Dr. John Archer who treated him in May 1773 and May 1775 and a child in June 1774; Samuel, Jr. was visited by Dr. John Archer who treated his wife in Oct 1777, him in Jun and Oct 1779, Feb 1780 and May and Jun 1781, and Grace in Aug 1781, inoculated 6 of his family in Sep 1781 and treated him in Jun and Sep 1782; Samuel, son of Samuel, was treated by Dr. John Archer in Sep 1787 (Ledger B, pp. 85, 88; Ledger C, p. 96) [continued in Ledger E, which is missing]; Ledger F, pp. 222, 230)

Webster, Samuel, Sr., was treated by Dr. John Archer in Jan 1777, Jul 1779, Apr 1780, Jan 1784 and Nov 1785 and the £7.10.9 medical bill was paid in full in cash by John Lee Webster on 27 Jan 1794 (Ledger C, p. 41; Ledger D, p. 61)

Webster, Samuel (tanner), was visited by Dr. John Archer who treated him and daughters Aliz., Mary and Marian or Mariam [name spelling unclear] in June and July 1788 (Ledger F, pp. 42, 354)

Webster, William, see Richard Webster, q.v.

Weems, Betsy, see John Weems and Philip Thomas, q.v.

Weems, Eliza, see Philip, Thomas, q.v.

Weems, John (colonel), "trans fluis" [i. e., "across the water," meaning across the Susquehanna River in Cecil County], was visited by Dr. John Archer who treated him and his daughter Betsy in Mar 1787 (Ledger F, p. 247)

Weems, William (major), was visited by Dr. Matthew J. Allen in Calvert County who treated him and a child in 1823 and him [William] in 1832 (pp. 6b, 17); see Jane A. Allen, q.v.

Weir, Thomas, son of Thomas, was visited by Dr. John Archer who treated him and his wife in Dec 1787 (Ledger F, p. 55)

Welch, Betsy, see William Welch, q.v.

Welch, Henry, see William Welch, q.v.

Welch, James, see William Welch, q.v.

Welch, John, was treated by Dr. John Archer in Sep and Oct 1779 (Ledger D, p. 27, noted "debt forgiven as before") [John Welch was a Revolutionary War veteran.]

Welch, Sarah, see William Welch, q.v.

Welch, Mrs., was mentioned by Dr. Robert H. Archer in non-medical matters from 21 Sep 1822 to 15 Sep 1826 and the ledger noted that she did the washing for Dr. Thomas Archer's sons John and Robert H. (Ledger F, p. 147); see John Archer (minor), q.v.

Welch, William, was visited by Dr. John Archer who treated him in 1772 [no dates and details were given] and is son in Apr 1774 (Ledger B, p. 77)

Welch, William, was visited by Dr. Robert H. Archer who treated his wife in Nov 1822 and Jul 1823, an infant in May 1823, a child from Aug to Dec 1823, and also mentioned William F. Miller in 1823; William was treated at various times in 1824 and 1825 by Dr. Alonzo Preston who also treated his wife and family in 1825 (Dr. Archer, p. 48, and Ledger F, p. 63, listed him as William Welsh, blacksmith; Dr. Preston, pp. 35, 75, 89)

Welch, William, was visited by Dr. Matthew J. Allen who treated children James, Henry, Betsy and William in May 1844 and one of his sons was treated for a broken arm in Aug 1845; daughter Sarah was treated 19 times between Jul 1847 and Jul 1848; account also noted that Mr. Lilly paid part of the bill in Nov 1848 and W. H. Dallam paid part in Jul 1850 and Oct 1850 (pp. 35, 52, 58, 88, and spelled name once as Welsh) [William Welsh was a Revolutionary War veteran.]

Wells, James, was visited by Dr. John Archer who treated him in Oct and Dec 1781 and him and his wife in Jul 1783 (Ledger D, p. 105) [account continued in Ledger E, which is missing]

Wells, James, at B. Friar [i. e., Bald Friar landing on the Susquehanna River] near M. Sweney's Mill [Matthew Sweeney's Mill], was treated by Dr. John Archer in Jan 1791 (Ledger F, p. 336)

Wells, Mrs., was prescribed medicine for her child by Dr. Robert H. Archer on 17 Nov 1804 (Rx Book, 1802-1804, p. 61); see Mrs. Jessop, q.v.

Wells, Rachel, Miss, was prescribed medicine by Dr. Robert H. Archer on 6 Sep 1804 (Rx Book, 1802-1804, p. 57)

Wells, Richard, was visited by Dr. John Archer who treated him and his pregnant wife on 12 Jan 1789 (Ledger F, p. 27)

Wells, Widow, see Ezekiel Barnes, q.v.

Wells, William, was visited by Dr. John Archer who treated his daughter in Sep 1772, him in June 1775 and William Wells, Sr. and his wife in Oct 1788 (Ledger B, p. 7; Ledger F, p. 90) [account continued in Ledger G, which is missing] [William Wells was a Revolutionary War veteran.]

Welsh, Mr., see Edward Flanagan, q.v.

Welsh, William, see William Welch, q.v.

West, Enoch, near Coop Town, was treated by Dr. John Archer in Jul and Aug 1782 (Ledger D, p. 13, noted "debt forgiven as before")

West, Enoch, "near stone house," was visited by Dr. John Archer who treated him and a child in July 1788 (Ledger F, p. 121); see James Ford, q.v.

West, James, near T. Gash, was visited by Dr. John Archer who treated him and his wife in June 1791 (Ledger F, p. 10)

West, Joseph (wheelwright), was treated by Dr. John Archer in Nov 1781 (Ledger D, p. 91, noted "debt forgiven as before")

West, Michael, was visited by Dr. John Archer who treated his mother in Jul 1775 and him and a child in Feb 1790 (Ledger B, p. 46; Ledger F, p. 344) [Michael West was a Revolutionary War veteran.]

West, Mr., was prescribed medicine for his wife by Dr. Robert H. Archer on 21 Nov 1804 (Rx Book, 1802-1804, p. 66)

West, Nathaniel, was visited by Dr. John Archer who treated him in May and June 1779 and his wife in July 1779 (Ledger C, p. 91, noted "debt forgiven by order of testator") [Nathaniel West was a Revolutionary War veteran.]

West, Stacy, was prescribed medicine by Dr. Robert H. Archer on 18 Oct 1802 (Rx Book, 1802-1804, p. 22)

West, Thomas (breeches maker), was visited by Dr. John Archer who inoculated 9 of his family in 1777 and treated him in Jul 1780 and Mar and Apr 1783 (Ledger C, p. 73; Ledger D, p. 82, noted "debt forgiven as before")

West, Thomas (miller), was visited by Dr. John Archer who treated him in Apr 1781 and his wife in Mar 1784 (Ledger D, p. 6, noted "debt forgiven as before") [Thomas West was a Revolutionary War veteran.]

Western, Mrs., High Street [in Baltimore City], was prescribed medicine by Dr. Robert H. Archer on 16 May 1798 (Rx Book, 1796-1801, p. 11)

Wetherel (Wetherall), James, see William Kitely and Capt. John Hall, q.v.

Whan, John (wheelwright), was treated by Dr. John Archer between 1794 and 1800 (Ledger I, which is missing, was abstracted by Dr. George W. Archer circa 1890; his notes are in Archives of the Historical Society of Harford County folder "Archer, G. W. Coll. – Ledgers and Day Books")

Whann, Mr. (turner), near Michael's, was treated by Dr. Robert H. Archer in Oct 1825 and Oct 1826 (p. 160; Ledger F, p. 46)

Wharton, Rev. Charles H. (D. D.), was treated and medicated by Dr. John Archer on 6 Dec 1796 (Ledger I, which is missing, was abstracted by Dr. George W. Archer circa 1890 and noted the debt was "forgiven;" Dr. George W. Archer's notes are in the Archives of the Historical Society of Harford County folder "Archer, G. W. Coll. – Ledgers and Day Books")

Wheeler, ---- [blank] &ca (sic), was treated by Dr. Robert H. Archer in Baltimore before 1822 [no dates or details were given] (Dr. Archer's "Alphabet to Ledger H" is his booklet [filed in the Archives of the Historical Society of Harford County] that contains his index to Ledger H [which is missing] for his patients in Baltimore City before 1822 and in Harford County after 1822, according to a notation by Dr. George W. Archer.)

Wheeler, Austin W., was prescribed medicine by Dr. Robert H. Archer on 16 Apr 1834 (Rx Book, 1825-1851, p. 111)

Wheeler, Benjamin, was visited by Dr. John Archer who treated him in Apr 1781 and Jun and Jul 1783 and him and son Benjamin in 1789 (Ledger D, p. 15 [account continued in Ledger E, which is missing]; Ledger F, p. 74, called him Sr.) [account continued in Ledger G, which is missing]; see Robert Boarman and Thomas Wheeler, of Benjamin, q.v.

Wheeler, Bennett [1784-1866], son of Ignatius, was treated by Dr. John Archer in 1791 and at times between 1795 and 1797 (Ledger F, p. 102, spelled his first name Bennit) [account continued in Ledger H, which is missing] (Ledger I, which is missing, was abstracted by Dr. George W. Archer circa 1890; his notes are in the Archives of the Historical Society of Harford County file "Archer, G. W. Coll. – Ledgers and Day Books") [Bennett Wheeler was a War of 1812 veteran.]; see Mrs. McGibbons (McCubbins?), q.v.

Wheeler, Caroline, see Henrietta Wheeler, q.v.

Wheeler, E., Miss, was prescribed medicine by Dr. Robert H. Archer on 16 Apr 1834 (Rx Book, 1825-1851, p. 111)

Wheeler, Francis I. [1782-1863], appeared on a list of debts dated 26 Dec 1822 and titled "A List of Allen's Claims" that were due and payable to Dr. Richard N. Allen for services rendered [no dates] to him (Document in Historical Society of Harford County Archives folder "R. N. Allen") [His full name was Francis Ignatius Wheeler, nicknamed Frank or Franky, and he was a War of 1812 veteran.]; see Ignatius Wheeler, q.v.

Wheeler, George, appeared on a list of debts dated 26 Dec 1822 and titled "A List of Allen's Claims" that were due and payable to Dr. Richard N. Allen for services rendered [no dates were given] by him to said Wheeler (Document filed in Historical Society of Harford County Archives folder "R. N. Allen"); George was later visited by Dr. Alonzo Preston who treated Washington Wheeler twice in April 1826 (p. 74)

Wheeler, George M., was treated by Dr. Matthew J. Allen in Aug 1847 for an eyelid problem (p. 63)

Wheeler, Harry, see Henrietta Wheeler, q.v.

Wheeler, Henrietta, widow of Ignatius, was treated by Dr. John Archer from 1794 to 1806 and many of her slaves were noted from 1794 to 1798, but not identified (Ledger I, which is missing, was abstracted by Dr. George W. Archer circa 1890; his notes are in the Archives of the Historical Society of Harford County folder "Archer, G. W. Coll. – Ledgers and Day Books"); she also appeared on a list of debts dated 26 Dec 1822 and titled "A List of Allen's Claims" that were due and payable to Dr. Richard N. Allen for services rendered [no dates were given] by him to said Henrietta (Document in Historical Society of Harford County Archives folder "R. N. Allen"); Mrs. Henrietta Wheeler was later visited by Dr. Robert H. Archer who treated son

Harry, also called Henry, in Oct 1824, Sep 1825, Jan 1827 and Mar 1827, daughter Caroline, also called Cary, in Nov 1825 and Nelly, a negro woman, in Mar 1827 (pp. 122, 156, 170; Ledger F, p. 64)

Wheeler, Henry, see Henrietta Wheeler, q.v.

Wheeler, Ignatius [c1714-1786] (esquire), was visited by Dr. John Archer who treated him in Dec 1774 and Jun 1775 and Apr 1777, a child in Feb 1778, his wife in Apr 1778, a child in Jul 1779, him in Sep 1779. Apr and Aug 1780, Richard Vogan in Feb 1780, him [Ignatius] in Jun 1780, a child and an infant in Aug 1780, a negro in Jan 1781, him [Ignatius] in Feb, Mar, May and Aug 1781, him, a child and Franky in Apr 1783, him in Mar 1783, a daughter in Jul 1783 and him in May 1786 (Ledger B, p. 96; Ledger C, p. 2; Ledger D, pp. 26, 46 [continued in Ledger E, which is missing]; Ledger F, p. 278); see Mr. Watters, Henrietta Wheeler and Joseph Wheeler, q.v.

Wheeler, Ignatius, Jr. [1744-1793] (esquire), was visited by Dr. John Archer who treated a daughter in Feb 1777, Negro and Negro wench in Apr 1777, son Joseph in Sep 1777, a negro in Mar 1778, a negro wench in Apr 1778, him [Ignatius] in Oct 1778, his daughter Maria in Apr 1779, him in Oct and Nov 1780 and Jan 1781, Miss Mocky in Sep 1782 and Mar 1783, a negro and Miss Mocky and him [Ignatius] in Sep 1783, him in Jan 1788 and Oct 1789 and daughters Monica and Mocky [misspelled Mauky] in Oct 1789 (Ledger C, p. 89; Ledger F, pp. 192, 228) [account continued in Ledgers E and G, which are missing] [Ignatius Wheeler, Jr. was a Revolutionary War veteran.]; see Bennett Wheeler, Mrs. Wheeler, George Macatee and John Smith, q.v.

Wheeler, Jacob [1740-1799], brother of Velinda Sanders, was visited by Dr. John Archer who treated him and a child in 1789 (Ledger F, pp. 32, 97); see Velinda Sanders, q.v.

Wheeler, Jacob, was treated by Dr. Robert H. Archer in Baltimore before 1822 [no dates or details were given] (Dr. Archer's "Alphabet to Ledger H" is his booklet [filed in the Archives of the Historical Society of Harford County] that contains his index to Ledger H [which is missing] for his patients in Baltimore before 1822 and Harford County after 1822, according to a notation by Dr. George W. Archer.)

Wheeler, Jacob, Mrs. (widow), was treated by Dr. Robert H. Archer in Baltimore before 1822 [no dates or details were given] (Dr. Archer's "Alphabet to Ledger H" is his booklet [filed in the Archives of the Historical Society of Harford County] that contains his index to Ledger H [which is missing] for his patients in Baltimore before 1822 and Harford County after 1822, according to a notation by Dr. George W. Archer.)

Wheeler, John, was prescribed medicine by Dr. Robert H. Archer on 22 Jan 1832 (Rx Book, 1825-1851, p. 104)

Wheeler, John F. [c1792-1833], appeared on a list of debts dated 26 Dec 1822 and titled "A List of Allen's Claims" that were due and payable to Dr. Richard N. Allen for services rendered [no dates were given] to said Wheeler (Document filed in the Archives of the Historical Society of Harford County folder "R. N. Allen"); John was also visited by Dr. Robert H. Archer who treated Negro woman Clare in Nov 1825, him in Mar 1826, mentioned John Judd in 1826, and treated John and prescribed medicine for him on 1 Sep 1832 (Ledger F, p. 70; Rx Book, 1825-1851, p. 107) [His full name was John Forwood Wheeler and he was a War of 1812 veteran.]

Wheeler, Joseph, was treated by Dr. Robert H. Archer in Baltimore before 1822 [no dates or details were given] (Dr. Archer's "Alphabet to Ledger H" is his booklet [filed in the Archives of the Historical Society of Harford County] that contains his index to Ledger H [which is missing] for his patients in Baltimore before 1822 and Harford County after 1822, according to a notation by Dr. George W. Archer.)

Wheeler, Joseph [1755-c1806], son of Ignatius, was treated by Dr. John Archer in Jun 1778, Aug, Oct and Nov 1779, Aug and Sep 1783 and May 1789 (Ledger C, p. 60; Ledger F, p. 191) [account continued in Ledger G, which is missing] [Joseph Wheeler was a Revolutionary War veteran.]; see Ignatius Wheeler, q.v.

Wheeler, Joseph (captain), was visited by Dr. John Archer who treated him, his wife and children at times between 1794 and 1797 (Ledger I, which is missing, was abstracted by Dr. George W. Archer circa 1890; his notes are in the Archives of the Historical Society of Harford County folder "Archer, G. W. Coll. – Ledgers and Day Books"); see Richard O. Brooks, q.v.

Wheeler, Josias, was treated by Dr. John Archer in Sep 1777, Nov 1781 and May 1783 (Ledger C, p. 93) [Josias was a Revolutionary War veteran.]; see Mrs. Wheeler and Edward Moore, q.v.

Wheeler, Maria, see Ignatius Wheeler, q.v.

Wheeler, Mocky, Miss, was treated by Dr. John Archer in Mar 1788 (Ledger F, p. 13); see Ignatius Wheeler, q.v.

Wheeler, Monica, Miss, was treated by Dr. John Archer in Jul 1788 (Ledger F, p. 129); see Ignatius Wheeler, q.v.

Wheeler, Mr., Jr., see William Betts, q.v.

Wheeler, Mrs. (widow), in the Necks, was treated by Dr. John Archer in 1786 (Ledger F, p. 47, indicated "now married to Robert Taylor," but no date of marriage was given)

Wheeler, Mrs., widow of Josias, was treated by Dr. John Archer in 1796 (Ledger I, which is missing, was abstracted by Dr. George W. Archer circa 1890; his notes are in Archives of the Historical Society of Harford County folder "Archer, G. W. Coll. – Ledgers and Day Books")

Wheeler, Mrs., [widow], "of Ignatius," was treated by Dr. John Archer in 1794 (Ledger F, p. 147)

Wheeler, Mrs., was mentioned in Dr. Robert H. Archer's ledger in a non-medical matter in Jan 1827 and he also mentioned, or possibly treated, her son Harry (p. 213)

Wheeler, Mrs., sister of C. Green, was treated by Dr. Robert H. Archer in Apr 1823 (p. 69)

Wheeler, Thomas [1755-1809], was treated by Dr. John Archer in June 1790 (Ledger F, p. 184) [continued in Ledger G, which is missing] [Thomas Wheeler was a Revolutionary War veteran.]

Wheeler, Thomas, of Benjamin, was treated by Dr. John Archer in 1794 and 1803 (Ledger I, which is missing, was abstracted by Dr. George W. Archer circa 1890; his notes are in Archives of the Historical Society of Harford County file "Archer, G. W. Coll. - Ledgers and Day Books")

Wheeler, Thomas, Mrs. (widow), was treated by Dr. John Archer in Sep and Oct 1778 and Aug 1779 (Ledger C, p. 124, noted "debt forgiven by order of testator")

Wheeler, Washington, see George Wheeler, q.v.

Wheeler, Widow, was treated by Dr. John Archer in Jul and Aug 1776 (Ledger C, p. 61); see James McGaw, Solomon Hillen, Mrs. Wheeler (widow) and Mrs. Thomas Wheeler (widow), q.v.

Wheeler, William, was visited by Dr. Robert H. Archer who treated a child in May 1823 (p. 75)

Wheeler, William, was treated by Dr. Matthew J. Allen in Jun, Jul, Oct and Nov 1847 (p. 57)

Whitaker, A., see Thaddeus Jewett, q.v.

Whitaker, Dorsey H., appeared on a list of debts dated 26 Dec 1822 and titled "A List of Allen's Claims" that were due and payable to Dr. Richard N. Allen for services rendered [no dates] to him (Document filed in Historical Society of Harford County Archives folder "R. N. Allen")

Whitaker, Howard [1790-1879], was visited by Dr. Alonzo Preston who treated him in 1825 and 1827 and a child on 25 Dec 1825 (p. 53, noted bill was "paid in full with 25 cts. int." on 29 Jun 1831 and the entry was signed by William B. Bond [referring to Dr. William B. Bond) [Howard Whitaker was a War of 1812 veteran.]

Whitaker, Isaac, was visited by Dr. John Archer who treated an infant in Dec 1781, a child in Jan 1782 and him in Aug 1786 (Ledger D, p. 111, spelled his name Whitecar; Ledger F, p. 375) [Isaac Whitaker (c1735-c1800), son of Charles, and Isaac Whitaker (c1758-c1806), son of Peter, were both Revolutionary War veterans.]

Whitaker, J., see Aquila Howard, q.v.

Whitaker, John [1753-1833], was visited by Dr. John Archer who treated him and a child in Jul 1787 (Ledger F, p. 359, listed as Jno. Whitacer) [John Whitaker was a Revolutionary War veteran.]

Whitaker, Joshua [1795-1861], was visited by Dr. Alonzo Preston who treated him in 1823 and Josh, Mater [mother], Rutha, Matilda and Susan in 1826 and 1827, and "Jno. wife in nocte" [John's wife at night] on 5 Apr 1827 (p. 31) [Joshua Whitaker was a War of 1812 veteran.]

Whitaker, Platt, at Samuel Bailey's, was treated by Dr. John Archer in Nov 1789 (Ledger F, p. 375)

Whitaker, Ruth, appeared on a list of debts dated 26 Dec 1822 and titled "A List of Allen's Claims" that were due and payable to Dr. Richard N. Allen for services rendered [no dates] to Whitaker (Document filed in Historical Society of Harford County Archives folder "R. N. Allen")

Whitaker, Thomas [1778-1860], was prescribed medicine for his wife by Dr. Robert H. Archer on 5 Aug 1802, medicine for his child on 7 Jul and 8 Jul 1803 and on 19 Nov 1804, and medicine for him [Thomas] on 28 Nov and 14 Dec 1804 (Rx Book, 1802-1804, pp. 8, 48, 49, 62, 66)

White, ---- (daughter), see John Cavenaugh, q.v.

White, Budd, was visited by Dr. John Archer, Jr. who treated his wife and child in May 1828 and mentioned T. Huggins and J. Cavenaugh in June 1818 and "cash paid at P. Deposit" [Port Deposit in Cecil Co.] on 10 May 1819 (p. 62); Dr. Archer received $15 "for rent" from Buddy White (no date – note was written on the inside of the back cover of his Ledger F)

White, Captain, see John Gregg & Co., q.v.

White, Elizabeth, was prescribed medicine by Dr. Robert H. Archer on 22 Jul 1829 (Rx Book, 1825-1851, p. 95)

White, James, was visited by Dr. John Archer who treated him and a child in 1802 (Ledger F, p. 327); see Cyrus Osborn, q.v.

White, Jonathan, was treated by Dr. John Archer in Sep 1787 (Ledger F, p. 302) [Jonathan White was a Revolutionary War veteran.]

White, Mr., "son of Mrs. Bailey, Charlestown" [in Cecil Co.], was visited by Dr. John Archer, Jr. who treated a child in Feb 1816 (p. 39)

White, Richard (shoemaker), was treated by Dr. John Archer in Mar 1773, Jan 1775, May 1778, Aug 1783 and him, his wife and child in 1788 (Ledger B, p. 75; Ledger C, p. 112) [account continued in Ledger E, which is missing]; Ledger F, p. 61) [account continued in Ledger G, which is missing] [Richard White was a Revolutionary War veteran.]

White, Thomas [1708-1779] (colonel), was visited by Dr. John Archer who treated a negro in Jan 1776 (Ledger C, p. 24, noted "by order of William Wilson" and the "debt forgiven by order of testator"); see Negro Rose and Negro Sam, q.v.

Whiteford, see John Mun, q.v.

Whiteford, Hugh, Sr. (tanner), was visited by Dr. John Archer who treated him and his wife in Feb 1787 (Ledger F, p. 326)

Whiteford, Hugh, "of Michael, or Swamp Hugh," was treated by Dr. John Archer in Dec 1786. Swamp Hugh Whiteford was treated by Dr. John Archer in 1795. (Ledger F, p. 47; Ledger I, which is missing, was abstracted by Dr. George W. Archer circa 1890; his notes are in the Archives of the Historical Society of Harford County file "Archer, G. W. Coll. – Ledgers and Day Books"); "Hugh Whiteford at the Swamp" was treated by Dr. John Archer in Sep 1801. (Ledger F, p. 208); see Nathaniel Wiley, q.v.

Whiteford, Hugh, Jr. [c1754-c1812], at Slate Ridge, was visited by Dr. John Archer who treated him in May 1775 and May and Jun 1781, his wife, his brother in Feb 1785 and a child in Jul 1785, and as Hugh Whiteford, of Hugh, was treated in Aug 1794 (Ledger B, p. 100; Ledger C, p. 61; Ledger D, p. 43; Ledger F, pp. 47, 326) [Hugh Whiteford was a Revolutionary War veteran.]

Whiteford, John, see Mrs. Park, q.v.

Whiteford, Michael, see Hugh Whiteford, q.v.

Whitesides, Andrew, at H. Kirkpatrick's, was treated by Dr. John Archer in 1774 (Ledger B, p. 29)

Whitlock, James, see Moses Whitlock, q.v.

Whitlock, John, see Moses Whitlock, q.v.

Whitlock, Moses, was visited by Dr. John Archer, Jr. who treated his wife in Dec 1816, son James in May 1817, son Samuel in Sep 1819, son John on Oct 1819, daughter Patty in Jul 1820 and mentioned L. Touchstone, Richard Barnes and William Williams in 1816 (p. 61)

Whitlock Patty, see Moses Whitlock, q.v.

Whitlock, Samuel, see Moses Whitlock, q.v.

Whitney, E., was treated by Dr. Robert H. Archer in Baltimore before 1822 [no dates or details were given] (Dr. Archer's "Alphabet to Ledger H" is his booklet [filed in the Archives of the Historical Society of Harford County] that contains his index to Ledger H [which is missing] for his patients in Baltimore City before 1822 and in Harford County after 1822, according to a notation by Dr. George W. Archer.)

Whitson, David, "near White Hall," was treated by Dr. John Archer in 1795 (Ledger I, which is missing, was abstracted by Dr. George W. Archer circa 1890; his notes are in the Archives of the Historical Society of Harford County folder "Archer, G. W. Coll. – Ledgers and Day Books")

Whittimore, Henry, was treated by Dr. Matthew J. Allen in Jun 1845 (p. 51, noted the bill was paid "by cash in full" in Oct 1848); see Joseph Madden, q.v.

Whord, Thomas, was treated by Dr. John Archer in May 1786 and his security was Benjamin Everist (Ledger F, p. 265)

Wiggins, James, was treated by Dr. John Archer in Jul 1782 and May 1785 (Ledger D, p. 55, noted "debt forgiven as before")

Wiggins, Joseph, was visited by Dr. John Archer who treated his child in Apr 1780 (Ledger D, p. 59, noted "Gerard Hopkins, security") [account continued in Ledger G, which is missing)

Wilds, John, on Jos. Dallam's place, was treated by Dr. John Archer in Sep 1791 (Ledger F, p. 168) [John Wild was a Revolutionary War veteran.]

Wiles, John, at Richard Webster's, was treated by Dr. John Archer in Sep 1788 (Ledger F, p. 290)

Wiley, see Robert Gordon, q.v.

Wiley, Katherine, see Nathaniel Wiley, q.v.

Wiley, Nathaniel, near Hugh Whiteford's, was visited by Dr. John Archer who treated him and his son [no name was given] and daughter Katherine in 1786 (Ledger F, p. 358, spelled his name Weily and spelled his daughter's name Katherin)

Wilgis, George, was treated by Dr. Matthew J. Allen in Jul 1848 (p. 90) [This statement was written on a separate page dated 24 Nov 1853 and inserted in the back of Dr. Allen's ledger. The note, addressed to Major Bond, was signed by I. Day and stated, "I have just returned after 3 days ride to look up the Drs. [debtors] of Dr. Allen and the following is the result." It mentioned several patients and included this: "Geo. Wilges *(sic)* says he does not owe nor never did owe the Dr."]

Wilkins, Elizabeth M., was treated by Dr. John Archer in Oct 1772 and Sep 1773 (Ledger B, p. 18)

Wilkins, Master, see Reuben H. Davis, q.v.

Wilkisson, Ann, was treated by Dr. John Archer in Aug 1786 and the bill for services was charged to Harford County (Ledger F, p. 160) [account continued in Ledger G, which is missing]

Willet, Cassey, see Samuel Willet, q.v.

Willet, Mr., was prescribed medicine by Dr. Robert H. Archer on 1 Jul 1803 (Rx Book, 1802-1804, p. 46)

Willet, Mrs., was prescribed medicine by Dr. Robert H. Archer on 25 Sep 1802 (Rx Book, 1802-1804, p. 6)

Willet, Peter, see Samuel Willet, q.v.

Willet, Samuel, was visited by Dr. John Archer who treated him in 1795 and inoculated his wife and eight of his family members, namely, William Irwin, James Irwin, Sarah Houston, Peter Willet, Thomas Willet, John Houston, James Dickson, Benjamin Dickson and Cassey Willet; Samuel Willet was prescribed medicine for his wife by Dr. Robert H. Archer on 4 Jul 1803 and Samuel Willets *(sic)* was prescribed medicine for a child on 7 Jul 1803 (Ledger F, p. 366; Rx Book, 1802-1804, pp. 47, 48)

Willet, Thomas, see Samuel Willet, q.v.

Willets, Samuel (blacksmith), was treated by Dr. John Archer in Aug 1772 (Ledger B, p. 4, spelled his name Willits and noted "run away to Georgia and is poor")

Willey, Henry, was prescribed medicine by Dr. Robert H. Archer for his child circa Dec 1804 (Rx Book, 1802-1804, p. 67); Henry Willey &ca *(sic)* was treated by Dr. Archer in Baltimore before 1822 [no dates or details were given] (Dr. Archer's "Alphabet to Ledger H" is his booklet [filed in the Archives of the Historical Society of Harford County] that contains his index to Ledger H [which is missing] for his patients in Baltimore before 1822 and Harford County after 1822, according to a notation by Dr. George W. Archer.)

Willey, Mary, Mrs., in Baltimore, was prescribed medicine by Dr. Robert H. Archer on 27 May 1799 (Rx Book, 1796-1801, p. 16, spelled her name Willy; Mrs. Willey was treated by Dr. Robert H. Archer in Baltimore before 1822 [no dates or details were given] (Dr. Archer's "Alphabet to Ledger H" is his booklet [filed in the Archives of the Historical Society of Harford County] that contains his index to Ledger H [which is missing] for his patients in Baltimore City before 1822 and in Harford County after 1822, according to a notation by Dr. George W. Archer.)

Williams, Edwin, see James W. Williams, q.v.

Williams, Griffin, was visited by Dr. John Archer, Jr. who treated his son Griffin in Jun 1816 (p. 55)

Williams, Hannah, was treated by Dr. John Archer in Aug 1774 and Feb 1775 and who also treated her mother in Jun 1774 (Ledger B, p. 55)

Williams, Isaac, near the Falls Quaker Meeting House, was treated by Dr. John Archer in Sep 1788 (Ledger F, p. 347)

Williams, Jacob, appeared on a list of debts dated 26 Dec 1822 and titled "A List of Allen's Claims" that were due and payable to Dr. Richard N. Allen for services rendered [no dates were given] by him to the said Williams (Document filed in Historical Society of Harford County Archives folder "R. N. Allen")

Williams, James, see James W. Williams, q.v.

Williams, James W. [1792-1842], was visited by Dr. Robert H. Archer who treated his wife and rendered obstetrical services on 14 Oct 1822 (p. 28 listed him only as James Williams); James W. was visited by Dr. Archer who treated Negro "Rache" in Sep 1822, [James W.'s] daughter Rosa, and an unnamed infant in Oct 1822, Negro Jane in March and July 1823, an unnamed infant and Mr. McAdow's Negro in Apr 1823, Negro Ned in May 1823, [James W.'s] daughter Mary in Sep 1825, Negro Peter in Oct 1825, Negro John in July 1825, James W., his wife and sons John and James in July 1825, cook Rachel and Negro Judie (Sudie?) in Sep 1725, Negro Peter in Oct 1825, [James W.'s] daughter Rosa in Dec 1825, his [James W.'s] wife "in partu" [in childbirth] in the night of 1 Apr 1826 and visited again on 3 Apr 1826, Negro Milley in Mar and Apr 1826, Negro Jane in May 1826, Negro Peter in June 1826, [James W.'s] son Edwin in Oct 1826, [James

W.'s] daughter Rosa in May 1826 and Feb 1827, Negro Jane in June 1827, [James W.'s] son John in Sep 1827 and Jan 1828, was prescribed medicine for Negro Milly on 12 Jan 1826 and Negro Jane on 1 Apr 1830, and treated daughter Priscilla in Mar 1835 (pp. 16, 29, 61, 64, 67, 73, 85, 155, 161, 173, 178, 179, 206, 216, 236, 247, 258; Rx Book, 1825-1851, pp. 86, 100; Ledger F, pp. 40, 147); see Mr. Gill, q.v.

Williams, John, "near the lower ferry" [now Havre de Grace], was visited by Dr. John Archer who treated his wife, his sister-in-law, and William Barnes in Feb 1777 (Ledger C, p. 31) [John Williams was a Revolutionary War veteran.]

Williams, John, overseer to J. Wilson, was treated by Dr. John Archer in Mar 1788 (Ledger F, p. 106) [John Williams was a Revolutionary War veteran.]

Williams, John, see James W. Williams, q.v.

Williams, Mary, see James W. Williams, q.v.

Williams, Priscilla, see James W. Williams, q.v.

Williams, Rosa, see James W. Williams, q.v.

Williams, Thomas, was visited by Dr. John Archer who treated him in Aug 1781 and him and his wife in Nov 1787 (Ledger D, p. 59, noted "debt forgiven as before;" Ledger F, p. 51)

Williams, William, see James Kent and Moses Whitlock, q.v.

Williams, William (carpenter), at Susquehanna, was visited by Dr. John Archer who treated him in Jul 1782 and his wife in Mar 1784 (Ledger D, p. 40, noted "debt forgiven as before")

Williams, William (schoolmaster), was treated by Dr. John Archer in 1794 (Ledger I, which is missing, was abstracted by Dr. George W. Archer circa 1890; his notes are in the Archives of the Historical Society of Harford County folder "Archer, G. W. Coll. – Ledgers and Day Books")

Williamson, John, at Samuel Wilson's, was treated by Dr. John Archer in 1787 (Ledger F, p. 260)

Williamson, Robert, was treated by Dr. John Archer in Jul 1775 and Oct 1777 (Ledger B, p. 103; Ledger C, p. 53, noted "debt forgiven by order of testator")

Williamson, William, at Bald Friar [a landing on the Susquehanna River], was treated by Dr. John Archer in Feb 1787 (Ledger F, p. 202) [William Williams was a Revolutionary War veteran.]

Willson, Mr., "son-in-law to Dˡ. Kenly" [Daniel Kenley], was treated by Dr. John Archer in Aug 1782 (Ledger D, p. 45, noted "debt forgiven as before")

Willson, Thomas, in the Barrens [an area in the northwestern part of the county near Pennsylvania], was visited by Dr. John Archer who treated his child in Mar 1782 and him in May 1783 and Aug 1784 (Ledger D, p. 125) [account continued in Ledger G, which is missing]

Wilmer, Lambert, at G. P. Neck [Gunpowder Neck], was treated by Dr. John Archer in March 1788 (Ledger F, p. 318) [Lambert Wilmer was a Revolutionary War veteran.]

Wilmott, Richard, was visited by Dr. John Archer who treated him in Dec 1776 and Jan 1777, negroes Hagar, Deb and Sall in Jan and Feb 1777, him in Feb 1780, May 1781 and Apr 1782, Miss ---- [illegible] in Apr 1782, a negro in Aug 1782 and him in Dec 1782 and Jul and Sep 1783; inoculated 7 of his family and treated his wife in Dec 1783, a negro in Jan 1784, an infant in Jan 1784 and him in Jun 1788 (Ledger C, p. 67; Ledger D, p. 57 [account continued in Ledger E, which is missing]; Ledger F, p. 364) [Richard Wilmott was a Revolutionary War veteran.]

Wilsa, Mrs., was prescribed medicine by Dr. Robert H. Archer on 27 Jul 1841 (Rx Book, 1825-1851, p. 115)

Wilson, A., Mrs., was prescribed medicine by Dr. Robert H. Archer on 24 Jan and 27 Jan and 30 Jan and 31 Jan 1801 (Rx Book, 1796-1801, pp. 27, 29, 30, 31)

Wilson, Alizana, see Christopher Wilson, Sr., q.v.

Wilson, Andrew, was visited by Dr. John Archer who treated him in Jun and Aug 1773 and Apr 1774, Elizabeth Golden in Apr 1775, him and his wife in Aug 1782 and also inoculated his wife and six children (Ledger B, p. 91; Ledger D, p. 119 [continued in Ledger G, which is missing) [Andrew Wilson was a Revolutionary War veteran.]

Wilson, Benjamin (merchant), Bel Air, was treated by Dr. John Archer at various times between 1798 and 1805 (Ledger I, which is missing, was abstracted by Dr. George W. Archer circa 1890; his notes are in Archives of the Historical Society of Harford County file "Archer, G. W. Coll. - Ledgers and Day Books")

Wilson, Benjamin, was treated by Dr. Robert H. Archer in Baltimore before 1822 [no dates or details were given] (Dr. Archer's "Alphabet to Ledger H" is his booklet [filed in the Archives of the Historical Society of Harford County] that contains his index to Ledger H [which is missing] for his patients in Baltimore before 1822 and Harford County after 1822, according to a notation by Dr. George W. Archer.)

Wilson, Benjamin, son of John, was visited by Dr. John Archer who treated his wife and infant in 1787 and him in 1790 (Ledger F, p. 137) [Benjamin Wilson was a Revolutionary War veteran.]

Wilson, Betsy, see Samuel Wilson, q.v.

Wilson, C., see Thomas Jay, q.v.

Wilson, Cassandra, was visited by Dr. John Archer who treated a negro in Jun 1782, and inoculated her and 8 of her family in Sep 1782 (Ledger D, p. 78, noted "debt forgiven as before")

Wilson, Cassy, see Joseph Wilson and Samuel Wilson, q.v.

Wilson, Christopher [1762-1846], was visited by Dr. John Archer who treated him and his wife in Feb 1791 and he was prescribed medicine by Dr. Robert H. Archer on 1 Jun 1796 (Ledger F, p. 342 [account continued in Ledger G, which is missing]; Rx Book, 1796-1801, p. 5); Christopher Wilson, Sr., was visited by Dr. Robert H. Archer who treated his daughter Alizana in Oct 1825 and him and his wife in Sep 1827 (pp. 164, 246; Ledger F, p. 148); Christopher Wilson, Sr., died on 11 Jul 1846, age 84 years ("True Book, 1845, 46, 47" filed in the Archives of the Historical Society of Harford County folder "Archer, Dr. Robert H., 1775-1857, Day Book, 1845-47"); see John Wilson, q.v.

Wilson, Christopher, Jr., was visited by Dr. Robert H. Archer who treated a negro in Aug 1823, him [Christopher] in Sep 1827 and his wife in Apr 1828 (pp. 88, 89, 246, 247, 271; Ledger F, p. 59)

Wilson, Dr., see Alonzo Hollis, q.v.

Wilson, Edward, was treated by Dr. John Archer, Jr. in 1820 in Harford County (p. 38)

Wilson, Edward, was treated by Dr. Matthew J. Allen in 1823 in Calvert County (p. 13b)

Wilson, George H. [1792-1834], was treated by Dr. Robert H. Archer in Oct, Nov and Dec 1825 (pp. 166, 171, 172, 173; Ledger F, p. 138) [George H. Wilson was a War of 1812 veteran.]

Wilson, Hugh, was treated by Dr. John Archer five times in June 1774 (Ledger B, p. 97)

Wilson, Humphrey [1759-1843], was treated at various times from 1822 to 1825 [no details were given] by Dr. Alonzo Preston who also treated Josias Wilson in 1825 (p. 25, noted that part of bill was paid in cash and the rest paid in full on 22 Dec 1827; payment received and initialed by "W.B.B.") [referring to Dr. William B. Bond]

Wilson, Irish John, see Michael Wilson, q.v.

Wilson, Isaac, was prescribed medicine for his wife by Dr. Robert H. Archer on 1 Jun 1796 and 18 Aug 1802 and for his child on 1 Jan 1803 (Rx Book, 1802-1804, pp. 5, 15, 29)

Wilson, Isaac, was prescribed medicine for his wife by Dr. Robert H. Archer on 27 Jul 1841 (Rx Book, 1825-1851, p. 114) [Isaac Wilson was a War of 1812 veteran.]

Wilson, Isaac, Jr., was prescribed medicine for his wife by Dr. Robert H. Archer on 29 Jun 1841 (Rx Book, 1825-1851, p. 114)

Wilson, J., see John Williams, q.v.

Wilson, J., Mrs., was prescribed medicine by Dr. Robert H. Archer on 6 Sep 1804 (Rx Book, 1802-1804, p. 57)

Wilson, James, near Bald Friar [landing on the Susquehanna River], was treated by Dr. John Archer in May and Jun 1779 (Ledger C, p. 112) [James Wilson was a Revolutionary War veteran.]

Wilson, James, near W. Barkley, Esq., was treated by Dr. John Archer in 1790 (Ledger F, p. 149) [James Wilson was a Revolutionary War veteran.]; see Samuel Corbett, q.v.

Wilson, James, was treated by Dr. Robert H. Archer in Baltimore before 1822 [no dates or details were given] (Dr. Archer's "Alphabet to Ledger H" is his booklet [filed in the Archives of the Historical Society of Harford County] that contains his index to Ledger H [which is missing] for his patients in Baltimore before 1822 and Harford County after 1822, according to a notation by Dr. George W. Archer.)

Wilson, Jane (negro), was treated by Dr. Robert H. Archer in Baltimore before 1822 [no dates or details were given] (Dr. Archer's "Alphabet to Ledger H" is his booklet [filed in the Archives of the Historical Society of Harford County] that contains his index to Ledger H [which is missing] for his patients in Baltimore before 1822 and Harford County after 1822, according to a notation by Dr. George W. Archer.)

Wilson, Jo., see Augustus J. Greme, q.v.

Wilson, Johana, see William Wilson, q.v.

Wilson, John, was visited by Dr. John Archer who treated him, his wife, little boy and daughter in Jun 1774, and him and wife in Jul 1774 (Ledger B, p. 103) [John Wilson was a Revolutionary War veteran.]

Wilson, John, son of Joseph, in the Barrens [area in northwest part of the county near Pennsylvania], was visited by Dr. John Archer who treated him in Apr, Jun and Aug 1781, his wife in Mar 1782, him in Jul 1782 and him and a child in Mar 1783 (Ledger D, p. 16) [account continued in Ledger E, which is missing] [John Wilson was a Revolutionary War veteran.]

Wilson, John, father-in-law to Joseph Miller, was visited by Dr. John Archer who treated him and his family at various times between 1796 and 1798 (Ledger I, which is missing, was abstracted by Dr. George W. Archer circa 1890; his notes are in the Archives of the Historical Society of Harford County folder "Archer, G. W. Coll. – Ledgers and Day Books")

Wilson, John (carpenter), on N. Gallion's place, was treated by Dr. John Archer in Aug 1778 and Oct 1778 (Ledger C, p. 121) [account continued in Ledger E, which is missing]

Wilson, John, "chair maker for Mr. Toberdier," was treated by Dr. John Archer in 1795 (Ledger I, which is missing, was abstracted by Dr. George W. Archer circa 1890; his notes are in the Archives of the Historical Society of Harford County file "Archer, G. W. Coll. – Ledgers and Day Books")

Wilson, John (joiner), was treated by Dr. John Archer in Nov 1786 (Ledger F, p. 130)

Wilson, John (weaver), near Bald Friar [landing on Susquehanna River], was treated by Dr. John Archer in Jun 1792 (Ledger F, p. 247)

Wilson, John, Rock (sic), was treated at Dr. John Archer in Feb, Mar, Jul and Aug 1781, May and Sep 1782 and Mar 1783 (Ledger D, p. 119) [account continued in Ledger E, which is missing]; John Wilson, at Rock Run, was visited by Dr. John Archer who treated him in 1788 and sons John and Christopher in 1789 (Ledger F, p. 48)

Wilson, John, near Blue Rocks, was treated by Dr. John Archer in June 1782 (Ledger D, p. 23, noted "debt forgiven as before")

Wilson, John, on Deer Creek, was treated by Dr. John Archer in Jul 1787 (Ledger F, p. 256) [account continued in Ledger G, which is missing]

Wilson, John, was visited by Dr. Robert H. Archer who treated a negro in Dec 1825 (p. 172)

Wilson, John, at Plumb Point, was visited by Dr. Robert H. Archer who treated his wife in Aug 1823 and him in Dec 1825 (p. 89; Ledger F, p. 61)

Wilson, John, see John Wilson, Michael Wilson, William Wilson and Robert Wilson, q.v.

Wilson, Joseph, was treated by Dr. John Archer in Nov 1802 (Ledger F, p. 110) [Two men named Joseph Wilson were Revolutionary War veterans in Harford County.]

Wilson, Joseph, was visited by Dr. Matthew J. Allen who treated his daughter Cassy three times in Jun 1847 for "reducing luxation" [dislocation] of both shoulder joints (p. 53, noted the $12 bill was reduced to $10 and it was paid 'by order on Mr. Greme")

Wilson, Joseph, see John Wilson, of Joseph, q.v.

Wilson, Josias, was treated by Dr. Robert H. Archer after 1822 [no dates or details were given] (Dr. Archer's "Alphabet to Ledger H" is his booklet [filed in the Archives of the Historical Society of Harford County] that contains his index to Ledger H [which is missing] for his patients in Baltimore before 1822 and Harford County after 1822, according to a notation by Dr. George W. Archer.); see Humphrey Wilson, q.v.

Wilson, Martha, Miss, was treated by Dr. John Archer in Jul 1793 (Ledger F, p. 321)

Wilson, Martha, Miss, at Thomas Jay's, was treated by Dr. Robert H. Archer in Nov 1823 (p. 93; Ledger F, p. 115)

Wilson, Michael, at Blue Rocks, was treated by Dr. John Archer in Jan 1786 and noted "his brother, Irish John Wilson, will pay" (Ledger F, p. 290)

Wilson, Mr., see Mr. Willson, q.v.

Wilson, Peter (storekeeper), was treated by Dr. John Archer between 1790 and 1799 and who stated that Wilson paid his account in 1795 and in 1799 "by boarding my two sons" (Ledger F, p. 288); visited by Dr. James Archer who treated him in January 1806 for dyspepsia (p. 29)

Wilson, Robert, son of John, near Bald Friar [a landing on Susquehanna River], was treated by Dr. John Archer in Jun 1789 (Ledger F, p. 332) [Robert Wilson was a Revolutionary War veteran.]

Wilson, Samuel, was visited by Dr. John Archer who treated him in Feb, Mar, Apr, May, and Sep 1780 and Jul 1781, him and a child in Aug 1781, son William in Sep 1781, inoculated 16 of his family in 1782 and treated him in Jan 1784 (Ledger D, p. 42) [account continued in Ledger E, which is missing] [Samuel Wilson, of William, was a Revolutionary War veteran.]; see John Williamson and William Smith, q.v.

Wilson, Samuel, was visited by Dr. John Archer at various times between 1794 and 1799 and treated him and daughters Betsy and Cassy (Ledger I, which is missing, was abstracted by Dr. George W. Archer circa 1890;

his notes are in the Archives of the Historical Society of Harford County folder "Archer, G. W. Coll. – Ledgers and Day Books")

Wilson, Samuel, was treated by Dr. Robert H. Archer in Baltimore before 1822 [no dates or details were given] (Dr. Archer's "Alphabet to Ledger H" is his booklet [filed in the Archives of the Historical Society of Harford County] that contains his index to Ledger H [which is missing] for his patients in Baltimore before 1822 and Harford County after 1822, according to a notation by Dr. George W. Archer.)

Wilson, Sarah, near J. Woolsey's, was treated by Dr. John Archer in Nov 1787 (Ledger F, p. 291); see Thomas Moore, q.v.

Wilson, Thomas, was treated by Dr. John Archer in 1796 and the bill was paid by Joseph Janney in 1802 (Ledger I, which is missing, was abstracted by Dr. George W. Archer circa 1890; his notes are in the Archives of the Historical Society of Harford County folder "Archer, G. W. Coll. – Ledgers and Day Books")

Wilson, William, see Robert Caruthers, Samuel Wilson, James Paca and Thomas White, q.v.

Wilson, William (silversmith), was visited by Dr. John Archer who treated him and his wife in 1788 and him and a child in 1791 (Ledger F, pp. 9, 278, 313)

Wilson, William, son of John, was visited by Dr. John Archer who treated a negro in Jul 1779, him [William] in Mar 1780, him, his wife and a negro in Apr 1780, a negro in Jun 1780, a child in Jan 1781, him in Jun 1781, a child in Jul, Aug and Sep 1782, a negro in Oct 1782, him and his wife Nov 1790 and him and a child in Jan 1792 (Ledger C, p. 97; Ledger D, p. 52, later noted "If this is overseer William it is settled." [account continued in Ledger E, which is missing]; Ledger F, pp. 15, 35) [account continued in Ledger H, which is missing]

Wilson, William, son of William, was visited by Dr. John Archer who treated him in Sep 1779, Mar and Apr 1780, sinet or semet(?) [an unclear Latin word] Johana in May 1781, him in Aug 1782 and him and his wife in Dec 1788 (Ledger D, p. 14) [account continued in Ledger E, which is missing]; (Ledger F, p. 71) [account continued in Ledger H, which is missing]

Wilson, William, was treated by Dr. Matthew J. Allen in 1823 in Calvert County (p. 3b)

Wilson, William, Jr. (overseer), was visited by Dr. John Archer who treated him in June and July 1774 and his child and his mother in June 1774 (Ledger B, p. 93)

Winchester, Samuel, was prescribed medicine by Dr. Robert H. Archer on 12 Mar 1803 (Rx Book, 1802-1804, p. 35)

Winfair, Aaron, at Samuel Webster, Sr.'s, was treated by Dr. John Archer in 1779 (Ledger C, p. 4) [Aaron Winfrey was a Revolutionary War veteran.]

Winks, ---- [blank], was visited by Dr. Alonzo Preston who treated him in Jun 1826 and a child in Dec 1827 (p. 79)

Wiser, Ellen, was treated by Dr. Matthew J. Allen in Jun, Jul and Aug 1847 (p. 54)

Wix, ---- [blank] (wheelwright), near J. Bull's Mill, was treated by Dr. John Archer in May 1788 (Ledger F, p. 171)

Wogan, ----, see Harford County for Pensioners, q.v.

Wolf, Jacob, was treated by Dr. Robert H. Archer in Dec 1821 (Ledger F, p. 27)

Wolrain, Peter, was treated by Dr. John Archer in Oct and Nov 1780 (Ledger D, p. 97, noted "debt forgiven as before")

Wood, John, on Thomas Durbin's place, was treated by Dr. J. Archer in Dec 1786 (Ledger F, p. 154)

Wood, Joseph, see Hollis Hanson, q.v.

Wood, Moses, was visited by Dr. John Archer who treated his wife in Apr 1781 and him in Feb and Sep 1785 (Ledger D, p. 18, noted "debt forgiven as before")

Woodland, Jonathan, was visited by Dr. John Archer who treated his wife in Aug 1778 and Aug 1780, him in Jan, Feb, Mar and Jul 1780 and Mar 1782, him and his wife in Oct 1782 and him and his daughter in Dec 1782 (Ledger C, p. 117, noted "debt forgiven by order of testator")

Woods, William, was treated by Dr. John Archer in Apr 1787 (Ledger F, p. 260)

Woolsey, see Sarah Wilson, q.v.

Woolsey, Debby, see Joseph Woolsey, q.v.

Woolsey, Henry (Henrie), see Joseph Woolsey, q.v.

Woolsey, Joseph, was visited by Dr. John Archer who treated him before 1773 [no dates or details were given], his wife in Sep 1773, him and his wife in Feb 1777, him in Apr 1777, May 1778, Jan 1779 and at various times between Mar 1780 and Dec 1780, son "Henrie" in Feb 1794, him [Joseph] in Aug 1794 and him, daughter Debby and son Henry at times between 1795 and 1799 (Ledger B, p. 70; Ledger C, p. 24; Ledger D, p. 94) [account continued in Ledger I, which is missing, but was abstracted by Dr. George W. Archer circa 1890; his notes are in the Archives of the Historical Society of Harford County file "Archer, G. W. Coll. – Ledgers and Day Books")

Woolsey, William, was prescribed medicine for his wife by Dr. Robert H. Archer on 5 Sep 1796 (Rx Book, 1796-1801, p. 9, listed his name as Wm. Wollsey)

Woolsey, William, was visited by Dr. Matthew J. Allen who treated "negro Aquilla, of Miss Amos" in Jun 1845 (p. 51, spelled his name Wolsey)

Worthington, Ann, Miss, was treated by Dr. Robert H. Archer in Oct 1825 in consultation with Dr. Worthington (p. 161; Ledger F, p. 38)

Worthington, Cassandra, Miss, was treated by Dr. Robert H. Archer in Nov 1826 (pp. 209, 210)

Worthington, Charles, was visited by Dr. John Archer who treated a negro girl in 1777, his daughter Maria in 1786 and him in Oct 1788 (Ledger C, p. 35; Ledger F, p. 131) [account continued in Ledger G, which is missing] [Charles Worthington was a Revolutionary War veteran.]; see Samuel Worthington, q.v.

Worthington, Dr., see George Courtnay, Isaac Coale, Mr. Jones, Henry O'Neil, John Quarles, Samuel Hopkins, James Coale, Joshua Husband, Joseph Husband, Joseph Husband, Jr., John Nevill, Mary Mifflin, Richard Dallam, Ann Worthington, Mrs. Leage, Mrs. Chew, Cassandra Chew, Richard Dallam and John Reese, q.v.

Worthington, John, was visited by Dr. John Archer who treated him in Jun 1781, inoculated daughter Prissy in Jan 1782, and treated a child in Jan, Feb, Mar and Apr 1785, his wife in Apr 1785, him in Jun 1788 and him and son Samuel at various times between 1795 and 1799 (Ledger I, which is missing, was abstracted by Dr. George W. Archer circa 1890; his notes are in the Archives of the Historical Society of Harford County folder "Archer, G. W. Coll. – Ledgers and Day Books") (Ledger D, p. 41; Ledger F, p. 148) [continued in Ledger G, which is missing]

Worthington, Maria, see Charles Worthington, q.v.

Worthington, Priscilla, see William Worthington, q.v.

Worthington, Prissy, see John Worthington, q.v.

Worthington, S., see Mrs. Chew, q.v.

Worthington, Samuel, see John Worthington, q.v.

Worthington, Samuel [1733-1815], was visited by Dr. John Archer who treated a negro in Jan 1777 and Charles Worthington paid the bill in May 1779 (Ledger C, p. 56) [Samuel Worthington was a Revolutionary War veteran.]

Worthington, Susan, see William Worthington, q.v.

Worthington, William, was visited by Dr. Robert H. Archer who treated his daughter Priscilla in May 1823 and his daughter Susan in June 1832 and April 1835 (p. 73; Ledger F, p. 32) [William Worthington was a War of 1812 veteran.]

Wren, William, was treated by Dr. John Archer in Nov and Dec 1781 and Oct 1782 (Ledger D, p. 99, noted "debt forgiven as before") [William Wrain or Wraine was a Revolutionary War veteran.]

Wright, W., see Charles S. Sewell, q.v.

Wyatt, Ann, had an account in Dr. John Archer, Jr.'s ledger that mentioned John N. Black in Nov 1816, R. Currier in Jan 1817 and noted "going to Charlestown" in Aug 1817 (p. 67)

Yarnall, Stephen (clockmaker), was treated by Dr. John Archer between 1794 and 1802 (Ledger I, which is missing, was abstracted by Dr. George W. Archer circa 1890; his notes are in Archives of the Historical Society of Harford County file "Archer, G. W. Coll. - Ledgers and Day Books")

Yeates, George, was visited by Dr. John Archer who treated an infant in Sep 1774 and him [George] in Oct and Nov 1774 and Jul 1779 (Ledger B, p. 103; Ledger C, p. 15, noted "debt forgiven by order of testator")

Yeates, Widow, was visited by Dr. John Archer who treated a negro in Jan 1777 (Ledger C, p. 63, noted the bill was paid by Joseph Miller in June 1777)

Yoe, Benjamin, was prescribed medicine for his wife by Dr. Robert H. Archer on 10 Feb 1803, medicine for a negro on 22 Feb 1803 and medicine for his child in Oct 1804, Nov 1804 and again later in 1804 [exact date was not given] (Rx Book, 1802-1804, pp. 32, 33, 58, 60, 64, 68)

York, Ben (negro), was treated by Dr. John Archer, Jr. at various times in 1817 and 1818 (p. 80); see George Jackson, q.v.

Young, Agness, Miss, was treated by Dr. John Archer in Feb 1782 (Ledger D, p. 120) [account continued in Ledger E, which is missing]

Young, Alexander, was visited by Dr. John Archer who treated him and daughter Hetty in 1789 and him, daughter Hetty and son Jefferson at various times between 1797 and 1802 (Ledger F, p. 336) [account continued in Ledger G, which is missing]; Ledger I, which is also missing, was abstracted by Dr. George W. Archer circa 1890; his notes are in the Archives of the Historical Society of Harford County folder "Archer, G. W. Coll. – Ledgers and Day Books")

Young, George, at Harford Town, was visited by Dr. John Archer who treated him in Sep and Nov 1778 and his wife in Sep 1782 (Ledger C, p. 124) [continued in Ledger E, which is missing]

Young, Harry, see Hugh Young, q.v.

Young, Hetty, see Alexander Young, q.v.

Young, Hugh, was visited by Dr. John Archer who treated him and his son Harry at various times in 1797 and 1798 (Ledger I, which is missing, was abstracted by Dr. George W. Archer circa 1890; his notes are in the Archives of the Historical Society of Harford County folder "Archer, G. W. Coll. – Ledgers and Day Books")

Young, Jacob, see Samuel Young, q.v.

Young, James (colored), was visited by Dr. Matthew J. Allen who treated his wife six times in Feb 1847, twice in Jul 1847 and once in Jul 1847, his son three times in Jul 1847 and seven times in Aug 1847 and three times in Sep 1847, and his wife in Apr, Jun and Aug 1848 (pp. 44, 55, 62, noted he paid part of the bill in May 1849 and the balance in full in 1850, exact date not given)

Young, Jefferson, see Alexander Young, q.v.

Young, John, was prescribed medicine for his wife by Dr. Robert H. Archer on 29 Jun, 11 Jul and 2 Aug 1803 (Rx Book, 1802-1804, pp. 45, 50, 52)

Young, John, was visited by Dr. Robert H. Archer who treated his daughter in Nov 1823, his wife in Sep 1825 and Jul 1827, his son Samuel in Sep 1827, a child in Apr 1828, his wife in Aug 1828 and him at various times between 1825 and 1828 (p. 93, 159, 237, 247, 271; Ledger F, p. 81)

Young, Robert, was treated by Dr. John Archer seven times from 19 Sep 1777 to 5 Oct 1777 and also mentioned Hugh Kirkpatrick (Ledger C, p. 77)

Young, Samuel, was visited by Dr. Matthew J. Allen who treated a child [name not given] from 13 to 15 Sep 1848, and extracted "a piece of glass 1¼ inches long and ¼ inch wide from Jacob's arm" on 18 Sep 1848, and treated his [Samuel's] wife on 24 Sep 1848 (p. 93); see John Young, q.v.

Young, Thomas (gardener), was treated by Dr. John Archer in Nov 1790 (Ledger F, p. 340)

----, Addy, see Jane A. Allen, q.v.

----, Adeline, see Gracey ----, q.v.

----, Almon, see Alms House, q.v.

----, Archy, see Aquila Paca, q.v.

----, Atleo or Atlas, see William Coale, q.v.

----, Beckey, at Thomas Giles', was treated by Dr. John Archer in Oct 1787 (Ledger F, p. 31)

----, Carolin, see James Moores (tanner), q.v.

----, Cleniss (black man), was visited by Dr. Alonzo Preston who treated his wife in Apr 1825 (p. 20)

----, Corbin (black man), see Bennett Love, q.v.

----, Elenor, see Capt. Sayre, q.v.

----, Eliza, at the Poor House, was treated by Dr. Matthew J. Allen in Dec 1847 (p. 71); see Trustees of the Poor, q.v.

----, Eliza, Miss, was treated by Dr. Birckhead in 1807 and the receipt stated: "1807, Dr. Wm. Hall to Dr. Birckhead, To medicine & attendance administered to Miss Eliza in Oct & Nov ... Ds. 20 ... Recd. payt. in full. Wm. Birckhead." On the reverse side of the paper was written "Mr. John Lewis." (Document in Archives of the Historical Society of Harford County folder "Birkhead")

----, Essex, see Matthew Ridley, q.v.

----, Frank, see James Allison, q.v.

----, Frisby, see Lloyd Bailey, q.v.

----, Gracey, "that lived here with Adeline," was treated by Dr. Matthew J. Allen in Aug 1848 (p. 91)

----, Hagan, see James Gillespie, q.v.

----, Hannah, see Jane Guyton, q.v.

----, Jimmy, see John Cretin, q.v.

----, Johana, see William Wilson, of William, q.v.

----, John, see Alms House, q.v.

----, Judie, see Richard Dallam, q.v.

----, Michael, see Mr. Whann, q.v.

----, Mahaley, see Joseph Gorrell, q.v.

----, Nat, see Henry Cooper, Sr., q.v.

----, Ned, see Joseph Brownlee, q.v.

----, Nelly, see Joseph Brownley, q.v.

----, Perry, see Harford County for Pensioners, q.v.

----, Petre, see Capt. John Hall, q.v.

----, Philip, at John Cretin's place, was treated by Dr. John Archer in Jul 1775 (Ledger B, p. 53)

----, Sam, see Henry G. Watters, q.v.

----, Vanclief, see Elizabeth Lee, q.v.

----, William (weaver), at Elisha Cook's, was visited by Dr. Robert H. Archer who treated his wife in Oct 1827 (p. 250)

www.ingramcontent.com/pod-product-compliance
Lightning Source LLC
Chambersburg PA
CBHW080237270326
41926CB00020B/4278